The
Orthopaedic
Physical
Examination

The
Orthopaedic
Physical
Examination

BRUCE REIDER, AB, MD

Professor of Surgery
Section of Orthopaedic Surgery and Rehabilitation Medicine
The University of Chicago
Pritzker School of Medicine
Director of Sports Medicine
The University of Chicago Hospitals
Chicago, Illinois

Photographs by David Christopher

Department of Audiovisual Communications
The University of Chicago
Pritzker School of Medicine
Chicago, Illinois

W.B. Saunders Company
A Division of Harcourt Brace & Company
Philadelphia London Toronto Montreal Sydney Tokyo

W.B. SAUNDERS COMPANY
A Division of Harcourt Brace & Company

The Curtis Center
Independence Square West
Philadelphia, Pennsylvania 19106

Library of Congress Cataloging-in-Publication Data

Reider, Bruce.
  The orthopaedic physical examination / Bruce Reider.—1st ed.

      p.   cm.

  ISBN 0–7216–7437–2

  1. Physical orthopedic tests.   2. Physical diagnosis.   I. Title.
  [DNLM: 1. Bone Diseases—diagnosis.   2. Joint Diseases—diagnosis.
  3. Physical Examination—methods.—WE 225R359o 1999]
  RD734.5.P58R45   1999

  616.7′0754—dc21

  DNLM/DLC   98–38025

THE ORTHOPAEDIC PHYSICAL EXAMINATION   ISBN 0–7216–7437–2

Printed in the United States of America.

Last digit is the print number: 9   8   7   6   5   4   3   2   1

This book is offered with thanks for
the wisdom of my teachers,
the enthusiasm of my students,
the gratitude of my patients,
and the love of my family.

Contributors

Michel A. Arcand, MD, FRCSC
Attending Physician, Oklahoma Orthopedic
Institute, Norman, Oklahoma
Shoulder and Upper Arm

Roderick Birnie, MBBCh, MMed, MD
Assistant Professor of Clinical Surgery, Section
of Orthopaedic Surgery and Rehabilitation
Medicine, The University of Chicago, Pritzker
School of Medicine, Chicago, Illinois
Elbow and Forearm

Michael E. Brage, MD
Assistant Clinical Professor, Department of
Orthopaedics, University of California—San
Diego, San Diego, California
Lower Leg, Foot, and Ankle

John M. Martell, MD
Assistant Professor of Clinical Surgery, Section
of Orthopaedic Surgery and Rehabilitation
Medicine, The University of Chicago, Pritzker
School of Medicine; Chicago, Illinois
Pelvis, Hip, and Thigh

Daniel P. Mass, MD
Professor of Clinical Surgery, Section of
Orthopaedic Surgery and Rehabilitation
Medicine, The University of Chicago, Pritzker
School of Medicine, Chicago, Illinois
Hand and Wrist

Frank M. Phillips, MD
Assistant Professor of Surgery, Section of
Orthopaedic Surgery and Rehabilitation
Medicine, The University of Chicago, Pritzker
School of Medicine; Attending Physician, The
University of Chicago Spine Center, Chicago,
Illinois
Lumbar Spine

Bruce Reider, AB, MD
Professor of Surgery, Section of Orthopaedic
Surgery and Rehabilitation Medicine, The
University of Chicago, Pritzker School of
Medicine; Director of Sports Medicine, The
University of Chicago Hospitals, Chicago,
Illinois
*Terms and Techniques; Shoulder and Upper
    Arm; Elbow and Forearm; Hand and Wrist;
    Pelvis, Hip, and Thigh; Knee; Lower Leg, Foot,
    and Ankle; Cervical and Thoracic Spine;
    Lumbar Spine*

F. Todd Wetzel, MD
Associate Professor of Surgery, Section of
Orthopaedic Surgery and Rehabilitation
Medicine; Associate Professor of Anesthesia and
Critical Care, The University of Chicago,
Pritzker School of Medicine; Chief, Section of
Orthopaedic Surgery, Louis A. Weiss Memorial
Hospital, Chicago, Illinois
Cervical and Thoracic Spine

I had barely begun a sports medicine research fellowship in 1976 when John Marshall asked me to give a lecture titled "The Sideline Evaluation of Knee Injuries" to a large group of physical educators and athletic trainers. Because I had not yet studied orthopaedics, the first thing I had to do was learn how to examine a knee myself. Since then, I have taught elements of the orthopaedic physical examination to medical students; orthopaedic and primary care residents and fellows; practicing physicians in orthopaedics, pediatrics, internal medicine, physiatry, and emergency medicine; physical therapists; athletic trainers; and laypeople. I have frequently found myself wishing that I had a text to reinforce my presentations. As the years have gone by and the orthopaedic physical examination has expanded to include many tests and techniques not covered in older references, this need has become more acute.

Then, in 1994, Eugene Geppert and Tracie DeMack asked me to teach the orthopaedic physical examination to the 2nd year medical school class at the University of Chicago. Teaching this course has helped me organize my thinking and refine my teaching methods and, finally, led to the decision to write this book.

The use of the physical examination continues to have a greater importance in orthopaedics than in most of the medical specialties. Orthopaedics is, in fact, one of the few specialties in which the physical examination is a large enough topic to serve as the subject matter for an entire textbook. Even more remarkable is the fact that the orthopaedic physical examination is in a state of continuing growth. Evolving clinical and biomechanical research, for example, has led to many new tests for abnormal joint laxity. Arthroscopy has led to the discovery of new conditions, and new clinical tests have been proposed to detect them. Some examination techniques have been discredited or fallen out of favor whereas others have arisen to replace or supplement them. The contents of this book represent a snapshot of the continually changing landscape of the orthopaedic physical examination.

This text is designed to satisfy a number of needs. By defining fundamental terms and describing the most basic tests, it seeks to serve the needs of individuals who are just beginning to learn the orthopaedic physical examination. At the same time, it includes many advanced or supplementary techniques that should make it a valuable resource for knowledgeable clinicians who wish to polish their skills or to review specific tests. As its title suggests, this text describes the examination of the musculoskeletal system from the perspective of the practicing orthopaedist.

This book may be used in different ways. The beginner should start with Chapter 1, which defines the basic terms and techniques of the orthopaedic physical examination, and continue through the remaining chapters in numeric order. The more experienced clinician can brush up on a specific anatomic area by reading the relevant chapter in its entirety or may focus on a specific test or group of tests by using the index.

Photographs were chosen to illustrate the text to give the reader a more realistic representation of the living patient than line drawings can afford. This is particularly true in the case of surface anatomy: patients rarely appear in the examination room with the underlying deep structures carefully drawn on their skin. Multiple figures have been used where necessary to convey the nature of movement in dynamic or manipulative tests.

It is somewhat artificial to approach the orthopaedic physical examination as an isolated body of information. A working knowledge of the relevant anatomy as well as of the pathophysiology and natural history of orthopaedic conditions will greatly enhance the information that can be obtained from the physical examination. This text acknowledges this interdependence in several ways. First, each chapter begins with a review of the relevant surface anatomy. Second, the text has been liberally spiced with clinical tidbits to give the reader a taste for the pathologic conditions that may be associated with different abnormal physical findings. Finally, the tables at the end of each chapter summarize the most common physical findings in a number of clinical conditions. Although the amount of such material that could be included was necessarily limited, it is hopefuly sufficient to indicate the role of various tests in clinical diagnosis and the potential significance of different physical findings. The newcomer to orthopaedics will find that a good anatomy atlas and a textbook of clinical orthopaedics are valuable companions for this text.

Acknowledgments

The author would like to recognize the following individuals whose contributions were vital to the realization of this volume:

David Christopher, for his skill and attention to detail in providing the photographs.

My early mentors, John Marshall, Russ Warren, and Bill Clancy, and the attending staff of the Hospital for Special Surgery, for the many things they taught me by word and example.

My models, Chris Stroud, Amy Williams, Brian Coan, Eric Barua, Dorothy Kelley, Maria Anderson, Armand Abulencia, and Aaron Horne, for their good-natured cooperation during the many hours necessary to achieve these photographs.

Dorothy Kelley, who typed the many revisions of the manuscript with thoughtful precision.

The many patients who consented to be photographed for this book.

My editors, Richard Lampert, Dolores Meloni, and Amy Cannon, who helped develop this project from the initial planning through to the final proofs.

Contents

Chapter 9

Bruce Reider

1

Terms
and
Techniques

The body of this book is divided into chapters, each focused on an anatomic segment including a major joint or portion of the spine. This division is somewhat arbitrary because anatomic structures and patients' symptoms often overlap adjacent body segments. For example, the hip joint and the lumbar spine are both intimately related to the pelvis, and the thigh could be included with the hip or the knee. To minimize redundancy, the material from such overlap areas is assigned to one chapter and cross-referenced in other chapters in which it is relevant.

Some confusion can arise owing to conflicts between the anatomic and the common names for the limb segments. Anatomists use the terms *upper extremity* and *upper limb* to describe the structure popularly known as the arm, and *lower extremity* and *lower limb* are used to identify what is commonly known as the leg. The confusion is greater when the individual segments of the limbs are identified. Anatomically, the terms *forearm* and *thigh* correspond to their popular meanings, whereas *arm* is used to describe the segment of the upper limb between the shoulder and the elbow and *leg* for the segment of the lower limb between the knee and the ankle. Because this usage conflicts with the popular meanings of these terms, the contributors chose to use the term *upper arm* for the limb segment between the shoulder and the elbow and *lower leg* for the limb segment between the knee and the ankle (Fig. 1–1) in an attempt to avoid confusion.

In general medicine, the physical examination is usually divided into sections: inspection, palpation, percussion, auscultation, and manipulation or special tests. This structure has been modified for this text. Auscultation and percussion were eliminated as major components of the examination process for various reasons. Auscultation is rarely used in the orthopaedic examination, except to detect bruits due to vascular constrictions or aneurysms. Similarly, because limbs are not hollow, percussion is not useful, as it is for delineating the size of organs in the chest and abdomen. When percussion is used, it is primarily to elicit a Tinel sign from a peripheral nerve.

Each chapter, therefore, is designed to follow a general organization: **Inspection:** Surface Anatomy, Alignment, Gait, Range of Motion; **Palpation**; and **Manipulation:** Muscle Testing, Sensation Testing, Reflex Testing, Stability Testing, and Miscellaneous Special Tests, the last of which focuses on tests for nerve compression, joint contracture, tendonitis, and other conditions particular to each body segment.

Inspection

The first part of any physical examination is a visual inspection of the area of the patient's complaint. This is so immediate and automatic that it is often done almost unconsciously. The examiner observes the outward appearance of the body part, how it is carried or aligned, how it is used in functional activities such as walking, and the range through which it is able to move, if applicable. The Inspection section of each chapter presents an organized mental checklist, because the more that this process is conducted consciously, the more valuable the information that is obtained from it will be.

SURFACE ANATOMY

Each Surface Anatomy section takes the reader on a visual tour of the surface of the area to be examined. Most chapters describe the appearance of the body part from each of the traditional anatomic perspectives: anterior, posterior, lateral, and medial. The exact order varies according to the requirements of the particular body part described. These terms are applied with the assumption that the patient is in the classic anatomic position (see Fig. 1–1). When they are used to describe relative position, **anterior** means toward the front of the body, **posterior** toward the rear of the body, **medial** toward the midline of the body, and **lateral** away from the midline of the body. Although these same four terms can be applied to the wrist and hand,

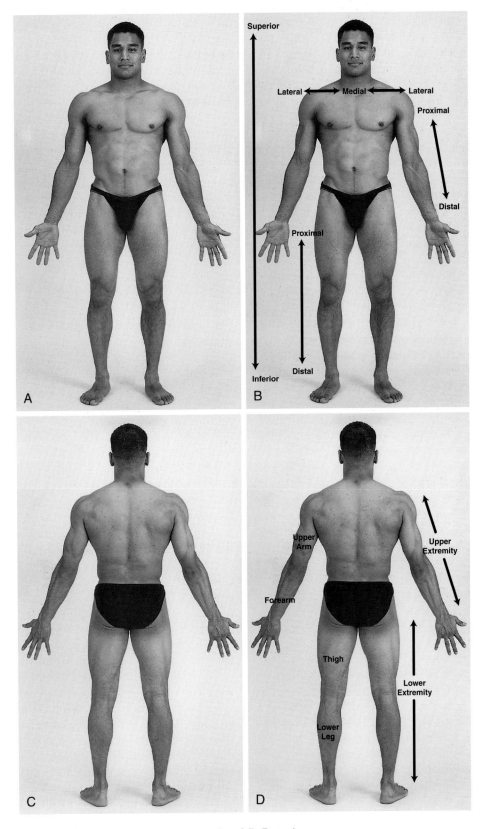

Figure 1–1. The anatomic position. *A* and *B,* Anterior. *C* and *D,* Posterior.

their use in that portion of the anatomy can be confusing owing to the forearm's ability to rotate and thus change the orientation of structures within the distal forearm, hand, and wrist in relationship to the rest of the body. The terms **dorsal, volar, radial,** and **ulnar,** therefore, are used for the hand and wrist. These terms are explained in Chapter 4, Hand and Wrist. In the foot, a description of the **plantar** surface is required.

The terms proximal and distal are also used to describe the relative position of structures. In the limbs, **proximal** means closer to the trunk, and **distal** means away from it. In the spine, **proximal** means toward the head, and **distal** means toward the sacrum. Some clinicians prefer to say **cephalad** or **rostral** when they mean toward the head and **caudad** when they mean toward the sacrum. In the trunk or the limbs, **superior** is often used as a synonym for proximal or cephalad and **inferior** as a synonym for distal or caudad.

The Surface Anatomy sections help orient the reader within the body part to be examined by pointing out anatomic landmarks that are visible in many or most patients. In addition, the location of other structures that are not normally visible is described to guide in palpation and other portions of the physical examination. Photographs, rather than line drawings, are used to give the reader an experience closer to that which will be encountered when examining an actual patient. At the same time, relatively well-defined models were chosen to increase the usefulness of the surface photographs.

In these photographs, the models are exposed for optimal visualization. In a clinical situation, the examiner should also strive for optimal exposure of the body part in question but may need to make compromises when necessary to preserve the comfort and modesty of the patient. Often, the area to be inspected can be exposed when necessary, then covered for the rest of the examination.

As the reader is guided around the surface anatomy, common visible deformities and abnormalities, except for congenital anomalies, are described. The examiner should always be on the lookout for such visible abnormalities. Gross departures from the realm of the normal may be quite obvious, but subtler deformities often require comparison with the patient's opposite side to verify that an abnormality exists. So much variation in appearance is possible among individuals that mild deformities can be overlooked. Comparison with the patient's other side is the best way to evaluate a potential abnormality, in order to differentiate between a subtle deformity and a normal variant.

ALIGNMENT

The Alignment section of each chapter describes the relationships of structures or body segments to one another. In each case, the criteria for normal alignment are described first. Possible variations or abnormalities, whether congenital, developmental, or acquired, are then discussed. As in most aspects of human anatomy, the range of normal varies considerably among individuals. Often, the distinction between a normal variant and an abnormality is arbitrary. The reader must remember that few individuals possess ideal skeletal alignment; the existence of a normal variant should be noted but not equated with pathology. For example, individuals with patellofemoral pain are more likely to have an increased Q angle, but individuals with an increased Q angle do not necessarily experience patellofemoral pain.

In the limbs, the most common types of malalignment are axial and rotational. **Axial alignment** refers to the longitudinal relationships of the limb segments. Often, axial alignment is described in terms of the angle made by the segments in relationship to a straight line. When such deviations are toward or away from the midline, the terms *valgus* and *varus* are usually employed to describe the alignment. These two terms are commonly used but often confused. In **valgus alignment,** the two limb segments create an angle that points toward the midline. In **hallux valgus,** for example, the two segments that constitute the angle are the first metatarsal and the great toe. Instead of forming a straight line, these two segments are angulated with respect to each other and the angle points toward the midline. Another way to define valgus is to say that the distal segment forming the angle points away from the midline. In the example just given, the great toe deviates away from the midline. In **genu valgum,** the angle formed at the knee between the femur and the tibia points toward the midline, and the tibia angles away from the midline (Fig. 1–2*A*).

Varus alignment is the opposite of valgus. In varus alignment, the angle formed by the two segments points away from the midline, and the more distal of the two segments points toward the midline. For example, in **genu varum,** the angle formed by the femur and the tibia at the knee points away from the midline, and the tibia angles back toward the midline (Fig. 1–2*B*). Angulation does not have to occur at a joint for these terms to be used. For example, in **tibia vara,** the angle occurs within the shaft of the tibia. In this case, the proximal and distal por-

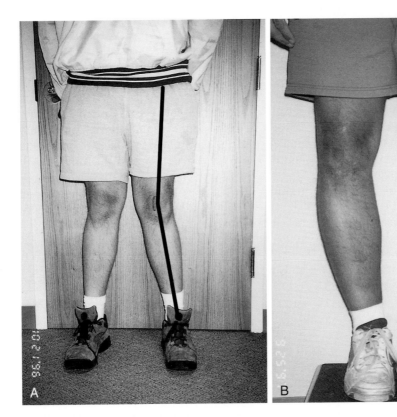

Figure 1–2. *A,* Genu valgum. *B,* Genu varum.

tions of the tibia are considered the two segments that constitute the angle.

Rotational alignment refers to the twisting of the limb around its longitudinal axis. Nomenclature for rotational alignment is less standardized. In the tibia, for example, the term **torsion** is usually used to describe the rotational relationship between the flexion axis of the knee at the proximal end of the tibia and the flexion axis of the ankle at the distal end of the tibia. A normal individual has about 20° of external **tibial torsion** (Fig. 1–3); the flexion axis of the ankle is rotated outward about 20° compared with the flexion axis of the knee. In the femur, the term **version** is more commonly used to describe the rotational relationship between the axis of the femoral neck and the plane of the femur as defined by the flexion axis of the knee. In the normal individual, the femoral neck points anterior to this plane, and normal **femoral anteversion** is present. When the angle between the femoral neck and the plane of the knee's flexion axis is less than the average amount, decreased femoral anteversion or **femoral retroversion** is said to be present.

A number of other terms are used to describe rotational alignment in different areas of the body. For example, when ideal alignment is present, an individual's patellas point forward when the feet are pointing forward. When the kneecaps angle inward, they may be said to be **in-facing;** when they angle outward, they may be said to be **out-facing.** Similarly, the term **in-toeing** is generally used when an individual stands or walks with the medial border of the foot pointing inward; if the foot points outward, the term **out-toeing** is commonly used. The colloquial equivalents of these two terms are *pigeon-toed* for intoeing and *slew-footed* for out-toeing. In the hand and forearm, rotational abnormalities that mimic

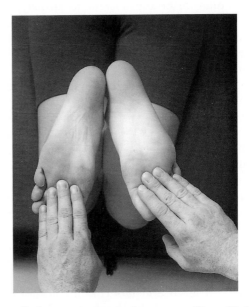

Figure 1–3. Examination in the prone position with knees flexed demonstrates external tibial torsion.

the natural direction of **pronation** are often described as pronation deformities; those that mimic the opposite direction, **supination,** are described as supination deformities. The terms *pronation* and *supination* are sometimes used analogously in the foot and toes, although the leg cannot truly supinate and pronate in the same manner possible in the forearm.

The spine, being a midline structure, has its own set of terms to describe alignment. These are defined in Chapter 8, Cervical and Thoracic Spine, and Chapter 9, Lumbar Spine. Because evaluation of alignment is such an intimate part of spine inspection, the surface anatomy and alignment sections are combined in these chapters.

GAIT

One of the most valuable components of the musculoskeletal examination is observation of the motion of the body segment in question while it is functioning dynamically. The most basic function of the lower extremities is ambulation; therefore, a vital part of the evaluation of any lower extremity disorder is to observe how the problem affects the patient's *gait,* or habitual pattern of ambulation.

The examiner must make a conscious effort to include the examination of gait in the office evaluation of musculoskeletal problems. Although traditionally the examiner might have observed the patient's gait as the patient was walking into the examination room, nowadays the clinician is more likely to walk into an examination room after the patient is already there. This means that the examiner often does not see the patient walk unless he or she makes a conscious effort to include this observation in the examination.

The material presented in each Gait section is by no means a description of laboratory gait analysis. Instead, these sections highlight details that can be detected by inspection and have a specific diagnostic significance. For example, the examiner's attention may be directed to anomalous motion of the affected body part during ambulation or the way a particular orthopaedic abnormality may influence the overall gait pattern.

To understand or detect these abnormalities, a detailed knowledge of the science of gait analysis is not necessary. Most clinicians possess an intuitive understanding of normal gait patterns. In order to observe and describe abnormalities of gait, however, it is helpful to be familiar with the terms used to describe the normal phases of a gait cycle. A complete **gait cycle** is considered to be the series of events that occur between the time one foot contacts the ground and the time the same foot returns to the same position.

Although ambulation is a continuous process, a gait cycle is arbitrarily said to begin when one foot strikes the ground (Fig. 1–4). Because first contact normally is made with the heel, this point in the gait cycle is described as **heel strike.** As the individual continues to move forward, the forefoot makes contact with the ground. The point at which both the forefoot and the heel are in contact with the ground is called **foot flat.** At the same time, the opposite foot is pushing off the ground and beginning to swing forward. The point at which the swinging limb passes the weight-bearing limb is the point of **midstance** for the weight-bearing limb. This is an extremely helpful point in the gait cycle to look for abnormalities, because the limb that is in midstance is temporarily bearing all the weight of the individual's body. As the opposite limb continues to move forward, weight is transferred from the standing limb to the swinging limb and the standing limb begins to push off. The process of **push-off** provides much of the propulsive energy used for ambulation. It is sometimes divided into **heel-off,** the point at which the heel leaves the ground, and the **toe-off,** the point at which the forefoot leaves the ground. The portion of the gait cycle just described, from heel strike to toe-off, is known as the **stance phase** of gait. Most abnormalities are evident during this gait phase because the involved limb is bearing weight and thus under stress. After toe-off, the limb passes through the **swing phase** of gait as it is advanced forward toward the next heel strike. During this time, the opposite limb is progressing through the same components of stance phase just described. When the first heel strikes the ground again, one entire gait cycle has been completed. Each lower limb spends about 60% of the gait cycle in stance phase because there is a portion of the cycle during which both feet are in contact with the ground. The portion of the cycle during which both lower limbs are weight-bearing is called **double leg stance,** whereas the portions during which only one limb is weight-bearing is called **single leg stance.**

In the upper extremity, there is no such standardized way of evaluating the dynamic function of the limb. Much of this information is therefore obtained during the **active range of motion (ROM)** examination. At times, however, it may be helpful for the clinician to ask the patient to perform certain tasks, particularly in the evaluation of the hand.

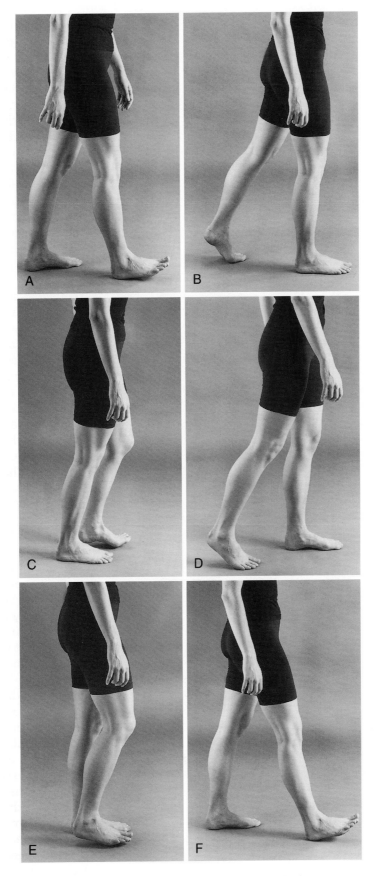

Figure 1–4. The normal gait cycle (right foot). *A,* Heel strike. *B,* Foot flat. *C,* Midstance. *D,* Push off. *E,* Swing phase. *F,* Heel strike.

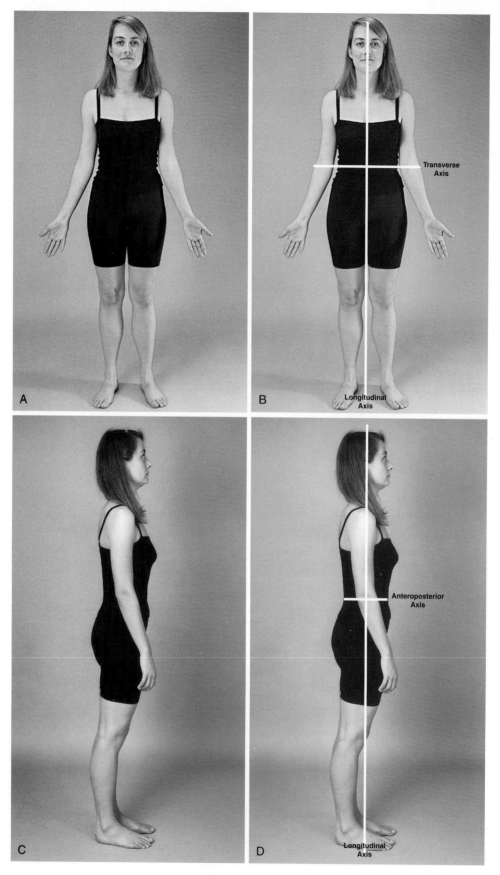

Figure 1–5. Planes and axes of movement. *A* and *B*, Coronal plane. *C* and *D*, Sagittal plane.

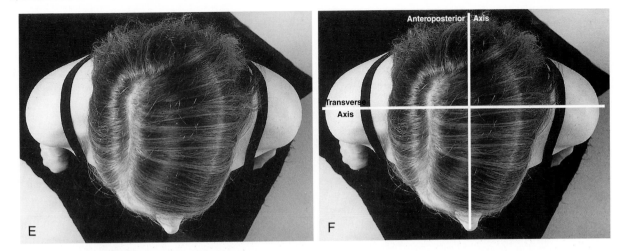

Figure 1–5 *Continued.* E and *F,* Transverse plane.

RANGE OF MOTION

The Range of Motion section of each chapter teaches the reader how to observe and quantitate the amount of motion possible in each joint. Traditionally, joint motion is assessed within three planes of movement, each described with a pair of terms: flexion/extension, abduction/adduction, and external rotation/internal rotation.

Each pair of terms describes movement that takes place in one of the body's cardinal planes when the body is in the anatomic position (Fig. 1–5). **Flexion** and **extension,** for example, describe motion that occurs in the sagittal plane. These movements could also be described as occurring around a transverse axis. This description is sometimes only approximate. For example, as already noted, the flexion axis of the ankle is externally rotated compared with the true sagittal plane.

The exact meaning of the terms *flexion* and *extension* varies depending on the nature of the joints in question. In the elbows, knees, and digits, flexion means movements that tend to bend the joint, and extension means movements that tend to straighten it. In the shoulder and hip, *flexion* refers to movements that bring the involved limb anterior to the coronal plane, whereas *extension* refers to movements that bring the limb posterior to the same plane (Fig.

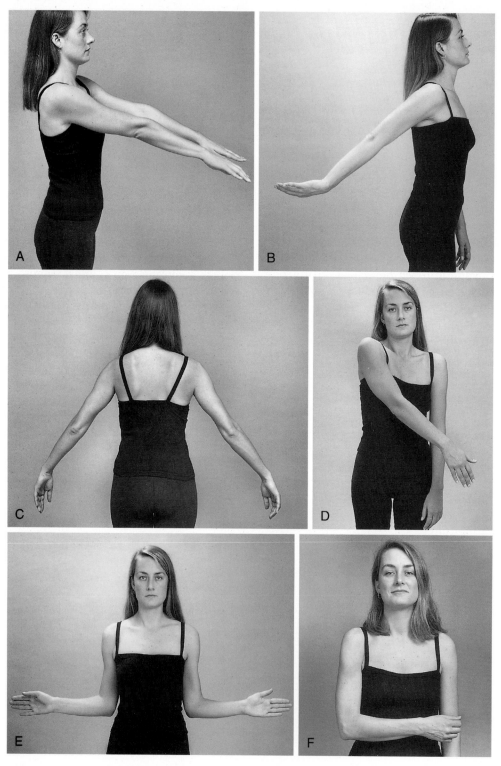

Figure 1–6. Paired motions in the shoulder. *A,* Flexion. *B,* Extension. *C,* Abduction. *D,* Adduction. *E,* External rotation. *F,* Internal rotation.

1–6*A* and *B*). In the wrist, these terms are further modified to **dorsiflexion** and **volar flexion;** in the ankle, they are modified to **dorsiflexion** and **plantar flexion.**

Abduction and **adduction** refer to motion within the coronal plane of the body, which may also be described as motion about an anteroposterior axis (Fig. 1–6*C* and *D*). Abduction describes movements that take the limb away from the midline of the body, whereas adduction describes movements that bring the limb back toward the midline. The spine is a midline structure; therefore, similar movements in the spine are described as right and left **lateral bending.**

External rotation and **internal rotation** describe movements that take place within the transverse plane, that is, motion about a longitudinal axis (Fig. 1–6*E* and *F*). External rotation describes movements in which the limb rotates away from the midline when viewed from an anterior perspective, whereas internal rotation describes movements in which the limb rotates toward the midline when viewed from an anterior perspective. In the spine, similar movements are described as right and left **lateral rotation.**

Needless to say, this method of analysis is a simplification of the complex motion possible at many joints. In the hip and shoulder, motion is possible in an infinite variety of planes; the three-plane method of motion analysis merely serves to simplify and therefore summarize the motions possible. Several joints are capable of movements that resist being forced into this system of classification. This has given rise to other descriptive terms particular to specific parts of the anatomy, such as **opposition, inversion/eversion,** and **pronation/supination.**

For most movements, an attempt should be made to quantitate the amount of motion. This can be estimated or measured. For many routine purposes, estimation is satisfactory. Most examiners can learn to estimate flexion angles fairly accurately by comparing the angle being measured with an imaginary right angle, which is 90°. When greater accuracy is necessary, a pocket goniometer is aligned with the axis of the limb segments that constitute the joint and a reading is obtained (Fig. 1–7). The reader must remember that normal ROM varies considerably, especially in particular joints. In each chapter, the average ROM is described and movements that show substantial variation among individuals are identified.

In any given joint, ROM may be measured both actively and passively. **Active range of motion** refers to the range through which the patient's own muscles can move the joint; **passive range**

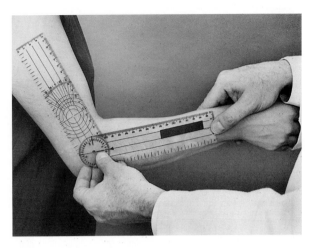

Figure 1–7. Use of the goniometer to measure elbow motion.

of motion refers to the range through which an outside force, such as the examiner, can move the joint. In the interests of time and patient comfort, it is not always necessary to measure both active and passive motion in every given situation. For example, if active flexion and extension of the knees appear full and symmetric, measuring passive ROM is probably superfluous. In general, active ROM is evaluated first, and passive ROM is assessed if the active ROM appears to be deficient.

The ROM examination is not just a time to systematically record numbers, it is a time to obtain valuable diagnostic information. Differences between active and passive ROM raise diagnostic questions that require further evaluation. For example, the inability of the patient to fully extend the knee against gravity may be due to a mechanical block, quadriceps weakness or injury, tendon rupture, or patellofemoral pain. Additional tests allow the examiner to determine which cause pertains in a particular patient. In the Range of Motion section of each chapter, the text describes the possible implications of decreased motion and alludes to supplementary tests that can be performed to further define the diagnostic significance of the lost motion.

Excessive joint motion has traditionally been described as a sign of ligamentous laxity. This may not be strictly accurate because factors other than ligaments may contribute to the joint motion. These factors include morphology of the bones involved and tightness of the muscle-tendon units that cross the joint. Nevertheless, the term *ligamentous laxity* enjoys broad usage.

Four specific tests are widely used to evaluate **generalized ligamentous laxity** (Fig. 1–8): (1) ability to hyperextend the elbows, (2) ability to passively touch the thumb to the adjacent fore-

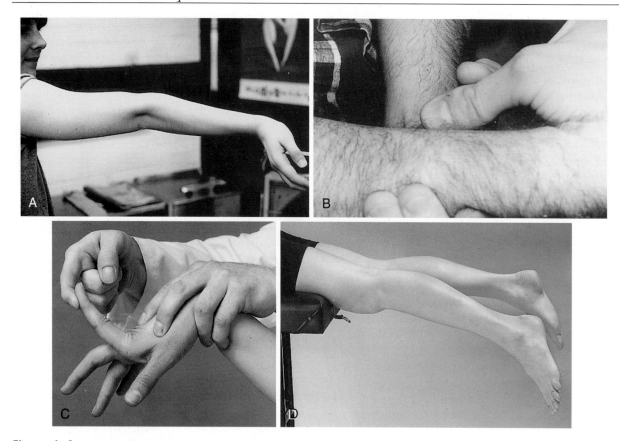

Figure 1–8. Tests of ligamentous laxity. *A,* Elbow hyperextension. *B,* Thumb to forearm. *C,* Index finger metacarpophalangeal joint hyperextension. *D,* Knee hyperextension.

arm, (3) ability to passively hyperextend the index finger metacarpophalangeal joint more than 90°, and (4) ability to hyperextend the knees. A person who can perform three or four of these tests is usually considered ligamentously lax.

Palpation

Palpation is the process of examining a body part by pressing on it, usually with the fingertips. Palpation has many purposes. First, it can be used for orientation. Careful palpation can help the examiner identify the location of specific anatomic structures. This, in turn, can aid in the interpretation of symptoms or facilitate the performance of other portions of the physical examination. By determining the location of specific easily recognizable structures, or **landmarks,** the examiner can estimate the location of other structures that are not otherwise identifiable. Of-

ten, the distinction between inspection of surface anatomy and palpation is somewhat arbitrary because many structures can be seen only in learner patients and must be palpated in others. In this way, the processes of inspection and palpation intermingle in a continuous give and take.

The second purpose of palpation is to elicit tenderness. **Tenderness** is a semi-objective finding. It requires the patient to inform the examiner verbally or physically that palpation of a given structure is painful. Tenderness must therefore always be interpreted with the knowledge that conscious deception or unconscious overreaction may be playing a role in the patient's response. Nevertheless, the identification of point tenderness is one of the most powerful tools in the clinician's armamentarium. Point tenderness can confirm or strongly corroborate such diagnoses as stress fracture, tendinitis, ligament sprain, or abscess. Careful palpation can refine a diagnosis of sprained ankle to one of sprained anterior talofibular ligament.

The third purpose of palpation is to verify the

continuity of anatomic structures. Careful palpation of an injured Achilles tendon, for example, will often allow the examiner to identify the discontinuity that confirms the diagnosis of Achilles' tendon rupture. In the same way, palpation can help assess the severity of an injury. For example, palpating an identifiable divot in a strained quadriceps muscle documents the presence of a severe muscle injury.

During palpation, the **temperature** of the area being examined can be assessed. In this manner, the warmth associated with infection or posttraumatic inflammation can be detected. Conversely, the coldness caused by vascular compromise or the transient vasoconstriction of reflex sympathetic dystrophy can be detected. Changes in temperature can often be quite subtle, so the examiner should always palpate the opposite limb simultaneously when a temperature change is suspected.

Palpation has special uses in the examination of neurovascular structures. By palpating **pulses,** the continuity of major arteries can be verified. Pressure on peripheral nerves can elicit or amplify pain or paresthesias, thus confirming the diagnosis of a nerve injury or entrapment. Percussion of the peripheral nerves can yield similar information and is also described in the Palpation sections.

The question is often asked, "How much pressure should be applied during palpation?" In general, palpation should be initiated with minimal pressure, especially if tenderness is anticipated. The amount of pressure can then be progressively increased when the examiner is assured that light pressure does not cause excessive discomfort. In general, the deeper the structure, the greater the pressure necessary to palpate it.

The contents of the Palpation section of each chapter are not exhaustive. In truth, the number of structures that can be palpated is legion. Any anatomic structure that is identifiable by touch or that may become tender may be palpated. The structures described in each Palpation section should serve as a basic framework for the clinician. As a clinician's knowledge of anatomy grows, the usefulness of palpation expands as well. For reasons of visual economy, common areas of palpation are identified on the surface anatomy photographs. Additional photographs that show the palpation of specific individual landmarks are included. In some of these photographs, the hand placement of the examiner is modified to avoid obscuring the anatomy.

Manipulation

The Manipulation section of each chapter contains a wide variety of material. Any examination technique that did not seem to fit readily under the rubrics of inspection or palpation is included here. The passive ROM examination can certainly be considered to involve manipulation, but it has been included with the Active Range of Motion section under Inspection for continuity and coherence.

MUSCLE TESTING

Each chapter that deals with the examination of the limbs contains the section Muscle Testing. This section describes ways to evaluate the strength of the major muscles or muscle groups used to move the joint or joints described in that chapter. For this reason, testing of the biceps and triceps brachii is included in Chapter 3, Elbow and Forearm, and testing of the quadriceps and hamstrings is included in Chapter 6, Knee. This method is thought to provide the most logical grouping of tests, although it serves to point out the arbitrary and somewhat artificial nature of dividing the limbs into segments. When possible, the isolated testing of individual muscles is described. Often, it is not possible to fully isolate a particular muscle, and it must be tested in concert with other muscles that perform a similar function.

Traditionally, muscle strength has been evaluated by assigning the muscle a grade from 0 to 5. **Grade 0** indicates that no contraction of the muscle is detectable. **Grade 1** is assigned to a muscle in which a contraction can be seen or palpated but strength is insufficient to move the appropriate joint at all, even with gravity eliminated. **Grade 2** is assigned to a muscle that can move the appropriate joint if the limb is oriented so that the force of gravity is eliminated. **Grade 3** is assigned to a muscle that is strong enough to move a joint against the force of gravity but is unable to resist any additional applied force. **Grade 4** is assigned to a muscle that is capable of moving the appropriate joint against the force of gravity and additional applied resistance but is not felt to be normal. **Grade 5** means that the muscle strength is considered normal; it is capable of moving the appropriate joint against gravity and against the normal amount of additional resistance.

The vast majority of muscles that the clinician encounters has at least grade 3 strength. Therefore, the technique described for each muscle group requires movement of the joint against the force of gravity, except a few cases in which such testing is awkward. If the muscle being tested is not capable of moving the appropriate joint against the force of gravity, the examiner should turn the patient so that the equivalent test can be performed with the force of gravity eliminated. For example, the usual method of testing the quadriceps femoris is with the patient seated on a table so that the knee is extended against the force of gravity (Fig. 1–9A). If the patient is unable to execute this maneuver, it means that the effective strength of the quadriceps is grade 2 or less. To further grade the muscle, the patient is instructed to lie on his or her side on the examination table with the knee flexed. The patient is then instructed to attempt to extend the knee with the lower leg and thigh supported by the examination table (Fig. 1–9B). In this fashion, the plane of motion is parallel to the ground and the force of gravity is thus eliminated. If the patient can extend the knee in this position, the quadriceps has grade 2 strength. If the patient is still unable to extend the knee, it means that the effective strength of the quadriceps is either grade 1 or grade 0. To distinguish between these two possibilities, the examiner again asks the patient to attempt to extend the knee with gravity eliminated while the examiner palpates the patient's quadriceps. If a contraction of the mus-

cle is felt or seen, grade 1 strength is present. Otherwise, the muscle is graded as 0.

The distinction between grade 5 and grade 4 muscle strength is somewhat arbitrary. In general, a muscle is graded 4 when it is capable of contracting against gravity and additional resistance but weaker than the corresponding muscle on the other side of the body. Although this is a valuable rule of thumb, the examiner should remember that, in the upper extremities, strength of corresponding muscles can vary between the dominant and the nondominant limbs.

Normal muscle strength varies tremendously among individuals depending on body habitus, occupation, and prior conditioning. The relative strength and size of the patient and the examiner also influence the ability of the examiner to overpower a given muscle group. Nevertheless, for each muscle or muscle group, the authors indicate the general amount of resistance that an average examiner can expect to feel while examining an average patient.

The examiner should keep in mind that manual testing measures the effective strength of the muscle group and can thus be diminished by factors, such as joint pain, which are extrinsic to the physiologic state of the muscle being tested.

Resistive testing can also yield additional diagnostic information. In particular, reproduction of the patient's pain during resistive testing of a particular muscle suggests a diagnosis of tendinitis, muscle strain, or contusion of the muscle-tendon unit being tested. Resisted contraction of a muscle that crosses a painful joint can often elicit or exacerbate the associated joint pain.

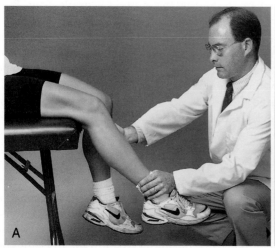
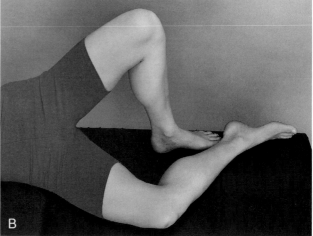

Figure 1–9. *A,* Testing quadriceps strength against gravity and resistance. *B,* Testing quadriceps strength with gravity eliminated.

SENSATION TESTING

The chapters that deal with the extremities contain sections entitled Sensation Testing. These sections describe the testing for sensory deficits associated with peripheral nerve compression or injury in the segment of the limb under discussion. Only the most commonly affected peripheral nerves are described in each chapter. The reader should remember that peripheral sensory nerve anatomy is highly variable and that the exact boundaries of altered sensation vary considerably from one individual to another.

The most common way to define peripheral nerve deficits is to map out the area of altered sensation using light touch or sharp/dull discrimination testing. To test **light touch,** the examiner may use specially designed filaments or everyday objects such as an artist's paintbrush, wisp of cotton, or rolled-up tissue. The patient is instructed to close his or her eyes and to notify the examiner when a touch is felt. The examiner can then begin touching the patient in the area of suspected hypoesthesia or anesthesia and move outward until the patient feels the touch normally. The border between altered or absent and normal sensation can be marked with a pen (Fig. 1–10). The examiner again starts touching in the abnormal area and proceeds outward in different directions, eventually mapping the entire anesthetic area. The area supplied by an injured peripheral nerve may be only hypoesthetic or even hyperesthetic, so the examiner should ask the patient to describe the quality of the sensation experienced, not just the presence or absence of tactile stimulation, in response to light touch. Because the distribution of peripheral nerves may overlap, a transition zone between normal and abnormal areas usually is appreciated.

Sharp/dull discrimination testing can also be used to confirm the findings of light touch examination. In this case, the patient is asked to close his or her eyes and tell the examiner whether the sharp or dull end of a specially designed tester or an ordinary safety pin is touched to the patient's skin. In areas of peripheral nerve injury, the patient may still be able to feel the touch of a pinpoint but not be able to distinguish it as sharp.

The tactile ability of the fingertips is so refined that a specialized method of testing, **two-point discrimination,** is generally used for peripheral nerve injuries or radiculopathies that involve the fingertips. Although specialized calipers, called two-point discriminators, are available, the examiner can improvise a serviceable device by

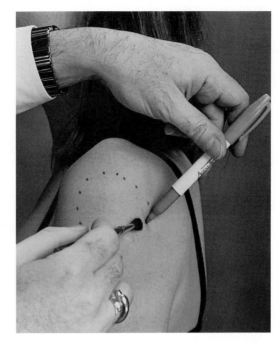

Figure 1–10. Delineating an area of altered sensation.

straightening out a paper clip and bending it over so that the two ends are separated by a defined distance (Fig. 1–11). Because an average individual should be able to distinguish between two points separated by 5 mm, the paper clip is usually configured so that the ends measure 5 mm apart. The patient is instructed to close his or her eyes and notify the examiner whether the finger in question is being touched by one or two points. The examiner then touches the fingertip with the device a number of times, sometimes with only one end of the paper clip and sometimes with both simultaneously. If two-point discrimination is impaired, the patient perceives the simultaneous touch of both ends of the paper clip as only one end. If this is the case, the examiner can gradually spread apart the ends of the paper clip until the distance between the points that is required for the patient to distinguish two separate points is determined.

Because of the intimate relationship between the spine, the spinal cord, and its nerve roots, the neurologic examination is an integral part of the physical examination of the spine. For this reason, the evaluation of motor, sensory, and reflex deficits by dermatome is included in Chapter 8, Cervical and Thoracic Spine, and Chapter 9, Lumbar Spine. For each dermatome, the evaluation of one or a few representative muscles, rather than all muscles innervated by that particular nerve root, is described. In the Sensory Testing sections, the average dermatomal distri-

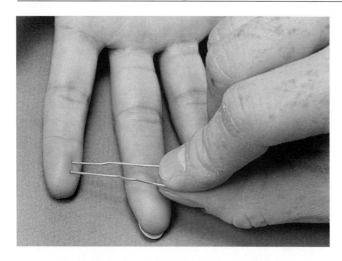

Figure 1–11. Testing for two-point discrimination.

butions of the appropriate sensory nerve roots are illustrated. Because the exact distribution of a given dermatome varies from one individual to another, suggested sites to screen for altered sensation are illustrated for each cervical, lumbar, and sacral dermatome. A description of sensory testing that is particularly relevant to the evaluation of spinal injuries, such as **proprioception** and **vibration** sense, is included in these last two chapters. Finally, the most commonly tested **peripheral reflexes** are described. Reflexes that are obscure or difficult to elicit are generally omitted.

STABILITY TESTING

In all the chapters that deal with the extremities, the Stability Testing section describes tests for abnormal joint laxity. The authors tried to avoid using the term *instability* to describe abnormal joint laxity. Although these two terms are often used interchangeably in the literature, the authors tried to restrict the use of the term *instability* to signify clinical episodes of a joint giving way, subluxing, or dislocating. Instead, terms such as *increased translation* and *abnormal laxity* are used to describe the physical finding of increased play in a given joint.

It is important that any examination for abnormal joint laxity be conducted as gently and painlessly as possible. The patient should be encouraged to relax so that the limb being tested feels completely limp in the hands of the examiner. When this state is obtained, very little force is

necessary to detect abnormal joint laxity. When the test is being performed, the examiner should note whether *pain* is induced, how much *excursion* (play or laxity) is perceived, and what sort of *end point* is felt. These data are often used to establish the anatomic severity of a ligament injury. In a **grade 1 ligament injury,** individual fibers of the ligament are injured but the structural integrity of the ligament is not affected. Stressing such a ligament should induce pain but not reveal any abnormal play in the joint. If the ligament is superficial enough to be palpated, tenderness of the injured ligament is also identifiable. In a **grade 2 ligament injury,** partial structural failure of the ligament has occurred. Such ligaments are elongated but not completely disrupted. Stability testing of such ligaments reveals increased laxity compared with the other side. Classically, a firm end point is still felt when the increased laxity is taken up, although this may be difficult to discern in the face of an acute injury because the stress testing still induces pain in the injured ligament. In a **grade 3 ligament injury,** the structural integrity of the injured ligament is completely disrupted. Often, the joint opens widely in response to stability testing, and the examiner feels a very indefinite resistance or end point, even after the abnormal laxity is taken up. Stress testing of grade 3 ligament injuries can actually be less painful than stress testing of grade 2 injuries because the continuity of the injured structure is completely disrupted. In the presence of a grade 3 injury of one ligament, associated injuries to other ligaments of the same joint are often detected because these other ligaments function as secondary stabilizers or backups to the ligament that has been totally compromised.

MISCELLANEOUS SPECIAL TESTS

In each chapter, miscellaneous special tests for nerve compression, joint contracture, tendinitis, or other conditions particular or unique to each body segment are included. The number of special tests that have been described over the years is enormous, and it was not possible to include every one that can be found in the literature. The goal was to include the tests that the authors themselves have found valuable in their own clinical practices, especially those tests whose anatomic or clinical significance has been established in the medical literature. Some classic tests that have been surpassed by more recent ones or whose reliability remains unproved are included for their historical interest. Finally, newer tests that currently enjoy an expanding popularity are described. Although some of these newer tests may not prove to have staying power, they are valuable for an understanding of current orthopaedic thought and literature.

Over time, clinicians often modify the technical details of specific tests. Sometimes this modification is done consciously to improve the usefulness of the test and sometimes it happens inadvertently. Some tests have an identifiable original description, whereas others have evolved with their origins shrouded in the mists of time. In this text, the contributors describe each test in the manner which is most useful. Usually, this follows the original description, but sometimes modifications were preferable. In certain cases, more than one technique is described. Some of the techniques originated with the contributors or were absorbed from colleagues through clinical interactions. Although most tests have a standard descriptive name or eponym, some do not. In these cases, the authors chose a name from available options or coined one, when necessary.

The terms *positive* and *negative* are traditionally used to report the results of tests. There can sometimes be confusion as to whether a positive result means that a test is normal or abnormal. For this reason, the authors chose the terms **normal** and **abnormal** to describe test results.

A text dedicated to the orthopaedic physical examination can never be truly complete; in practice, a thorough knowledge of anatomy and the pathogenesis, pathophysiology, and natural history of orthopaedic conditions is required to design and interpret the physical examination of each individual patient. The authors deal with this dilemma through a compromise, alluding briefly to relevant anatomy and the clinical implications of abnormal physical findings. In keeping with this desire to provide clinical relevance, each chapter concludes with a table summarizing the possible physical findings in several common or well-known conditions of the body segment being discussed. Table 1–1 on the following page summarizes the physical findings in general orthopaedic conditions.

Among the major joints, the shoulder is distinguished by its tremendous range of motion. (ROM). The shoulder's wide ROM allows humans to position their hands almost wherever desired and thus literally manipulate their environment. The shoulder's ROM is so great that an individual can lose much of it and still be able to perform most of the common tasks of daily living. Human ingenuity, however, has led to the development of sports such as baseball and gymnastics that require a great ROM, so that athletes are most sensitive to small losses of shoulder motion.

The price of this wide ROM is loss of stability. The shoulder is the most potentially unstable of all the major joints. Its anatomy is like a large golf ball balanced on a small tee, so that bony stability is poor compared with other joints such as the ankle or hip. Like other joints, the glenohumeral joint has ligaments to help hold its bony components together. These ligaments must be relatively lax, however, to allow the wide ROM present in the shoulder. Muscles and their associated tendons must, therefore, supply dynamic stabilization forces to supplement the static restraints provided by the ligaments.

To make matters more complicated, the shoulder is not a single joint but a complex of four joints. The main shoulder joint is the glenohumeral joint, the articulation of the round head of the humerus with the glenoid socket at the supralateral corner of the triangular scapula. The scapula itself is anchored to the thorax by a series of broad muscular attachments instead of a true synovial joint. The primary foundation of the upper limb is thus dependent on muscle tone and innervation. The only true articular attachment between the shoulder and the axial skeleton is provided anteriorly by the clavicle, which connects to the scapula at the acromioclavicular joint and to the thorax at the sternoclavicular joint.

When investigating shoulder complaints, it is important to remember the shoulder's intimate relationship to other parts of the body. What a patient perceives as shoulder pain may be caused by pathology in the cervical spine or chest.

Inspection

SURFACE ANATOMY

Anterior Aspect

Although the shoulder joint is covered with more muscle tissue than most of the other major joints except for the hip, several bony and soft tissue landmarks are easily identifiable. Muscle atrophy may make normal bony prominences more pronounced and may reveal some that are not normally visible. Although the general configuration of the shoulder is constant, the ease with which various anatomic structures may be seen or detected by superficial palpation varies considerably among individuals.

Changes in *pigmentation,* or skin color, may alert the examiner to underlying pathology. Ecchymosis is frequently seen about the shoulder following fracture or musculotendinous injury. Sometimes the ecchymosis helps identify the injured structure. An example is the discoloration overlying a fractured clavicle. Ecchymosis and associated swelling may sometimes migrate from the site of injury into the distal arm and elbow or adjacent chest wall, distracting the examiner from the location of the actual injury. Localized erythema and swelling are more suggestive of infection or inflammation. Such findings are most likely to be detectable in the superficial acromioclavicular and the sternoclavicular joints. In most patients, inflammation and even signs of infection of the glenohumeral joint may not be visible owing to the thickness of the overlying deltoid.

CLAVICLE. When the shoulder is viewed anteriorly (Fig. 2–1), the clavicle is the most recognizable landmark. Although ancient anatomists thought it resembled a key, most modern observers tend to describe it as a gracefully curving lazy S. It is virtually subcutaneous throughout its entire length, thus easily seen in most individuals. The clavicle is said to be the most commonly fractured long bone in the human body. Normally,

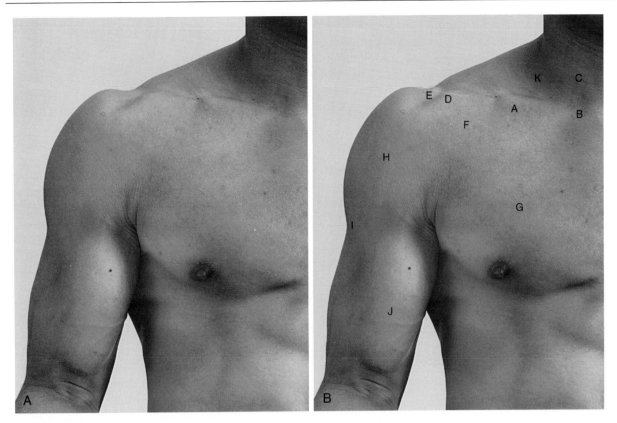

Figure 2–1. Anterior shoulder and upper arm. A, clavicle; B, sternoclavicular joint; C, sternocleidomastoid muscle; D, acromioclavicular joint; E, acromion; F, coracoid process; G, pectoralis major; H, deltoid; I, deltoid tubercle; J, biceps brachii; K, supraclavicular fossa.

the graceful curves of an individual's two clavicles are symmetric. Most fractures occur in the middle third of the clavicle and produce an obvious swelling or deformity (Fig. 2–2). Acute fractures or chronic nonunions can be distinguished from healed fractures by the accompanying tenderness. In the case of an acute injury, ecchymosis is usually present. At the medial end of the clavicle lies the **sternoclavicular joint,** a synovial articulation between the clavicle and the sternum. The **sternocleidomastoid muscle** connects the proximal clavicle and adjacent sternum with the corresponding mastoid processes of the skull. The two sternocleidomastoid muscles combine to produce the characteristic V shape seen in the anterior neck, with the superior sternal notch constituting the angle of the V (Fig. 2–3).

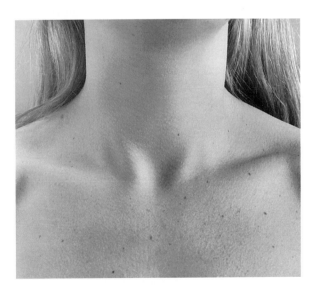

Figure 2–2. Fractured left clavicle.

Figure 2–3. Sternal notch.

STERNOCLAVICULAR JOINT. The sternoclavicular joint is bound together by strong ligaments. Considerable motion occurs here, particularly during active abduction of the shoulder. The joint is very superficial and easily seen in most patients. Swelling and deformity overlying this joint may signify a fracture of the medial clavicle near the joint, a dislocation of the joint itself, or an arthritis of various etiologies (Fig. 2–4). In an *anterior sternoclavicular dislocation,* the proximal clavicle is displaced anteriorly with respect to the sternum and becomes more prominent. This is usually obvious during visual inspection, although massive swelling may obscure the nature of the injury if the patient is examined on a subacute basis. In a *posterior sternoclavicular dislocation,* the medial clavicle is displaced posteriorly with respect to the sternum and becomes less prominent (Fig. 2–5). Such a dislocation may compress the patient's airway and produce respiratory distress. Degenerative arthritis of the sternoclavicular joint may produce visible enlargement owing to synovitis or osteophyte formation. Swelling accompanied by erythema suggests the possibility of infection or inflammatory arthritis.

ACROMIOCLAVICULAR JOINT. At the distal end of the clavicle lies the acromioclavicular joint, its articulation with the acromion process of the scapula. This joint has strong ligaments that prevent anterior and posterior displacement of the distal clavicle. Inferior displacement of the acromion from the clavicle is resisted by the coracoclavicular ligaments. The visibility of the acromioclavicular joint varies tremendously among individuals. In some patients, it appears as a marked bony prominence, whereas in others, it is hidden by adipose tissue and may even be difficult to palpate. In the normal individual, however, both acromioclavicular joints should

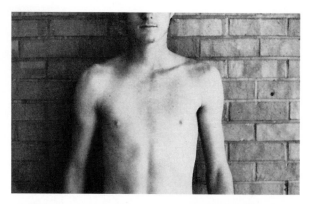

Figure 2–5. Posterior dislocation of the right sternoclavicular joint. (From Rockwood CA Jr, Green DP [eds]: Fractures, 2nd ed. Philadelphia, JB Lippincott, 1984.)

look the same. An asymmetric enlargement of the acromioclavicular joint may be due to acute or chronic inflammation, bony hypertrophy caused by degenerative arthritis, or acute ligamentous injury.

Ligamentous injuries, or sprains, of the acromioclavicular joint were divided by Rockwood into six types, which can often be distinguished by their clinical appearance. In a *Type I* injury, the acromioclavicular ligaments are damaged but not fully ruptured. There is, therefore, no relative displacement of the bones constituting the joint, but the prominence of the joint may be slightly increased due to intraarticular hemorrhage and edema. In a *Type II* injury, more severe damage to the acromioclavicular and coracoclavicular ligaments allows the joint to subluxate, subtly increasing the prominence of the distal clavicle (Fig. 2–6). The deformity is much more marked in the *Type III* injury, in which a complete rupture of the acromioclavicular and coracoclavicular ligaments allows the joint to dislocate completely (Fig. 2–7). The acromion and attached limb are pulled downward by gravity, giving the impression that the distal clavicle is displaced upward. The next step in this progression of injury is the *Type V,* in which tearing of the deltoid and trapezius attachments to the distal clavicle allow the distal clavicle to become so prominent that it appears to be in danger of poking through the skin (Fig. 2–8). This type is sometimes humorously described as an *ear tickler.* Types *IV* and *VI* are rare injuries in which the increased superior prominence of the distal clavicle seen in the other types is absent. In the *Type IV* injury, the distal clavicle is displaced posteriorly and lodged in the trapezius; in *Type VI,* it is displaced inferiorly and lodged beneath the coracoid process. The deformities in both these types may be more easily appreciated by palpation than by inspection.

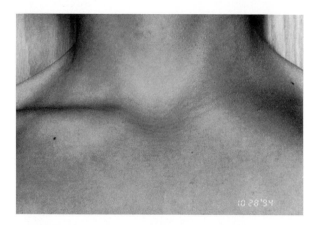

Figure 2–4. Swollen sternoclavicular joint due to a fracture of the medial end of the left clavicle.

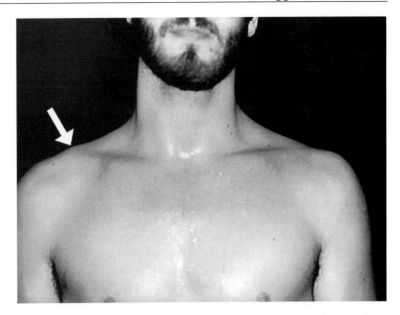

Figure 2–6. Type II acromioclavicular joint injury *(arrow)*.

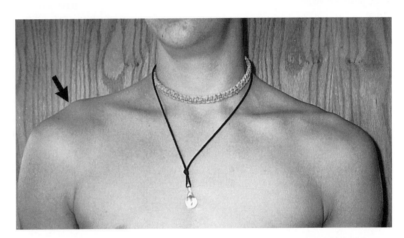

Figure 2–7. Type III acromioclavicular joint injury (right shoulder) *(arrow)*.

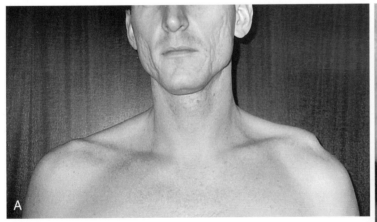

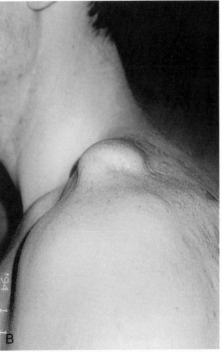

Figure 2–8. Type V acromioclavicular joint injury (left shoulder). *A*, Anterior. *B*, Lateral.

ACROMION. The acromion is a long flat process of the scapula that articulates with the distal clavicle. It serves as an origin for the middle portion of the deltoid muscle and overlies the rotator cuff tendon. Its flat superior surface is easily seen in many patients. The straight lateral edge of the acromion is usually palpable but rarely visible. This is because the round humeral head normally extends lateral to the acromion underneath the deltoid muscle to give the lateral border of the shoulder its rounded appearance. In anterior dislocation of the shoulder, the humeral head usually moves medially, increasing the visibility of the lateral edge of the acromion and converting the rounded contour to a straight one (Fig. 2–9). Axillary nerve injury, which is sometimes seen as a complication of acute shoulder dislocation, can lead to deltoid atrophy and also give the shoulder a straight-edged appearance.

CORACOID PROCESS. The coracoid process is a deep scapular apophysis that is palpable but not normally visible. It serves as the origin for the short head of the biceps and coracobrachialis and the insertion for the pectoralis minor. This landmark may occasionally be seen in very thin patients, or in patients with significant deltoid atrophy. It can also be visible in patients with a posteriorly dislocated shoulder. In this case, the anterior and lateral deltoid heads are flattened against the front of the glenoid rim, making the coracoid prominent. The coracoid can usually be palpated at a point about 2 cm inferior to the junction of the middle and lateral thirds of the clavicle.

PECTORALIS MAJOR. The muscles that are most prominent when the shoulder is viewed anteriorly are the pectoralis major, deltoid, and biceps brachii. The pectoralis major is a triangular muscle that originates broadly on the sternum, clavicle, and ribs and tapers to a flat tendon about 2.5 cm to 3 cm wide that inserts on the proximal humerus just lateral to the bicipital groove. The pectoralis major is a powerful adductor, flexor, and internal rotator of the arm. It constitutes the primary contour of the chest, particularly in the male, and forms the anterior border of the axilla. Ruptures of the pectoralis major are not common, but they seem to be occurring with greater frequency as weight training increases in popularity. They usually occur at or near the tendinous insertion into the humerus. When a rupture occurs, it produces a characteristic clinical appearance of an abnormal anterior axillary crease (Fig. 2–10). Unilateral absence of all or part of the pectoralis major is a relatively common congenital abnormality.

DELTOID. The deltoid is a superficial muscle that gives the shoulder its normal rounded contour. As its name implies, it is triangular. Its broad origin begins anteriorly along the lateral third of the clavicle and continues across the acromioclavicular joint, along the lateral border of the acromion, and finally posteriorly along the scapular spine. These three segments, or heads, taper to a common tendon of insertion on the lateral aspect of the humerus. This point of insertion, the **deltoid tubercle,** is usually visible as a small depression in the lateral arm.

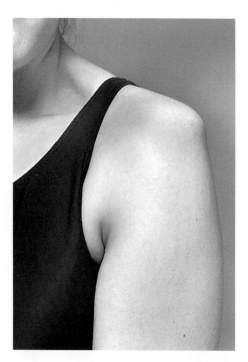

Figure 2–9. Lateral edge of the acromion is more visible when an anterior dislocation of the shoulder is present.

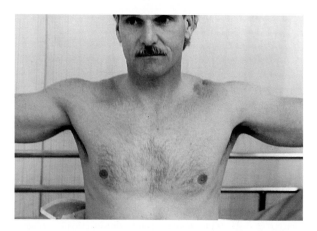

Figure 2–10. Rupture of the left pectoralis major tendon.

The deltoid is a major motor of the arm, producing abduction, flexion, and extension. Deltoid atrophy may occur as the nonspecific result of disuse of the shoulder or as the specific result of injury to the *axillary nerve.* As noted, deltoid atrophy increases visibility of underlying bony prominences such as the acromion, the scapular spine, the coracoid process, and humeral tuberosities. Rotator cuff pain is frequently referred to the deltoid insertion. Deltoid tendinitis, on the other hand, is extremely rare. Pain at the deltoid insertion is, therefore, almost always the result of rotator cuff pathology, although patients may be extremely skeptical of this assertion.

SUBACROMIAL BURSA. The subacromial bursa (subdeltoid bursa) lies deep to the acromion and deltoid and is therefore not normally visible. Because the subacromial bursa has a synovial lining, it may become inflamed in rheumatoid arthritis and cause swelling in the anterior superior shoulder (Fig. 2–11). Swelling related to subacromial bursitis or synovitis in the glenohumeral joint is more likely to be visible in the presence of disorders such as rheumatoid arthritis, owing to the deltoid atrophy that often accompanies these diseases.

BICEPS BRACHII. The biceps brachii is the most prominent muscle of the anterior arm. It is primarily a flexor of the elbow and supinator of the forearm, although its attachments to the glenoid and coracoid give it some limited function in shoulder flexion. True to its name, it has two heads and two proximal tendons. The first, or *long head tendon,* originates at the superior glenoid labrum, passes distally through the shoulder joint, then continues through the groove between the greater and the lesser tuberosities of the humerus. The second, or *short head tendon,*

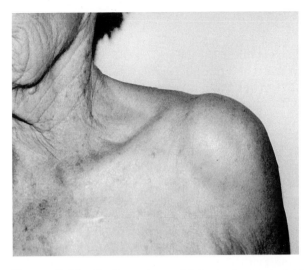

Figure 2–11. Swollen subacromial bursa in rheumatoid arthritis. (Courtesy Wayne Burkhead, Jr.)

originates from the coracoid process in a common tendon with the coracobrachialis muscle. The biceps is innervated by the *musculocutaneous nerve,* a nerve that is occasionally injured after shoulder dislocation or surgery.

The biceps is well known to the lay public because its muscle belly is quite prominent and contributes greatly to the appearance of muscularity. Rupture of the short head tendon of the biceps almost never occurs, but rupture of the long head tendon is common and often associated with rotator cuff injury. This injury is usually accompanied by pain and ecchymosis, which often accumulates distal to the site of injury. Rupture of the long head of the biceps causes a characteristic deformity, as the muscle belly bunches up distally when elbow flexion is attempted (Fig. 2–12). This is sometimes called a **Popeye deformity,** after the appearance of the biceps of the famous cartoon character.

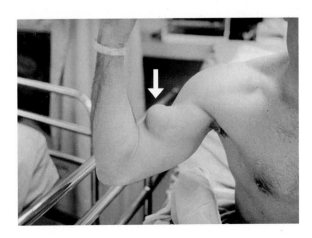

Figure 2–12. Rupture of the long head of the biceps tendon *(arrow).*

Lateral Aspect

Inspection of the lateral aspect of the shoulder provides a different perspective on several structures that have already been discussed: acromion, middle third of the deltoid, deltoid tubercle, and biceps brachii (Fig. 2–13). From this perspective, the biceps is seen in profile, along with the **triceps brachii,** the primary extensor of the elbow, which constitutes the bulk of the posterior arm. The triceps is innervated by the *radial nerve,* which it covers. As its name reflects, the triceps has three heads of origin. The medial and lateral heads arise from the humerus itself, whereas the long head arises from the inferior aspect of the posterior glenoid and is sometimes the site of painful tendinitis in throwing athletes.

Posterior Aspect

SCAPULA. Inspection of the posterior aspect of the shoulder provides a valuable perspective on shoulder anatomy and function (Fig. 2–14). From this viewpoint, the scapula can be seen as the foundation of the shoulder. The *scapula* is a flat triangular bone that is enveloped almost entirely by muscle. One side of this triangle, the medial border, is oriented parallel to the thoracic spine in a roughly vertical manner. The glenoid fossa is perched on the supralateral corner of the scapula opposite this medial border. The most visible bony feature of the posterior shoulder is the **spine of the scapula.** This spine is a ridge of bone oriented at right angles to the main plane of the scapula. It begins at the medial border of the scapula and proceeds toward the supralateral corner of the scapula, where it terminates in the acromion process. The spine divides the posterior scapula into two unequal portions, or fossae. The belly of the **supraspinatus** muscle fills the superior, or supraspinatus, fossa, and the **infraspinatus** and **teres minor** muscles lie in the inferior, or infraspinatus, fossa. The spine serves as the insertion site of the trapezius and the origin of the posterior third of the deltoid. Despite these muscular attachments, the spine is usually quite visible. It is usually slightly prominent, especially laterally where it joins the acromion. In a

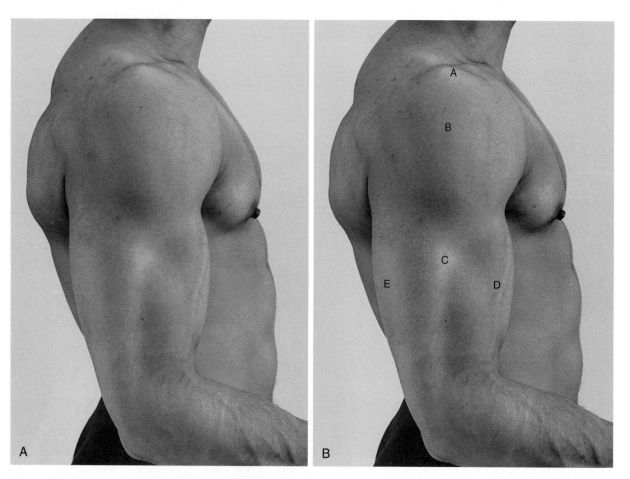

Figure 2–13. *A* and *B,* Lateral aspect of the shoulder and upper arm. A, acromion; B, deltoid; C, deltoid tubercle; D, biceps brachii; E, triceps brachii.

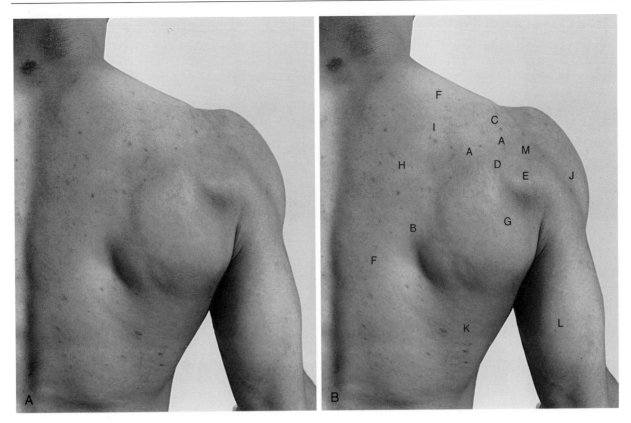

Figure 2–14. *A* and *B*, Posterior aspect of the shoulder and upper arm. A, spine of the scapula; B, medial border of the scapula; C, supraspinatus; D, infraspinatus; E, teres minor; F, trapezius; G, lateral border of the scapula; H, rhomboid muscles; I, levator scapula; J, posterior deltoid; K, latissimus dorsi; L, triceps brachii; M, soft spot.

muscular individual with a well-developed trapezius and deltoid, however, it may appear as a linear depression. Atrophy of the supraspinatus, infraspinatus, or trapezius can cause the spine to appear more prominent.

Of the three borders of the scapula, the *medial border* is most consistently visible. Hyperinternal rotation of the shoulder normally causes the medial border to stand out from the chest wall (Fig. 2–15). If this protrusion of the medial scapula occurs in situations in which the scapula should be stabilized against the chest wall, winging of the scapula is said to occur (Fig. 2–16). Winging is most commonly the result of weakness of the serratus anterior, but weakness of the rhomboids or trapezius may produce different types of winging. Even in the absence of winging, atrophy of the rhomboids may make the medial border of the scapula more visible.

The *lateral border* of the scapula is covered by the latissimus dorsi, but this border can be seen in some patients. Prominence of this part of the scapula may be the result of latissimus dorsi atrophy. The *superior border* of the scapula is

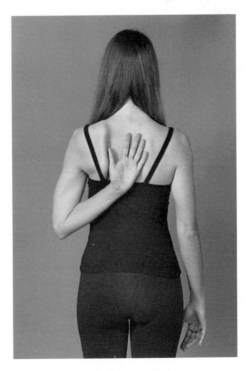

Figure 2–15. Medial border of the scapula becomes more prominent when the shoulder is internally rotated.

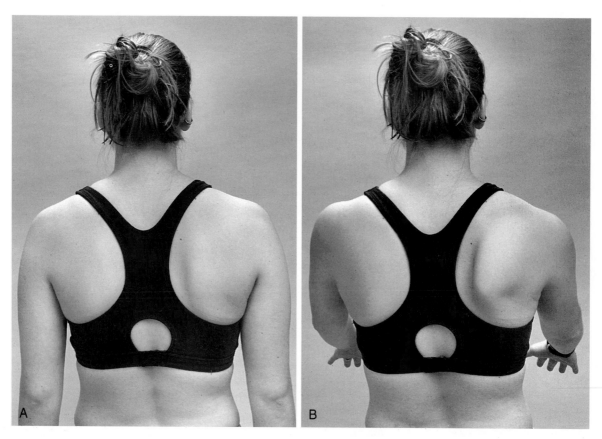

Figure 2–16. *A and B*, Winged right scapula.

covered by the trapezius and supraspinatus muscles and is not normally visible. It can be seen only when the trapezius is severely atrophied.

The posterior aspect of the shoulder displays the contours of a number of visible muscles. These include stabilizers of the scapula, elements of the rotator cuff, and major motors of the shoulder.

TRAPEZIUS. The trapezius originates from the occiput, the nuchal ligament, and the cervical and thoracic spinous processes and inserts on the spine of the scapula, acromion, and distal clavicle. It thus forms the superior border of the shoulder. Cervical spine pain is often referred to the upper trapezius and is perceived by the patient as upper shoulder pain. The trapezius helps to stabilize, lift, and retract the scapula. It is innervated by the *XIth cranial nerve,* which may be injured during biopsy of posterior lymph nodes. Injury to this nerve, also known as the *spinal accessory nerve,* can paralyze the trapezius, resulting in pain, drooping shoulder, and neurologic symptoms due to traction on the brachial plexus.

LEVATOR SCAPULA. The levator scapula is a small muscle that originates on the spinous proc-

esses of C1 through C4. It inserts on the superior angle of the scapula. It is innervated by the posterior roots of C2 to C4. The levator scapula raises the superior angle of the scapula. This muscle is not normally visible but may be seen in a patient with a spinal accessory nerve palsy. The **rhomboid muscles** arise from the nuchal ligament and spinous processes of C7 through T5 and insert on the posterior medial border of the scapular spine. They are innervated by the *dorsal scapular nerve* and function by elevating and adducting the scapula. The rhomboids are not normally distinctly seen but may be visible in a patient with spinal accessory nerve palsy. As noted, weakness or denervation of the rhomboids can produce a subtle winging of the scapula, resulting in increased visibility of the medial border.

SUPRASPINATUS. The supraspinatus arises from the supraspinatus fossa of the scapula, passing beneath the acromion to its insertion on the greater tuberosity of the humerus. Because it is covered completely by the trapezius, atrophy of the supraspinatus can be difficult to detect, unless it is profound (Fig. 2–17). Even then, only a subtle decrease in the fullness of the region superior to the scapular spine may be noted. Atrophy of the supraspinatus muscle is most com-

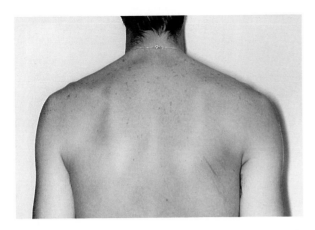

Figure 2–17. Left supraspinatus and infraspinatus atrophy due to a suprascapular nerve palsy.

monly the result of a rotator cuff tear but may occasionally reflect a *suprascapular nerve* palsy due to impingement of the suprascapular nerve at the suprascapular notch.

INFRASPINATUS. The infraspinatus arises from the superior portion of the infraspinatus fossa and also passes beneath the acromion to insert on the greater tuberosity of the humerus posterior to the supraspinatus insertion. Although it is covered by the posterior third of the deltoid, infraspinatus atrophy is more easily observed than atrophy of the supraspinatus. It can be atrophied in both rotator cuff tears and *suprascapular nerve* entrapment (see Fig. 2–17). If the suprascapular nerve is compressed before it enters the supraspinatus, both muscles are affected. If it is entrapped at the spinoglenoid notch distal to the innervation of the supraspinatus, only the infraspinatus is atrophied.

SERRATUS ANTERIOR. The serratus anterior arises from the outer surface of the upper eight or nine ribs and inserts on the deep surface of the medial scapula. Its serrated origins can be seen in the axilla of lean muscular individuals (Fig. 2–18). Although the serratus itself is not usually visible, the loss of its function is normally readily apparent. Weakness or denervation of the serratus due to *long thoracic nerve* injury results in the classic, most severe winging of the scapula. Dynamic tests to bring out this winging are described later in this chapter.

DELTOID. The posterior third of the deltoid, which originates from the lateral scapular spine, completes the rounded lateral border of the posterior aspect of the shoulder. In the case of posterior dislocation of the shoulder, the humeral head

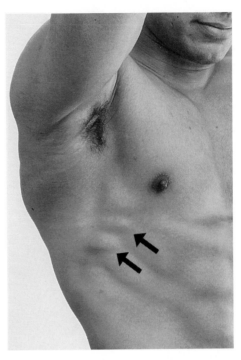

Figure 2–18. Prominent serratus anterior *(arrows)* in a muscular wrestler.

may be seen to bulge posteriorly toward the observer. Often, this posterior bulge is easier to see if the shoulder is viewed from a superior position. Thus, if the clinician suspects a posterior dislocation, the patient should be asked to sit on a chair or stool so that the examiner may view the shoulder from above (Fig. 2–19).

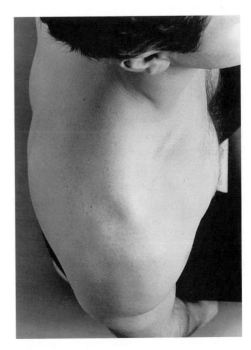

Figure 2–19. Overhead view of the normal right shoulder.

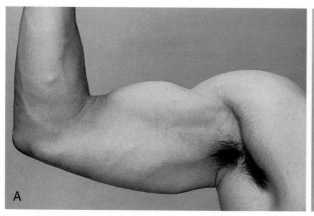 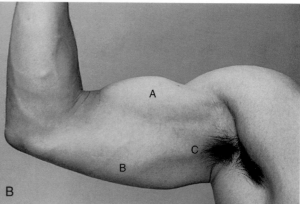

Figure 2–20. *A* and *B*, Medial aspect of the upper arm. A, biceps brachii; B, triceps brachii; C, axillary sheath.

Medial Aspect

The surface anatomy of the medial aspect of the upper arm is straightforward (Fig. 2–20). In most individuals, a longitudinal groove runs down the upper arm from the axilla toward the elbow. Anterior to this groove, the bulk of the arm is occupied by the biceps brachii, augmented by the coracobrachialis proximally and the brachialis distally. Posterior to this groove lies the muscle belly of the triceps brachii. The groove itself marks the location of the **axillary sheath,** which contains the brachial artery, basilic vein, and the ulnar and median nerves.

ALIGNMENT

Although the word *alignment* is not frequently used in conjunction with the shoulder, terms such as *carriage, attitude,* and *posture* are frequently employed to convey concepts of alignment. Whether the patient is viewed anteriorly or posteriorly, the two shoulders should appear symmetric. Imaginary lines drawn between paired landmarks such as the sternoclavicular joints or acromioclavicular joints should be horizontal. The inclination of the clavicles and scapular spines should be symmetric in both shoulders. Posteriorly, the visible medial borders of the scapulae should be roughly parallel and equidistant from the spinous processes of the thoracic spine. Although the orientation of the scapula on the thorax changes as the shoulder is abducted, the placement of the scapulae should be the same for identical positions during shoulder motion. The usual resting position can vary widely among individuals, however. Some people tend to carry their shoulders with their scapulae retracted to-

ward the "attention" position, whereas many other individuals habitually assume a protracted or round-shouldered position.

Differences between the two shoulders can exist. The patient may carry the dominant shoulder slightly lower than the nondominant one. In manual laborers and individuals who participate frequently in sports such as baseball or tennis, this difference in shoulder height may be more marked. When a shoulder is painful, the patient may tend to tighten the muscles of the shoulder girdle and support the forearm, so that the painful shoulder is carried higher than the normal one. In **Sprengel's deformity,** a well-known congenital malformation, the involved scapula is smaller and carried higher than on the uninvolved side (Fig. 2–21).

In throwing athletes, soft tissue contracture can draw the scapula of the dominant shoulder away from the midline. This has been called the **lateral scapular slide.** This abnormality can

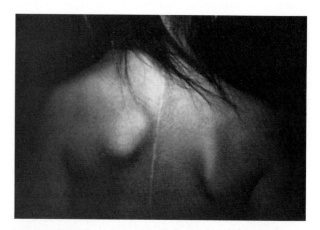

Figure 2–21. Sprengel's deformity (left shoulder). (From Rockwood CA Jr, Matsen FA III: The Shoulder, 2nd ed. Philadelphia, WB Saunders, p 110, 1996.)

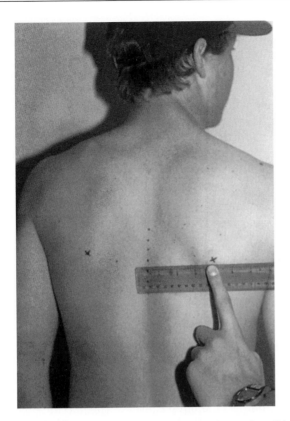

Figure 2–22. Measuring to detect a lateral scapular slide. (From Reider B: Sports Medicine: The School-Age Athlete, 2nd ed. Philadelphia, WB Saunders, p 516, 1996.)

be detected by measuring the distance from the inferior tip of the scapula to the midline (Fig. 2–22). A measurement from the inferior tip of the dominant scapula to the midline that is at least 1.5 cm greater than the same measurement on the nondominant side has been correlated, by Kibler, with posterior shoulder pain and anterior impingement symptoms.

RANGE OF MOTION

Evaluation of shoulder ROM is relatively complicated; motion is possible in so many directions. Active ROM is normally assessed first; passive ROM is then assessed in certain directions if active motion is abnormally limited. The normal range of some motions such as abduction and forward flexion is fairly consistent among normal individuals, but the magnitude of other motions such as internal and external rotation can vary widely from one individual to another. The patient's uninvolved side can normally be used as a normal control, although the examiner must remember that internal and external rotation usually differ between the dominant and the nondominant limbs.

ABDUCTION. To evaluate **abduction,** the clinician asks the patient to bring both arms up to the side as far as possible, indicating motion in the coronal plane. Often the patient will stop at 90° of abduction and need to be encouraged to continue until the arms are straight overhead (Fig. 2–23). At about 90° of abduction, the patient usually is observed to externally rotate the arms so that the greater tuberosity can pass under the acromion. Taking the starting position with the arms along the side as 0°, abduction can usually be obtained to at least 160°, if not a full 180°.

It is best to observe abduction from a posterior perspective so that the relative contributions of glenohumeral and scapulothoracic motion to shoulder abduction can be noted. The smooth coordination of these two components of abduction is often called the *scapulohumeral rhythm.* If glenohumeral motion is restricted by arthritis or a painful, weak, or torn rotator cuff, the pa-

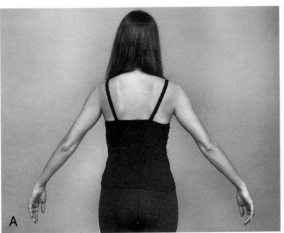

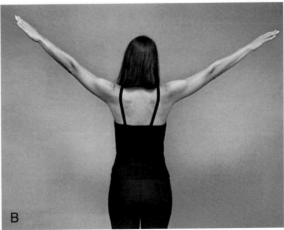

Figure 2–23. *A* and *B*, Active shoulder abduction.

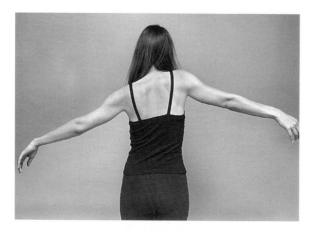

Figure 2–24. Shrugging of the scapula to increase abduction (right shoulder).

tient unconsciously tries to supplement the glenohumeral abduction by increasing the scapulothoracic movement (Fig. 2–24). This **shrugging** of the shoulder produces a characteristic appearance that is frequently seen in the presence of rotator cuff injury but may be observed in other conditions as well.

Another phenomenon that may be detected while testing active abduction is **painful arc syndrome.** In painful arc syndrome, the patient experiences no pain during the initial portion of abduction but begins to report pain as the abducted limb approaches shoulder level (Fig. 2–25). If the patient is able to continue abducting through the pain, he or she may actually report a decrease or resolution of the pain as the arm approaches full abduction. Sometimes the pain continues unabated to 180° of abduction. Although the patient often spontaneously reports

or reveals the pain by facial expression, the examiner should specifically inquire about the presence of pain during abduction if the history or abnormal scapulohumeral rhythm raises the suspicion of rotator cuff pathology. A painful arc phenomenon suggests the possibility of an impinged or torn rotator cuff.

If abduction is far from complete, the examiner should evaluate **passive abduction** (Fig. 2–26). The patient should be alerted before performing such a test, as the uninformed patient may instinctively try to prevent such a potentially painful motion. The examiner grasps the patient's limb at the elbow and slowly and gently abducts it past the limit of maximal active abduction. When passive abduction dramatically exceeds active abduction, a painful or torn rotator cuff is the most common cause.

FORWARD FLEXION. Forward flexion is usually the next motion to be measured. The patient is asked to lift his or her arms forward in the sagittal plane as far as possible (Fig. 2–27). Again, the patient may have to be prompted to continue past shoulder level to the maximal overhead position. With the resting position at the side considered 0°, usually 160° to 180° of forward flexion is possible. Forward flexion may also be limited in the presence of arthritis, adhesive capsulitis, or rotator cuff tears. Rotator cuff impingement is more likely to limit abduction than forward flexion, although very large rotator cuff tears may limit both. If forward flexion is significantly limited, **passive forward flexion** is then usually evaluated. Again, passive forward flexion that is significantly greater than active forward flexion is usually related to muscular weakness or tendon injury. This may mean injury to the

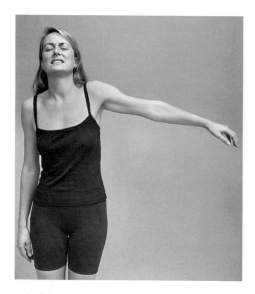

Figure 2–25. Painful arc of abduction.

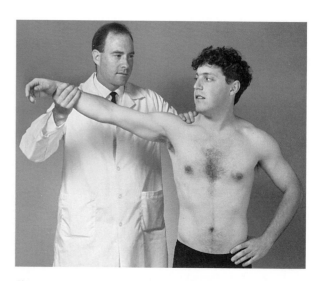

Figure 2–26. Passive shoulder abduction.

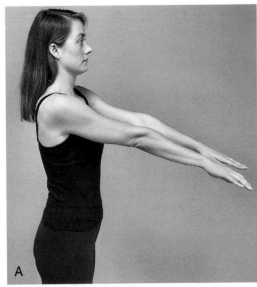

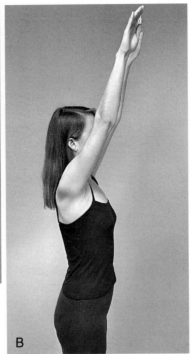

Figure 2–27. *A* and *B*, Active shoulder flexion.

rotator cuff tendons, although weakness or paralysis of the scapular stabilizers can also limit active forward flexion.

TOTAL ACTIVE ELEVATION. The Society of American Shoulder and Elbow Surgeons recommends measuring **total active elevation** rather than flexion or abduction. When total active elevation is assessed, the patient is instructed to raise the arm as far forward as possible in the plane that is most comfortable. This plane is usually somewhere between strict forward flexion and abduction, about 20° to 30° from the sagittal plane.

ROTATION. **Rotation** can be measured in two positions: with the arm at the side and with the arm abducted 90°. The elbow is flexed 90° so that the forearm indicates the amount of rotation. Whether measured at the side or in abduction, neutral (0°) rotation is present when the forearm is pointed directly forward. To assess **external rotation at the side,** the examiner stands directly in front of the patient. The patient is asked to place both arms firmly against the sides and flex both elbows to 90° (Fig. 2–28*A*). The patient is then instructed to externally rotate both forearms as far as possible while keeping the elbows firmly against the sides of the trunk (Fig. 2–28*B*).

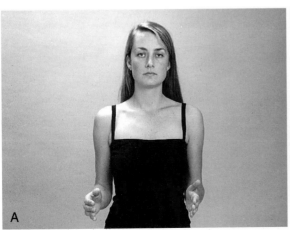

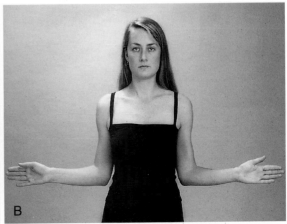

Figure 2–28. External rotation at the side. *A*, Neutral position. *B*, Externally rotated position.

Normal external rotation in this position may vary from 45° to 90°. It may be slightly greater on the dominant than the nondominant side. Massive tears that involve the posterior portion of the rotator cuff may compromise external rotation strength so severely that the patient is unable to externally rotate even to a neutral position. In this situation, the examiner is able to passively increase external rotation significantly by stabilizing the patient's elbow with one hand and gently externally rotating the forearm (Fig. 2–29). When the examiner releases the forearm, the patient is unable to hold the shoulder in external rotation and the limb drifts back into internal rotation.

External rotation in 90° abduction can also be measured. Functionally, this tends to be a more important motion than external rotation at the side because it simulates the motion required in overhead activities such as throwing, playing racquet sports, and swimming. Both limbs may be assessed simultaneously or in sequence. The patient is asked to abduct each arm to 90°. Again, the neutral position is with the forearm facing forward when the elbow is flexed (Fig. 2–30A). The patient is then asked to externally rotate the arm at the shoulder as far as possible (Fig. 2–30B). Normal external rotation in this position is 90° or more. When mea-

sured in this position, external rotation is usually about 20° greater on the dominant side than on the nondominant side. This is particularly true in throwing athletes, whose external rotation may easily measure 135° or more. When external rotation is limited, the patient may consciously or unconsciously try to compensate for the loss of motion by arching the upper back. It is important for the examiner to detect this tendency, which substitutes trunk motion for restricted shoulder motion. In the presence of anterior shoulder instability, the externally rotated abducted position puts the patient at risk for involuntary subluxation or dislocation. In such patients, external rotation may be falsely limited on the affected side because the patient is afraid to force the shoulder into this vulnerable position (see apprehension test under Stability Testing, in the Manipulation section).

Internal rotation may also be tested in both positions. **Internal rotation in 90° abduction** is easy to measure. The patient starts in the same neutral position as for external rotation and is asked to internally rotate the arm at the shoulder (Fig. 2–30C). Average internal rotation in this position ranges from about 30° to 45°. Internal rotation in this position, however, is not nearly as important functionally as internal rotation with the arm at the side.

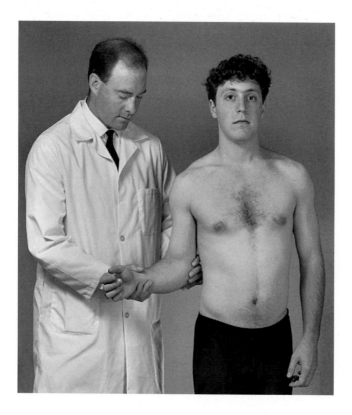

Figure 2–29. Passive external rotation.

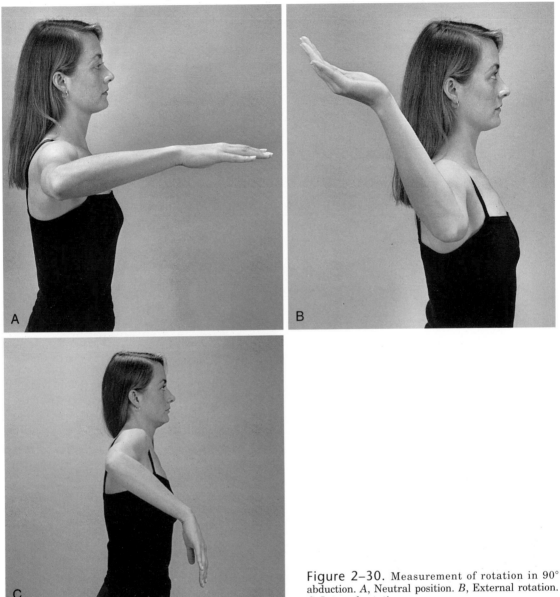

Figure 2–30. Measurement of rotation in 90° abduction. *A*, Neutral position. *B*, External rotation. *C,* Internal rotation.

To assess **internal rotation at the side,** the patient again starts with the elbow at the side of the trunk and this time turns the arm in (Fig. 2–31*A*). This measures pure internal rotation, but is limited to about 80° when the forearm contacts the abdomen. To measure full internal rotation, the patient is asked to reach behind his or her back as if trying to scratch an itch in midback (Fig. 2–31*B*). This maneuver is sometimes called the **Apley scratch test.** This is a complex motion, as some extension of the shoulder is necessary to move the hand into this position. It is a very functional motion, however, because it is required for daily activities such as reaching a back pocket, cleansing the perineum,

scratching the back, or fastening clothes. This motion is usually quantitated by identifying the spinous process of the highest vertebra reached. This is normally about T7 for women and T9 for men. Most individuals are able to reach about two levels higher with the nondominant limb (Fig. 2–31*C*). Remembering that the iliac crests mark the level of the L4–L5 interspace, the examiner can identify the L4 spinous process and count upward from there. Internal rotation is typically the first motion lost in adhesive capsulitis and the last to be regained. Patients with this condition are usually not able to reach even the lumbar spine. In these cases, the internal rotation is recorded by the nearest landmark

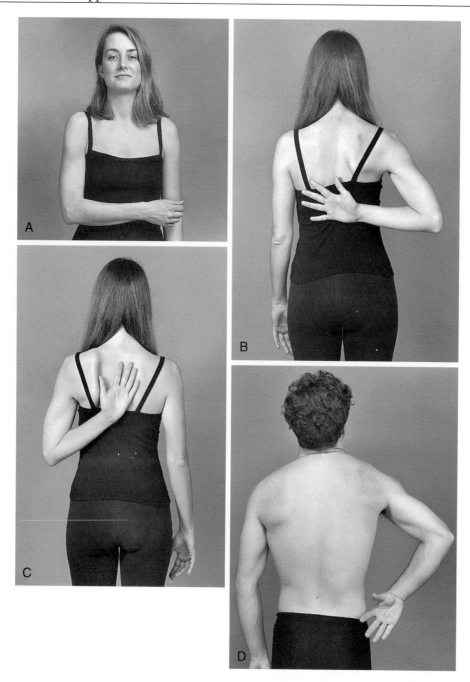

Figure 2–31. Internal rotation with arm at side. *A,* To abdomen. *B,* Behind the back (Apley's scratch test), dominant arm. *C,* Nondominant arm. *D,* Internal rotation limited to posterior iliac crest.

reachable: the greater trochanter, the posterior superior iliac spine, the sacrum, and so forth (Fig. 2–31*D*).

ADDUCTION. Adduction may also be measured in two different ways. The most direct is to have the patient start with the arm at the side and swing the upper extremity across the trunk while keeping the elbow straight (Fig. 2–32). Normal adduction in this position is about 30°. A more functional way to measure adduction is called **cross-chest** or **cross-body adduction.** In this test, the patient is asked to forward flex the shoulder 90°, then reach across the body and try to place the hand on or past the opposite shoulder as far as possible (Fig. 2–33). Patients

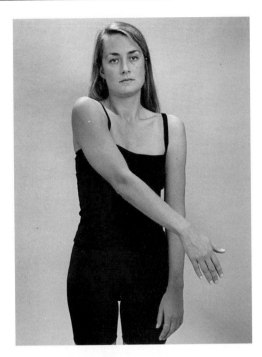

Figure 2–32. Adduction.

should normally be able to at least cup the hand over the opposite shoulder, and many can reach far past this. This motion may be quantitated if desired by measuring the distance from the antecubital fossa to the opposite acromion. This

motion may be painful or limited in patients with acromioclavicular joint pathology.

EXTENSION. Shoulder **extension** is tested in a manner opposite to that of shoulder flexion. The patient is asked to swing the upper limb as far posteriorly as possible in the sagittal plane while keeping the elbow straight (Fig. 2–34). Normal shoulder extension is much less than forward flexion, ranging from about 40° to 60° in the average subject. Because pure shoulder extension is not frequently used in daily activities, it is not always tested as part of a routine shoulder examination.

Protraction and retraction are movements that take place at the scapulothoracic interface, not the glenohumeral joint. They are usually not measured but observed in a qualitative way. To demonstrate **scapular retraction,** the patient is asked to pull the shoulders back in a position of attention. The scapulae are noted to approach each other as they move toward the midline (Fig. 2–35). In **scapular protraction,** this movement is reversed as the patient shrugs the shoulders forward in a hunched attitude. The scapulae are seen to slide away from the midline (Fig. 2–36). In the presence of *snapping scapula* syndrome, reciprocal retraction-protraction produces a palpable and often audible grating. This is most commonly felt best at the supramedial corner of the scapula.

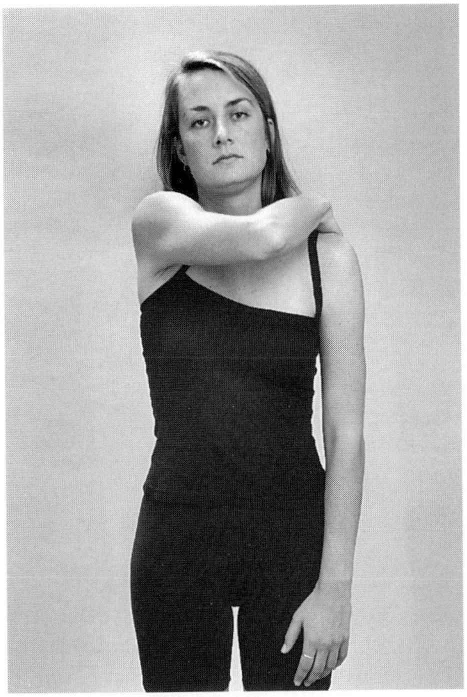

Figure 2–33. Cross-chest adduction.

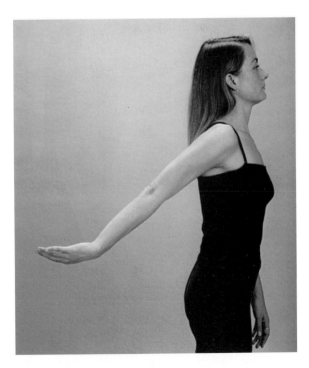

Figure 2–34. Extension.

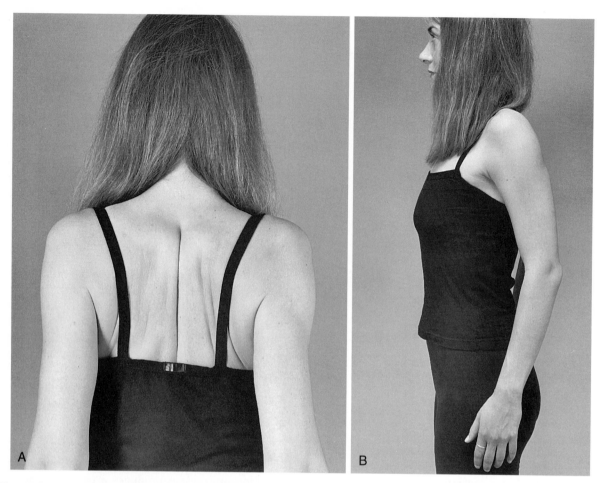

Figure 2–35. Scapular retraction. *A*, Posterior view. *B*, Lateral view.

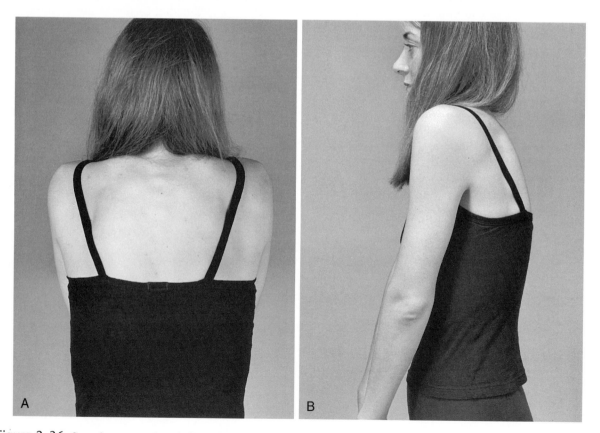

Figure 2–36. Scapular protraction. *A*, Posterior view. *B*, Lateral view.

Palpation

Many areas of possible palpation have already been mentioned in the Surface Anatomy section. These include landmarks that are occasionally visible, such as the coracoid process and the lateral border of the acromion. This section highlights areas in which palpation for tenderness or, occasionally, crepitus often helps lead to a diagnosis. Palpation should be avoided where inspection has already yielded a diagnosis and palpation would only cause the patient unnecessary pain, as in the presence of an acutely dislocated acromioclavicular joint or fractured clavicle.

Anterior Aspect

ACROMIOCLAVICULAR JOINT. Because the clavicle is so superficial, palpation is often helpful in evaluating possible disorders of this bone or its associated articulations. As noted, it is usually redundant as well as unkind to palpate an obviously dislocated acromioclavicular joint when the patient describes an acute injury. However, in the case of a Type I or mild Type II acromioclavicular joint injury, only a subtle swelling may be present. In such a case, lightly palpating the acromioclavicular joint to confirm the presence of tenderness allows the examiner to verify the diagnosis.

Palpation can also be helpful in the presence of a chronically enlarged acromioclavicular joint. It is not unusual for a patient to have a painless enlargement of the acromioclavicular joint due to the accretion of asymptomatic osteophytes. Eliciting tenderness at the joint suggests that the arthritic joint itself is contributing to the patient's pain and is not merely an incidental finding.

As noted, the prominence of the acromioclavicular joint varies greatly from one individual to another. When the location of the acromioclavicular joint line is obscure, the examiner can often identify it in the following manner: while the patient is standing or seated, the examiner grasps the patient's arm with one hand. The examiner then pushes upward on the arm while pushing downward on the clavicle with his or her other hand. The examiner looks for the site of motion between the clavicle and the acromion and may also palpate for it using the index finger (Fig. 2–37).

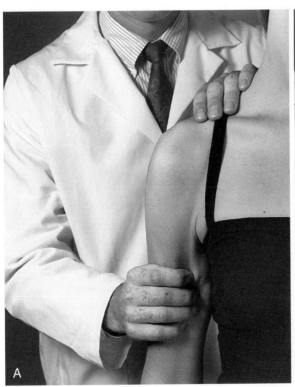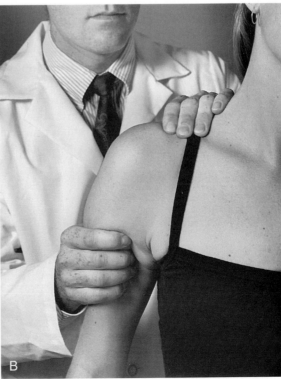

Figure 2–37. *A* and *B*, Pushing downward on the clavicle and upward on the arm helps identify the acromioclavicular joint.

Palpation can also help distinguish between Type I and Type II acromioclavicular joint injuries. Tenderness of the **coracoclavicular ligaments** is present in the Type II injury but not in the Type I injury. Although the examiner cannot distinguish the actual outlines of the coracoclavicular ligaments in a normal patient, tenderness over these ligaments can be determined. Knowing that the ligaments run from the coracoid superiorly to the overlying clavicle, the examiner first palpates the coracoid process about 2 cm inferior to the junction of the middle and lateral thirds of the clavicle. The examiner then palpates fairly deeply between the coracoid process and the clavicle (Fig. 2–38). Eliciting tenderness in this interval suggests injury to the coracoclavicular ligaments.

STERNOCLAVICULAR JOINT. It is not usually necessary to palpate an obviously deformed sternoclavicular joint when the patient gives a history of acute injury. However, when the diagnosis is uncertain, eliciting tenderness in the sternoclavicular joint can be very helpful. To palpate the sternoclavicular joint, the examiner locates the sternal notch, a landmark that should be evident in virtually all patients. The sternoclavicular joint line can usually be palpated approximately 1.5 cm to 2.0 cm lateral to the midline of the notch (see Fig. 2–1).

ACROMION. Other areas of bony palpation can be valuable when fracture is suspected but no definite deformity is seen. Palpation of the acromion (see Fig. 2–1), for example, is normally painless. However, in the condition known as *os acromionale,* a separate ossification center fails to unite to the main body of the acromion. Through overuse or trauma, the fibrous union of the two portions of the acromion may become painful. When the clinician identifies an *os acromionale* on a radiograph, palpating the acromion for tenderness helps to distinguish between a clinically significant condition and a painless incidental finding.

CLAVICLE. Gentle palpation of the clavicle for localized tenderness may be helpful if a fracture is suspected from the patient's history but no visible deformity is observed. Bony crepitus should never be actively sought during such palpation, but when it is detected incidentally a diagnosis of fracture is confirmed. Palpation can also be helpful when the clinician suspects a fracture in other bony structures such as the acromion, greater tuberosity, or coracoid process. Eliciting tenderness can be particularly crucial in the presence of nondisplaced fractures of these structures because radiographs may be difficult to evaluate unequivocally.

SUBACROMIAL BURSA. The subacromial bursa underlies the acromion and extends outward under the anterior and lateral deltoid. Its purpose is to help the rotator cuff glide under the acromion. When a full thickness tear of the rotator cuff is present, this bursa communicates with the shoulder joint. Occasionally, in patients with a large or massive rotator cuff tear, interarticular fluid can be distinctly palpated in the bursa. Otherwise, the margins of the bursa cannot be distinctly palpated. By default, tenderness just anterior to the acromion is usually assumed to be due to *subacromial bursitis.* Passively extending the patient's shoulder brings more of the subacromial bursa anterior to the acromion and increases the ease of palpation (Fig. 2–39). Tenderness of the subacromial bursa is frequently, but not always, present in cases of *rotator cuff impingement* or *tear.*

LONG HEAD BICEPS TENDON. *Biceps tendinitis* may sometimes cause anterior shoulder pain. The long head biceps tendon is typically affected where it passes underneath the acromion and enters the intertubercular groove between the greater and the lesser tuberosities. This groove usually faces anteriorly when the shoulder is in about 10° of internal rotation. To palpate the long head biceps tendon, the examiner holds the patient's shoulder in about 10° of internal rotation with one hand and palpates along a line running from 1 cm to 4 cm distal to the anterior acromion (Fig. 2–40). Except in cases of extreme deltoid atrophy, the biceps tendon itself cannot

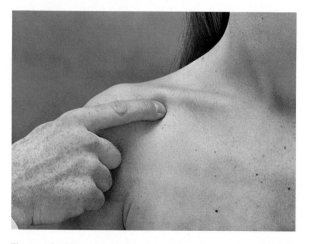

Figure 2–38. Palpation of the coracoclavicular ligaments.

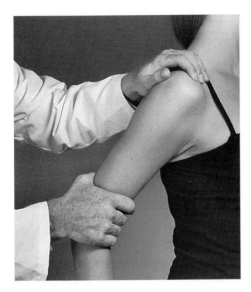

Figure 2–39. Palpation of the subacromial bursa.

be distinctly felt. Sometimes, the medial edge of the greater tuberosity can be appreciated, and this marks the *intertubercular groove.* Tenderness in the expected location of the long head biceps tendon is assumed to represent *biceps tendinitis,* although confirmation of the diagnosis through other tests adds confidence. In the presence of isolated biceps tendinitis, passive internal or external rotation of the patient's shoulder underneath the palpating finger should ease the pain as the intertubercular groove is rotated out from under the pressure of the examining finger. Frequently, biceps tendinitis exists concomitantly with rotator cuff disease. In this case, the rotator cuff disease may produce more widespread anterior tenderness, and the presence of biceps tendinitis as a distinct entity may be difficult to con-

firm. Special tests for biceps tendinitis are discussed in the Manipulation section.

BICEPS MUSCLE. Palpation of the biceps muscle belly is occasionally helpful. *Biceps ruptures* most commonly involve either the long head tendon proximally or the distal tendon insertion. This latter possibility is discussed in Chapter 3, Elbow and Forearm. However, tears of the muscle itself sometimes occur. These are most commonly situated at the distal musculotendinous junction. If such an injury is suspected, the examiner should ask the patient to flex the elbow against resistance with the forearm supinated. The examiner then identifies the biceps tendon distally and palpates along it proximally until the point of maximal tenderness is reached. Sometimes, an actual divot can be felt at the musculotendinous junction, although this is usually obscured by hematoma and edema if the injury is in a subacute phase.

Myositis ossificans can occur in the biceps or underlying brachialis following contusion. As in the thigh, myositis ossificans in the arm is usually presaged by a feeling of warmth and firmness in the affected muscle.

PECTORALIS MAJOR. Palpation can be helpful in the presence of a suspected pectoralis major rupture. To palpate the pectoralis major, have the patient set the muscle by isometrically pressing the palms together (Fig. 2–41). Starting palpation over the pectoralis major muscle belly, the

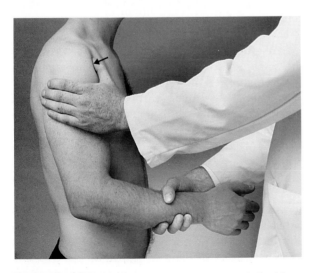

Figure 2–40. Palpation of the long head of the biceps tendon *(arrow).*

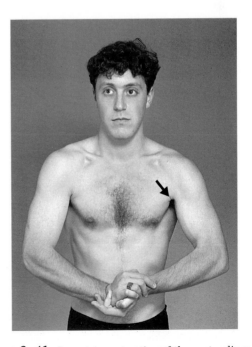

Figure 2–41. Isometric contraction of the pectoralis major facilities palpation of its tendon *(arrow).*

examiner should be able to follow the muscle as it tapers to a flat tendon in the axilla and inserts on the humerus. In the case of an *intratendinous tear* or *avulsion,* discontinuity is detectable.

When *traction injuries* of the **brachial plexus** occur, tenderness may be noted in the supraclavicular area lateral to the sternocleidomastoid. Mild injuries of this sort are common in sports, where they are referred to as *burners* or *stingers.*

Lateral Aspect

Palpation of the **deltoid** muscle can be helpful when an axillary nerve palsy is suspected. A clinical situation in which this is particularly useful is following acute dislocation or shoulder stabilization surgery. In these situations, it may be difficult for the examiner to distinguish between a deltoid whose contraction is present but weak owing to pain and a deltoid that is paralyzed owing to axillary nerve injury. To palpate the deltoid in such a situation, the examiner places one hand against the lateral aspect of the patient's distal arm at the elbow and asks the patient to isometrically abduct against this resistance. The index and long fingers of the examiner's other hand are placed with light to moderate pressure on the patient's deltoid approximately 1 cm lateral to the lateral border of the acromion (Fig. 2–42). The examiner should

be able to feel the deltoid tense as the patient abducts isometrically, even if the deltoid is very weak. Palpating a distinct deltoid contraction confirms that some motor activity of the deltoid is present, although it cannot distinguish between a partial neuropraxia and weakness owing to pain.

Posterior Aspect

What the patient describes as posterior shoulder pain may often be localized to the **trapezius** or upper **rhomboids.** Pain in these areas may represent a local muscle injury, although such pain is more likely to be referred from the cervical spine. Finding tenderness to palpation in these areas may not reliably distinguish between these two diagnostic possibilities. Even when the primary pathology appears to be in the cervical spine, pain radiating to the trapezius or upper rhomboids frequently is associated with a tender trigger point at the site of referred pain. However, palpation of the trapezius and rhomboids is useful for confirming the presence of such trigger points (see Fig. 2–14).

Palpation of the body or spine of the **scapula** is useful in cases of suspected scapular fracture. Finding tenderness of the bony scapula may alert the examiner to the possibility of a subtle fracture that could be overlooked on routine shoulder radiographs. Palpating while the patient is asked to alternately protract and retract the shoulders allows the examiner to detect the popping or grinding phenomenon that is known as *snapping scapula.* This distinct sensation, which is caused by the scapula rubbing over the underlying ribs, may occur for a number of reasons. It can most commonly be localized to the supramedial corner of the scapula (Fig. 2–43).

A useful landmark of palpation posteriorly is the so-called **soft spot** of the posterior shoulder. If the examiner palpates a point approximately 1 cm medial to the posterolateral corner of the acromion and 2 cm inferior to it, a soft spot approximately 1.5 cm in diameter is felt. This soft spot identifies the superior portion of the glenohumeral joint between the humeral head and the glenoid margin. This landmark is useful for injection of the glenohumeral joint. A needle inserted through this spot and aimed at the palpated tip of the coracoid process anteriorly usually enters the posterior superior glenohumeral joint between the head of the humerus and the glenoid fossa.

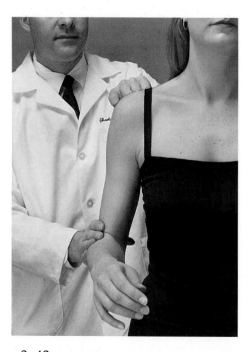

Figure 2–42. Palpation for lateral deltoid contraction.

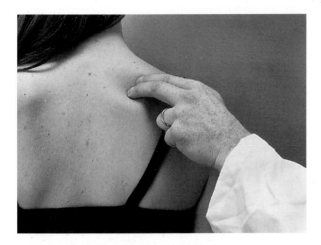

Figure 2–43. Palpation for snapping scapula.

Medial Aspect

As already noted, the **brachial artery** travels in the axillary sheath, which is located in the groove between the biceps and the triceps on the medial arm. Moderately firm palpation in this groove close to the axilla allows the examiner to appreciate the pulsations of the brachial artery. The median and ulnar nerves travel with the artery in this part of the arm, but they cannot be distinctly palpated. Firmer palpation along the groove allows the examiner to appreciate the bony resistance provided by the medial aspect of the humerus (see Fig. 2–20).

Manipulation

MUSCLE TESTING

Many muscles are active about the shoulder and arm, and they interact in a complex fashion. It is rarely possible to truly test a single muscle in isolation, so the resistance noted during strength testing may be due to more than one muscle. Within those limitations, this section describes methods for testing the major motor muscles of the shoulder and arm.

Scapular Stabilizers

Strong muscles are necessary to stabilize the scapula against the thorax and allow it to func-

tion as the foundation of the upper extremity. When these muscles are weak or denervated, the scapula may pull away from the thorax, a phenomenon known as *winging*. When scapular stabilization is ineffective, the function of the entire upper extremity is compromised.

SERRATUS ANTERIOR. The serratus anterior originates from the anterior ribs and inserts on the medial border of the scapula. Weakness of this muscle manifests itself as winging of the medial border of the scapula. The serratus anterior is innervated by the *long thoracic nerve,* which is subject to traction injury during weight lifting and other sports. If serratus anterior function is completely lost owing to a long thoracic nerve palsy, the winging is quite dramatic (see Fig. 2–16). In severe cases, this winging is obvious as soon as the patient attempts to flex the involved shoulder forward. The classic test for serratus anterior weakness is to ask the patient to perform a modified pushup against the wall. The examiner stands behind the patient in order to best observe winging and may provide additional resistance with the palm of the hand. If the weakness is subtle, asking the patient to perform the pushup with the arms at various heights above and below shoulder level may help to bring it out (Fig. 2–44). An alternative method for demonstrating serratus anterior weakness is to have the patient attempt to raise the arms from the 90° forward flexed position while the examiner or an assistant provides isometric resistance.

RHOMBOIDS. The rhomboids are responsible for retraction of the scapulae on the thorax. These are deep muscles that are covered by the trapezius. To look at the rhomboids, the examiner

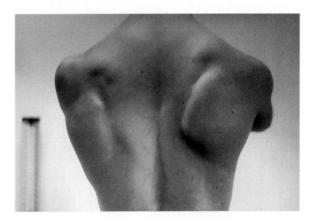

Figure 2–44. Demonstration of scapular winging (right shoulder).

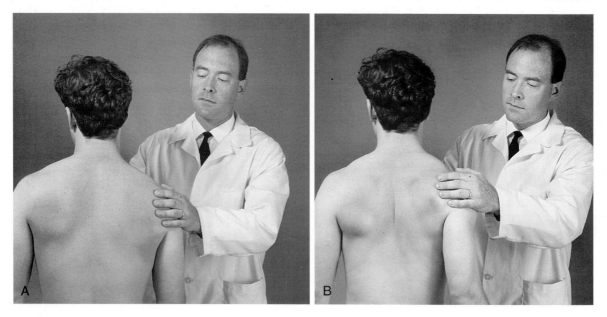

Figure 2–45. *A* and *B*, Assessing rhomboid strength (scapular retraction).

stands behind the patient and asks the patient to retract the scapula. This may be described to the patient as pulling the shoulders back or coming to "attention." The examiner presses on the spine of the scapula with the palm of one hand to provide resistance and may palpate the muscles medial to the scapula with the fingers of the other hand for evidence of contraction (Fig. 2–45). The rhomboids are innervated by the *dorsal*

scapular nerve. Isolated palsy of this nerve, an uncommon phenomenon, produces a scapular winging that is milder and more subtle than that produced by long thoracic nerve injury.

TRAPEZIUS. The trapezius is a large superficial muscle that dominates the junction of the posterior shoulder and adjacent neck. When the trapezius is weak, the resting position of the

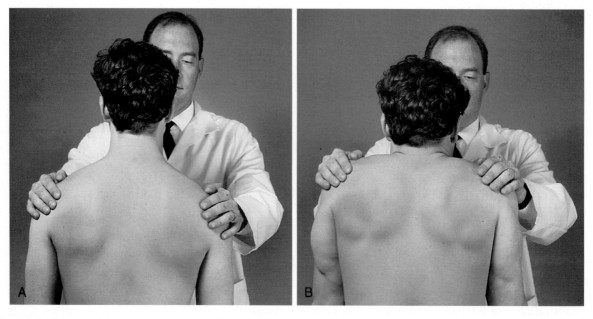

Figure 2–46. *A* and *B*, Assessing trapezius strength.

scapula may be more lateral than normal and its superior and medial borders have a tendency to wing when the arm is actively moved against resistance. To test the trapezius, the examiner stands behind the patient and asks him or her to shrug shoulders. One of the examiner's hands provides resistance through downward pressure on the acromion while the other can palpate the trapezius directly for evidence of contraction (Fig. 2–46). The trapezius is innervated by cranial nerve XI, the *spinal accessory nerve,* which may be injured during surgical procedures such as dissection of posterior cervical lymph nodes.

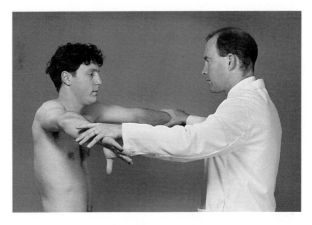

Figure 2–47. Supraspinatus isolation test.

Rotator Cuff

Despite its name, the rotator cuff complex functions not only to rotate but also to stabilize the humeral head in the glenoid fossa during abduction. The supraspinatus and subscapularis muscles are evaluated individually, whereas the infraspinatus and teres minor are graded together as a unit.

SUPRASPINATUS. The supraspinatus muscle lies deep to the trapezius in the supraspinatus fossa. Impingement or tearing of the rotator cuff tendon usually begins with the supraspinatus portion of the cuff. As a rotator cuff tear progresses, the infraspinatus becomes involved. Less commonly, the supraspinatus may be weakened by impingement of the suprascapular nerve at the superior scapular notch. In this case, the infraspinatus is also affected.

The supraspinatus is evaluated using the **supraspinatus isolation test (Jobe test).** To perform the test, the examiner stands in front of the patient, who is asked to abduct the arms to 90° with the elbows fully extended. The patient's arms are then brought forward to a position 30° anterior to the true coronal plane and maximally internally rotated so that the thumbs are pointing down. The patient is then asked to push toward the ceiling while the examiner provides resistance (Fig. 2–47). Weakness noticed during this test may signify muscle inhibition due to pain or true muscle dysfunction.

INFRASPINATUS. Isolated weakness of the infraspinatus may be caused by injury to the *suprascapular nerve* at the spinoglenoid notch because such a lesion affects the nerve after the supraspinatus has already been innervated. To test the infraspinatus, the patient is asked to place the arms tightly at the sides with the elbows flexed

to 90°. The patient is then asked to externally rotate the arms while the examiner provides resistance (Fig. 2–48). The **teres minor,** which constitutes the most posterior portion of the rotator cuff, is tested along with the infraspinatus. The teres minor would be involved in only the most massive rotator cuff tears. The teres minor is innervated by the *axillary nerve,* and thus is paralyzed if a complete axillary nerve palsy occurs. In this situation, however, the weakness of the teres minor is overshadowed by the profound loss of deltoid function.

SUBSCAPULARIS. Subscapularis strength can be graded in two ways. The first is the **subscapularis liftoff test,** described by Gerber. This test is described in the Manipulation section. In the second method, the patient is asked to stand with

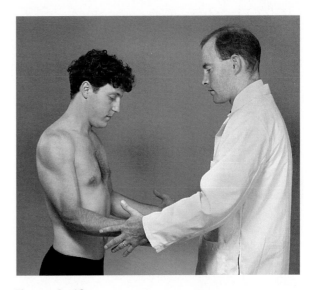

Figure 2–48. Assessing infraspinatus and other external rotators.

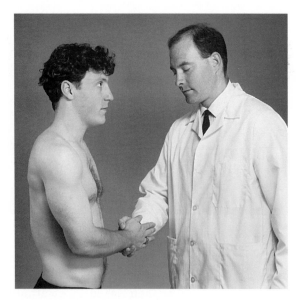

Figure 2–49. Assessing subscapularis and other internal rotators.

Humeral Adductor/Internal Rotators

PECTORALIS MAJOR. The humeral internal rotators are large and superficial, making them easy to examine. The pectoralis major is a large triangular muscle that adducts and internally rotates the arm at the shoulder. The pectoralis major can be observed for function and continuity by asking the patient to compress the hands together in front of the chest with the elbows and shoulders comfortably flexed (see Fig. 2–41). Pressing the hands together in this position causes an isometric contraction of the muscle that can be palpated in virtually all patients and seen in many. When overlying adipose or breast tissue obscures the bulk of the pectoralis major, its distal portion can still be palpated where it crosses the anterior axilla to insert on the humerus. As noted earlier, this is the place where the pectoralis major tendon is most likely to rupture. If a pectoralis major rupture is present in a lean male, the muscle belly will be observed to bunch up abnormally when the contraction is elicited. Pectoralis major muscle strength may be tested by asking the patient to forward flex the shoulder with the elbow slightly bent. The patient is then instructed to adduct the arm against the examiner's resistance (Fig. 2–50). The pectoralis major can be observed to contract and its strength may be estimated. The muscle is innervated by the *medial* and *lateral pectoral nerves* (see Fig. 2–10).

the elbow flexed to 90° and the hand on the abdomen. The patient is instructed to press the hand down against the abdomen while the examiner attempts to lift the patient's hand away from the trunk (Fig. 2–49). This method is particularly helpful in assessing the strength of the subscapularis in patients with restricted internal rotation, who cannot place their hands behind their backs to perform the liftoff test properly. The subscapularis is innervated by the *upper* and *lower subscapular nerves*.

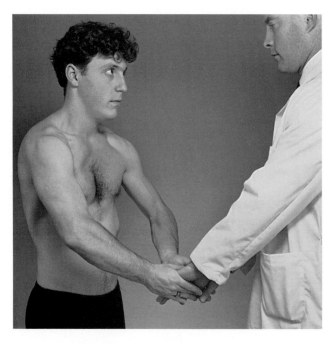

Figure 2–50. Assessing pectoralis major strength.

LATISSIMUS DORSI. The latissimus dorsi is a large internal rotator and extender of the arm. It arises from the back and constitutes the posterior border of the axilla as it courses to its insertion on the humerus. To test the latissimus dorsi, the patient is asked to flex the shoulder forward to 90° with the elbow flexed as well. The patient is then instructed to attempt to internally rotate and extend the arm at the shoulder as if attempting to climb a ladder (Fig. 2–51). The examiner may resist this motion with both hands while visually confirming the latissimus contraction or resist with one hand and use the other to palpate the latissimus contraction. The latissimus dorsi is innervated by the *thoracodorsal nerve*. Injury to this nerve results in a latissimus dorsi weakness (Fig. 2–52).

Humeral Abductors

The deltoid muscle is the principal abductor of the arm at the shoulder. The rotator cuff muscles assist the deltoid in this function by stabilizing the humeral head in the glenoid fossa, thus establishing a stable fulcrum. In the presence of a paralyzed deltoid, the rotator cuff can provide some weak abduction on its own.

The **deltoid** muscle is divided into three portions, or heads, each of which is innervated by

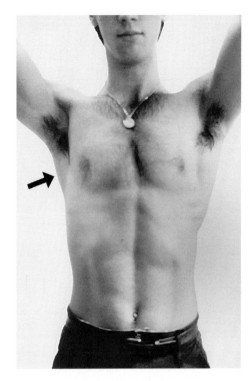

Figure 2–52. Latissimus dorsi atrophy (*arrow*).

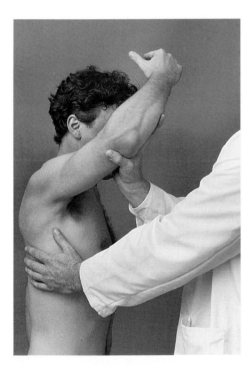

Figure 2–51. Assessing latissimus dorsi strength.

the *axillary nerve*. The axillary nerve is the most common peripheral nerve to be injured during shoulder dislocation or surgery. The primary function of each of the three deltoid heads can be predicted by its position: the *anterior deltoid* flexes the shoulder, the *middle deltoid* abducts the shoulder, and the *posterior deltoid* extends the shoulder. To test the anterior deltoid, the examiner stands in front of the patient, who is asked to slightly flex the arm. The patient is then instructed to attempt to further flex the arm while the examiner provides resistance at the distal arm. The examiner's other hand may be used to palpate and thus confirm the contraction of the deltoid just distal to the anterior acromion (Fig. 2–53*A*).

The middle head of the deltoid is tested in an analogous manner. The patient is asked to place the arm in a slightly abducted position. The examiner then provides isometric resistance to further abduction with the hand placed just above the elbow, while the examiner's other hand can palpate the deltoid for contraction just lateral to the lateral border of the acromion (Fig. 2–53*B*). Similarly, the posterior third of the deltoid is tested by asking the patient to extend one shoulder against resistance while palpating this portion of the muscle (Fig. 2–53*C*).

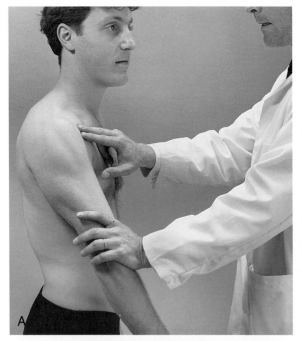

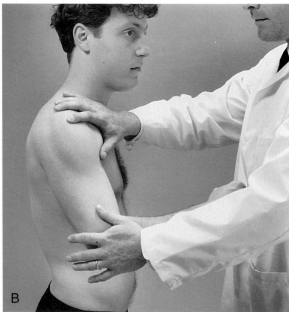

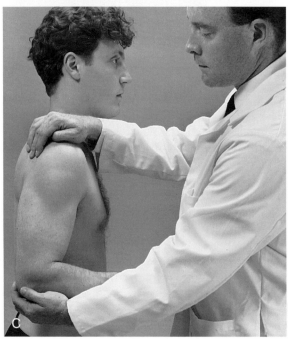

Figure 2–53. Deltoid strength testing. *A,* Anterior. *B,* Middle. *C,* Posterior.

Elbow Flexors and Extenders

Although the biceps and triceps cross the shoulder joint, their principal function is to move the elbow. Strength testing of the biceps and triceps is therefore described in Chapter 3, Elbow and Forearm.

SENSATION TESTING

The **axillary nerve** is the peripheral nerve at greatest risk for injury during shoulder trauma, especially dislocations. Its cutaneous branch supplies an area over the lateral deltoid sometimes described as a shoulder patch (Fig. 2–54). The

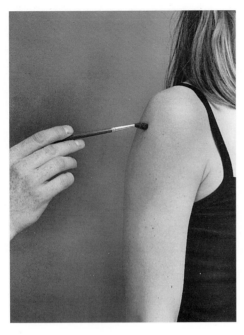

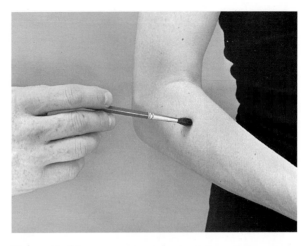

Figure 2-55. Testing for sensory deficit of the sensory branch of the musculocutaneous nerve (lateral cutaneous nerve of the forearm).

Figure 2-54. Testing for axillary nerve sensory deficit.

musculocutaneous nerve is also sometimes injured at the shoulder. Its sensory branch is the lateral cutaneous nerve of the forearm (lateral antebrachial cutaneous nerve), which supplies sensation to the lateral side of the forearm (Fig. 2-55).

SPECIAL TESTS

Rotator Cuff Disorders

Disorders of the rotator cuff complex are among the most common problems afflicting the shoulder. They may vary from reversible bursitis and overuse tendinitis to frank massive rupture of the tendinous cuff. Several findings frequently associated with rotator cuff disorders have already been discussed: tenderness in the subacromial bursa, a painful arc of abduction, abnormal scapulohumeral rhythm during abduction, a weak supraspinatus muscle-tendon unit, and a weak infraspinatus muscle-tendon unit. Several other manipulative tests have been described for detecting rotator cuff disease.

IMPINGEMENT SIGN. Charles Neer proposed the concept of the *impingement syndrome,* which states that most rotator cuff tears are part of a spectrum of rotator cuff tendinopathy that is caused by impingement of the rotator cuff and intervening subacromial bursa on the anterolateral acromion. Neer made the distinction between a rotator cuff impingement sign and an impingement test.

To elicit the **Neer impingement sign,** the examiner passively flexes the patient's shoulder to the position of maximal forward flexion while stabilizing the patient's scapula with the other hand. Reproduction of the patient's symptomatic pain at maximal forward flexion is designated a positive impingement sign and is considered evidence of impingement syndrome (Fig. 2-56A). This maneuver is thought to bring the pathologic anterolateral acromion into contact with the affected portion of the rotator cuff and greater tuberosity, thereby producing pain. The discomfort of impingement may often be increased by flexing the patient's elbow and internally rotating the shoulder before performing the impingement sign (Fig. 2-56B).

When the impingement sign is painful, Neer recommended injecting local anesthetic in the subacromial bursa and repeating the impingement sign. He named this procedure the **[Neer] impingement test.** Pain that is elicited by the Neer impingement sign and eliminated by the subacromial injection of local anesthetic is usually caused by rotator cuff impingement or tear. Present day clinicians are not always careful to make the distinction between the terms *impingement sign* and *impingement test* as Neer originally described them.

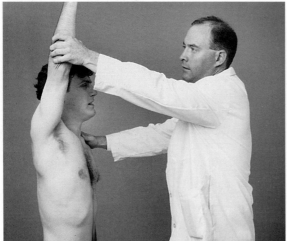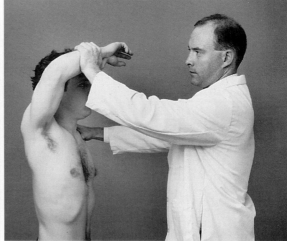

Figure 2–56. *A*, Neer's impingement sign. *B*, Modified Neer's impingement sign.

Another impingement test was described by Hawkins. The **Hawkins impingement reinforcement test** is performed by asking the patient to forward flex the shoulder 90° with the forearm parallel to the floor (Fig. 2–57). The examiner then passively internally rotates the shoulder while keeping the arm in the forward flexed position. This maneuver is felt to drive the greater tuberosity and associated rotator cuff into the acromion and coracoacromial ligament. The production of pain with this maneuver suggests pathology of the rotator cuff or subacromial bursa. As with the Neer impingement test, elimination of this pain by subacromial anesthetic injection strengthens the evidence for rotator cuff pathology. A similar maneuver has also been de-

scribed for eliciting pain in the rare syndrome of *coracoid impingement.*

The **droparm test** is useful when passive abduction greatly exceeds the patient's ability to actively abduct the shoulder. In this case, the examiner gently abducts the patient's shoulder to the maximal degree possible (Fig. 2–58). After warning the patient, the examiner releases the patient's arm and asks him or her to slowly lower the arm back to the side. When a droparm sign is present, the patient is able to lower the arm part way, usually to about 100° of shoulder abduction. The patient then loses control of the arm, which drops suddenly to the side. A **droparm sign** usually indicates a large rotator cuff-tear, although an axillary nerve palsy may pro-

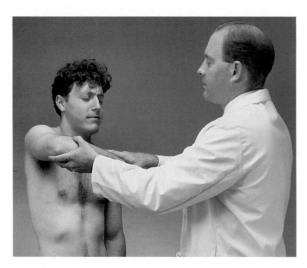

Figure 2–57. Hawkins' impingement reinforcement test.

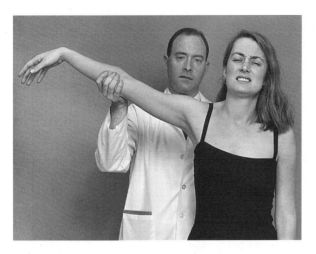

Figure 2–58. Droparm test.

duce the same sign. Improvement in the droparm sign following subacromial anesthetic injection implies that at least some of the dysfunction was due to pain.

SUBSCAPULARIS INJURY. Subscapularis injury is rare. Unlike the other three components of the rotator cuff, the subscapularis inserts on the lesser tuberosity. It is occasionally involved in the most massive rotator cuff tears and also

sometimes ruptured as an isolated injury. Gerber described the subscapularis liftoff test as a physical sign of subscapularis rupture. To perform the **subscapularis liftoff test,** the patient is asked to internally rotate the arm behind the back to the midlumbar region. The dorsum of the patient's hand rests on the back (Fig. 2–59A). The patient is then asked to lift the hand off the back (Fig. 2–59B). The ability to perform this maneuver is thought to require the presence of a functioning subscapularis. Subscapularis strength can also be evaluated by asking the patient to hold the arm in the lifted position while the examiner tries to force the patient's hand toward the back. Strength can be graded in the normal fashion.

PASSIVE ROTATION TEST. Passive rotation in the abducted position may provide supporting evidence for subacromial pathology. To perform this test on the left shoulder, the examiner stands behind the patient. The patient is asked to abduct the left shoulder to 90° with the elbow flexed. The examiner then grasps the patient's left elbow with his or her left hand, and asks the patient to relax control of the arm. The examiner's right hand is placed on the patient's shoulder. The examiner then rotates the patient's shoulder through as wide an arc of internal and external

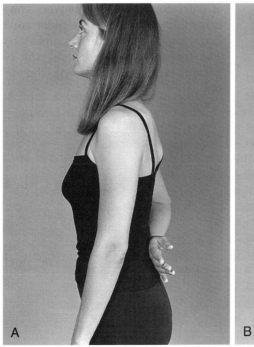
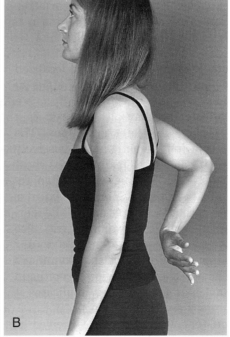

Figure 2–59. *A* and *B*, Subscapularis liftoff test.

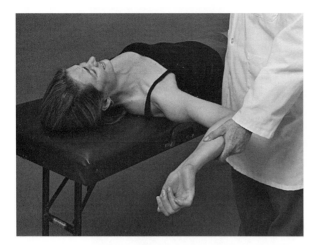

Figure 2–63. Apprehension test.

or apprehension (see Fig. 2–63). The examiner then applies a posteriorly directed force on the anterior aspect of the patient's shoulder with the examiner's free hand. The purpose of this force is to push the presumably subluxed humeral head back into the glenoid fossa. Reduction or resolution of the patient's pain or apprehension by this posteriorly directed force tends to confirm the impression of symptomatic anterior instability (Fig. 2–64A). The examiner may even be able to externally rotate and extend the shoulder several degrees further while maintaining the posteriorly directed force on the patient's humerus. Releasing or easing the posteriorly directed force at this point should cause the patient's pain or apprehension to return. This portion of the maneuver may be called the **release test** (Fig. 2–64B).

shoulder during this test. Although such an episode is pathognomonic of anterior instability, it is not normally considered desirable for this event to occur. The examiner should, therefore, move the patient's arm slowly and stop as soon as the patient indicates a feeling of apprehension or confirms that the test reproduces the position of instability.

In patients with subtle cases of recurrent anterior subluxation, the apprehension test may produce pain but no true apprehension. Pain in the apprehension position is suggestive, but not diagnostic, of anterior instability. The **relocation test** was developed to increase the specificity of the apprehension test for cases of subtle anterior instability. To perform this test, the examiner places the patient's arm in the apprehension position, abducting, extending, and externally rotating the shoulder until the patient feels pain

INTERNAL IMPINGEMENT. Internal impingement is a recently described syndrome in which the apprehension and relocation tests may also both be relevant. In this condition, the posterior rotator cuff impinges against the posterior lip of the glenoid fossa. Abduction–external rotation causes these two structures to come into contact while the relocation maneuver decompresses them. When this happens the patient experiences pain rather than apprehension in response to the apprehension test, and the pain is relieved by the relocation maneuver. This syndrome tends to be associated with more minor degrees of abnormal anterior laxity. The possibility of an internal impingement syndrome, although much less common than anterior instability, should therefore always be kept in mind in a patient, especially an athlete who throws, who experiences pain in response to the apprehension test.

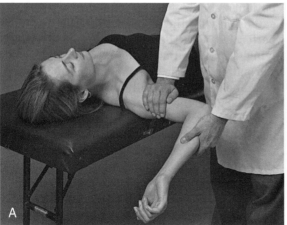
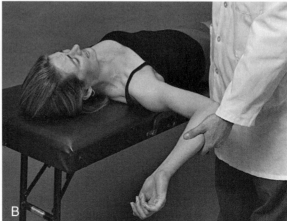

Figure 2–64. *A*, Relocation test. *B*, Release test.

ANTERIOR AND POSTERIOR LAXITY. The **drawer** and **load-and-shift tests** are two ways of quantitating the amount of anterior and posterior laxity present in a given shoulder. To perform the **drawer test,** the patient is asked to sit or stand in a comfortable position with the arm hanging loosely at the side. To examine the patient's right shoulder, the examiner stands behind the patient and grasps the patient's right scapula with the examiner's left hand. The examiner's left index finger is placed on the patient's coracoid process and the left thumb is placed on the scapular spine, allowing the examiner to control and stabilize the scapula and thus the glenoid fossa. The examiner then grasps the humeral head between the thumb and the fingers of his or her right hand (Fig. 2–65A). To assess anterior laxity, the examiner gently pushes the humeral head as far forward as possible, attempting to quantitate the amount of translation sensed (Fig. 2–65B). To assess posterior laxity, the examiner pushes in the opposite direction (Fig. 2–65C). Because considerable variation in shoulder laxity exists among individuals, it is important to examine and compare both shoulders. In fact, examining the normal shoulder first often allows the patient to relax better.

Most normal individuals exhibit greater posterior than anterior laxity with this test. In many normal patients, the humeral head can be translated anteriorly approximately 25% of the width of the glenoid and posteriorly about 50% of the

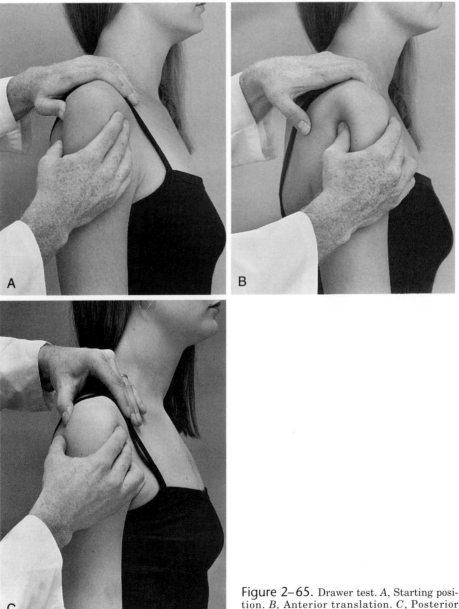

Figure 2–65. Drawer test. *A,* Starting position. *B,* Anterior translation. *C,* Posterior translation.

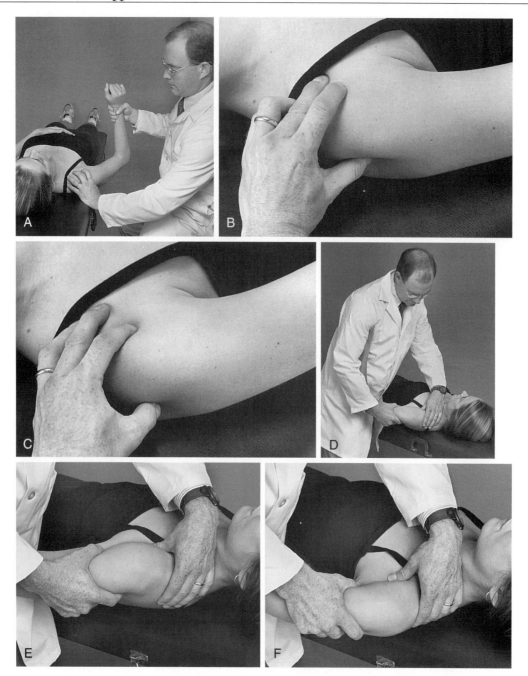

Figure 2–66. Load and shift test. *A*, Standard position. *B*, Anterior translation. *C*, Posterior translation. *D*, Alternative technique. *E*, Anterior translation. *F*, Posterior translation.

width of the glenoid. Translation greater than these amounts, particularly when increased compared with the asymptomatic shoulder, suggests the possibility of clinical instability in the associated direction. The examiner (and patient) may also note some grinding during this maneuver. Such grinding suggests degeneration of or damage to the glenoid labrum.

The **load-and-shift test** is similar in concept to the drawer test, but it is performed with the shoulder in a mildly abducted position. To perform this test, the patient is asked to lie on the

examination table in a supine position. Ideally, the patient's trunk should lie right along the edge of the table so that the shoulder extends slightly over the edge of the table. There are two techniques for performing the load-and-shift test. In the first, the examiner stands or sits comfortably next to the patient. To examine the patient's right shoulder, the examiner grasps the patient's right wrist with the examiner's right hand and supports it so that the entire limb feels limp and relaxed (Fig. 2–66*A*). To assess *anterior laxity,* the humeral head is grasped with the examiner's left index finger and thumb. At the same time, the examiner's left long finger is positioned over the anterior tip of the coracoid process. The examiner then pushes the humeral head forward with the thumb while stabilizing the scapula with the long finger (Fig. 2–66B). The amount of translation is assessed as in the drawer test. Obviously, complete patient relaxation is essential for the proper interpretation of this test. The test is initially performed with the shoulder in a position of neutral rotation, 30° flexion, and 30° abduction. The examiner may vary the position of the patient's shoulder until the position of greatest laxity is found. To assess *posterior laxity,* the examiner merely reverses the direction of the applied force to translate the humeral head posteriorly between the examiner's thumb and the index finger (Fig. 2–66C). In this case, the examination table itself serves to restrain the scapula, so that no additional stabilization of the scapula is required. Again, the exact position of the shoulder can be varied until the position of maximal posterior laxity is determined. As in the drawer test, translation in the normal and the symptomatic shoulder should be compared. The range of normal translation is similar to that found in the drawer test.

In the *alternative technique,* the examiner suspends the patient's limb by squeezing the patient's hand between the examiner's upper arm and chest. The advantage of this technique is that it frees both of the examiner's hands so that one hand may be used to control the patient's humeral head while the other hand is used to stabilize the scapula as in the drawer test (Fig. 2–66D–F). The disadvantage of this technique is that it is more difficult to control and vary the exact position of the patient's shoulder.

MULTIDIRECTIONAL INSTABILITY. Multidirectional instability occurs when the humeral head can be dislocated or subluxed in more than one direction. The sine qua non of multidirectional instability is inferior instability combined with instability in at least one other direction. Some, but not all, of these patients also have signs of generalized ligamentous laxity.

INFERIOR LAXITY. The **sulcus sign** demonstrates inferior laxity of the shoulder. The sulcus sign is usually elicited in the standing or sitting patient. The examiner stands at the patient's side and encourages the patient to relax. The examiner then grasps the patient's arm just above the elbow while looking at the lateral border of the patient's acromion. The patient's arm is then pulled downward. The purpose of this traction is to sublux the humeral head inferiorly in relationship to the glenoid fossa. In patients with greater degrees of inferior laxity, a hollow or sulcus is visible between the lateral edge of the acromion and the humeral head (Fig. 2–67). The size of the sulcus can be quantitated subjectively or estimated in millimeters or centimeters. The pres-

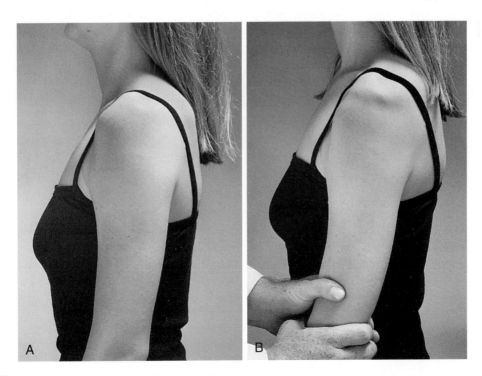

Figure 2–67. Sulcus sign. *A,* Starting position. *B,* Ending position.

ence of a sulcus sign identifies the patient who is at risk for multidirectional instability, but a sulcus sign does not conclusively indicate this diagnosis. The significance of the sulcus sign increases if the size of the sulcus is greater on the symptomatic than on the normal side. Patients with inferior instability often exhibit signs of apprehension when the sulcus test is performed.

POSTERIOR INSTABILITY. The **jerk** and **circumduction tests** are two provocative tests to reproduce symptoms of posterior instability. The **jerk test** is best performed in the supine, relaxed patient. The patient's shoulder is forward flexed 90° with the elbow flexed. The examiner then applies a posteriorly directed force at the elbow, attempting to push the humeral head out the back of the glenoid fossa (Fig. 2–68). A jerk or jump may be felt as the humeral head dislocates

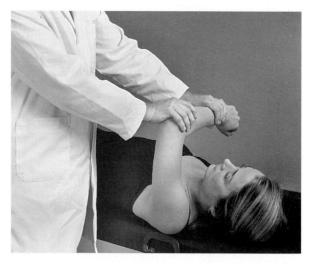

Figure 2–68. Jerk test.

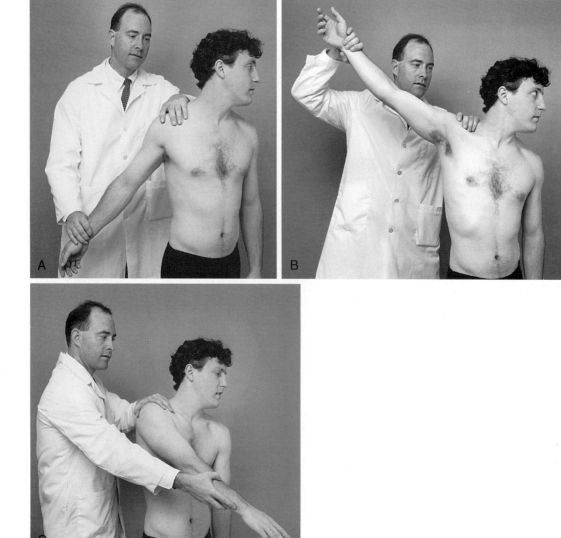

Figure 2–69. *A–C*, Circumduction test.

out of the glenoid posteriorly. Internal rotation and adduction of the shoulder may help the humeral head to dislocate. In the presence of more subtle posterior instability, the test may produce pain or apprehension without a palpable dislocation.

The **circumduction test** is performed in the standing position. To examine the right shoulder, the clinician stands behind the patient and grasps the patient's right forearm with the examiner's own right hand. The examiner initiates circumduction by bringing the patient's shoulder into an extended and slightly abducted position (Fig. 2–69A). The examiner then continues around, describing a complete circle with the patient's arm (Fig. 2–69B). After the patient's arm comes over the top, it continues down in front of the patient into a flexed and adducted position (Fig. 2–69C). The position of risk occurs when the patient's shoulder is flexed forward and adducted. In patients with recurrent posterior instability, the patient's humeral head can usually be felt and seen to sublux posteriorly. The examiner's free hand may be placed on the posterior aspect of the patient's shoulder to detect this subluxation. The patient should be asked if the maneuver elicits the patient's familiar symptoms.

VOLUNTARY DISLOCATION. Some patients are capable of **voluntary dislocation** of their own shoulders. Some of these are purely voluntary dislocators; the shoulder dislocates only when the patient initiates the phenomenon. Other patients are capable of voluntary dislocation, but present to the physician because they are troubled by episodes of involuntary dislocation. All patients being evaluated for shoulder instability should be asked if they can voluntarily reproduce their symptoms. If the response is affirmative, they should be asked to demonstrate this for the physician.

Voluntary dislocation may be anterior, posterior, or multidirectional. Most commonly, the patient dislocates the shoulder by placing it in a certain position and selectively contracting certain muscle groups (Fig. 2–70A). Other patients dislocate the shoulder solely through proper positioning of the arm. Some individuals have shoulders that are so unstable that they can grasp the humeral head with the opposite hand and push it out of the socket in the desired direction (Fig. 2–70B). The ability to voluntarily dislocate the shoulder is important to detect because it may be a sign of emotional illness. If there is suspicion that the patient is using the dislocations for secondary social or psychologic gain, a thorough psychologic evaluation should be conducted. In other cases, the ability to voluntarily dislocate the shoulder is merely a sign of the great degree of abnormal laxity present and not an indication of emotional illness.

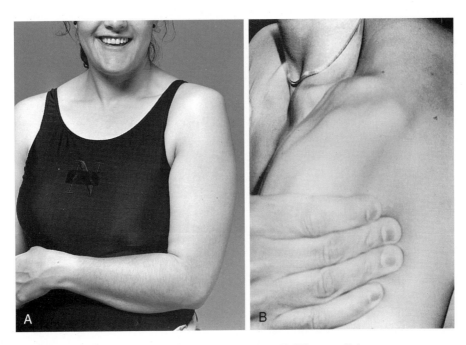

Figure 2–70. *A,* Voluntary dislocation by selective muscle contracture. *B,* Voluntary dislocation by self-manipulation.

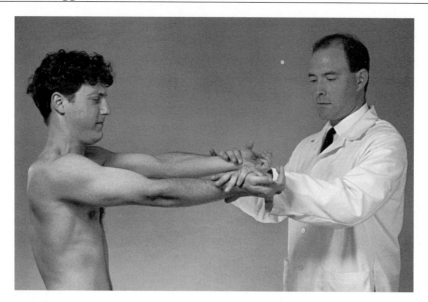

Figure 2–71. Speed test.

Biceps Tendon

TENDINITIS. In the past, biceps tendinitis was thought to be a very common cause of shoulder pain. Currently, isolated biceps tendinitis is considered to be much more uncommon than was originally believed. When it occurs, it almost always involves the long head tendon. Biceps tendinitis is frequently associated with signs of rotator cuff impingement or tear.

A number of tests have been described to elicit pain in the presence of biceps tendinitis. The **Speed test** is perhaps the most sensitive for provoking biceps tendon pain. It is performed by asking the patient to place the shoulder in the 90° forward flexed position with the elbow fully extended; the forearm is supinated. The patient is then instructed to resist as the examiner attempts to push the patient's arm downward (Fig. 2–71). The patient with biceps tendinitis tends to complain of pain with this maneuver and exhibits difficulty resisting the examiner's downward pressure.

To perform **Yergason's test,** the patient places the arm at the side with the elbow flexed 90° and the forearm pronated. The examiner then grasps the patient's hand and asks the patient to attempt to simultaneously flex the elbow and supinate the forearm while the examiner resists (Fig. 2–72). Flexion of the elbow and supination of the forearm are the primary functions of the biceps muscle. Pain in the anterior aspect of the shoulder produced by this maneuver is thought to reflect biceps tendinitis or instability. In the au-

thors' experience, it is less sensitive than the Speed test.

INSTABILITY. The **biceps instability test** was described by Abbott and Saunders to demonstrate instability of the long head biceps tendon in the intertubercular groove. This phenomenon is usually associated with a tear of the rotator cuff. To perform the test, the examiner grasps the patient's arm and brings it into abduction and external rotation (Fig. 2–73A). While palpating the bicipital groove, the examiner then internally rotates the shoulder in the scapular plane. Subluxation or dislocation of the tendon pro-

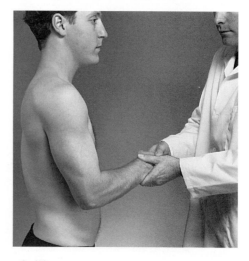

Figure 2–72. Yergason's test.

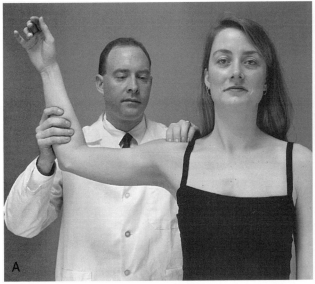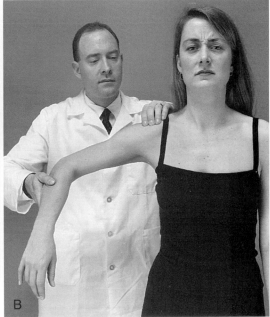

Figure 2–73. *A* and *B*, Biceps instability test.

duces a palpable and sometimes audible snap (Fig. 2–73*B*).

Thoracic Outlet Syndrome

Compression of the neurovascular structures as they exit the thorax above the first rib is known as thoracic outlet syndrome. It has many origins. Compression can cause pain and paresthesias in the arm and shoulder. This syndrome is part of the differential diagnosis of shoulder pain. Its symptoms can easily be confused with much more common disorders such as rotator cuff tendinitis. Several maneuvers have been described to help diagnose this condition.

Adson's test is the most well known of these maneuvers. The arm of the seated or standing patient is abducted 30° at the shoulder and maximally extended. The examiner grasps the patient's wrist, positioning the examiner's fingers to palpate the radial pulse. The patient is then asked to turn the head toward the injured shoulder (Fig. 2–74*A*). The patient may also be asked to take a deep breath and hold it. The examiner evaluates the quality of the radial pulse in this position and compares it with the quality of the pulse with the arm resting at the patient's side (Fig. 2–74*B*). Diminution or disappearance of the pulse in the test position suggests the possibility of a thoracic outlet syndrome, especially if the patient's symptoms are reproduced. Some clinicians have modified this test by having the pa-

tient turn the head away from the side being tested (Fig. 2–74*C*). A similar test, in which the shoulder is abducted to 90° and fully externally rotated, is known as **Wright's maneuver.**

In the **Roos test,** the patient is asked to abduct the affected shoulder 90° while flexing the elbow 90° as well. The patient is then asked to open and close the hand 15 times (Fig. 2–75). The patient is encouraged to describe any sensation felt during this process. Numbness, cramping, weakness, or an inability to complete the prescribed number of repetitions is suggestive of thoracic outlet syndrome. Symptoms that appear as the test progresses are more suggestive than symptoms that are present initially and do not change during the test.

Halsted's test is performed in the upright patient. The examiner palpates the radial pulse with the patient's arm at the side (Fig. 2–76*A*). The patient is asked to turn the head away from the involved shoulder and extend the neck while the examiner places downward traction on the arm and continues to palpate the pulse (Fig. 2–76*B*). Obliteration of the pulse by this maneuver is suggestive of thoracic outlet syndrome. A partial obstruction can be determined by the production of an auscultable bruit during testing.

In the **hyperabduction test,** the examiner fully abducts both arms simultaneously after verifying the patient's pulses with the arms at the sides. Diminution or obliteration of the pulse on the affected side compared with the normal con-

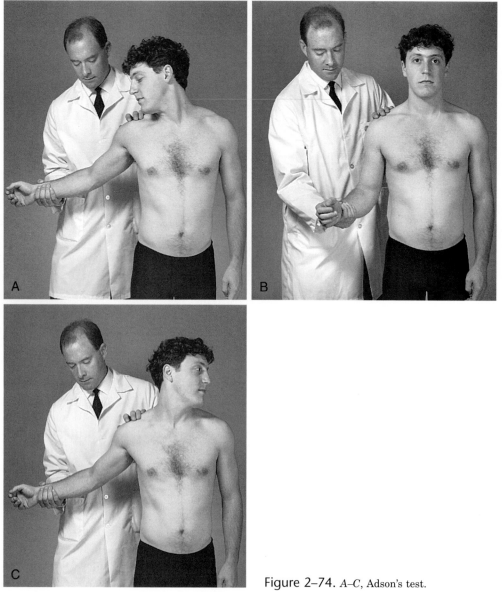

Figure 2–74. *A–C*, Adson's test.

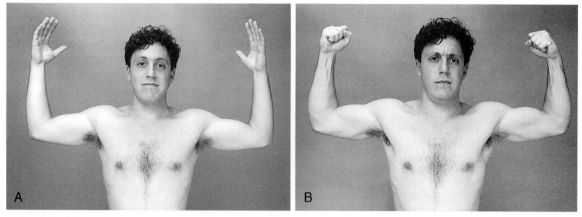

Figure 2–75. *A* and *B*, Roos' test.

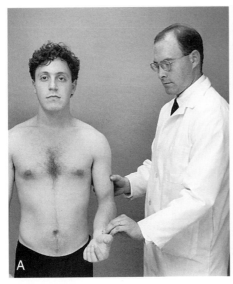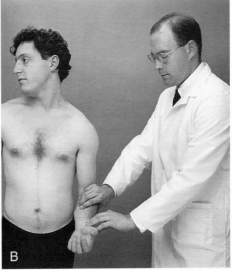

Figure 2–76. *A* and *B,* Halsted's test.

tralateral side is suggestive of thoracic outlet syndrome (Fig. 2–77). Of course, if the patient has bilateral involvement, the test is less helpful. Bilateral diminution of pulses may occur in some normal individuals.

Examination of Other Areas

Shoulder pain can be produced by pathology in other areas of the body, especially the neck. Cervical spine pathology can result in pain in several sites in the shoulder girdle, most commonly in the upper trapezius or rhomboid areas. Pain of cervical origin can often be distinguished by the fact that it is exacerbated by movement or manipulation of the neck rather than of the shoulder itself.

Disorders of the heart, lungs, and abdominal viscera may also produce shoulder pain. In such cases, the examiner usually observes that movement or manipulation of the shoulder has no reproducible effect on the pain, and the evaluation of the appropriate organ reveals related abnormalities

The physical findings in common conditions of the shoulder and upper arm are summarized in Table 2–1.

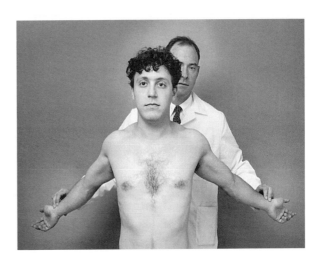

Figure 2–77. Hyperabduction test.

TABLE 2–1.
PHYSICAL FINDINGS IN COMMON CONDITIONS OF THE SHOULDER AND UPPER ARM

Impingement Syndrome

Hawkins' impingement reinforcement test abnormal
Neer impingement sign often present
Supraspinatus resistance testing often painful
Painful arc of abduction often present
Subacromial bursa tender (variable)

Rotator Cuff Tear

Hawkins' impingement reinforcement test abnormal
Neer impingement sign often present
Painful arc of abduction present
Supraspinatus resistance painful and often weak
Supraspinatus atrophy present (more severe cases)
Infraspinatus resistance painful and possibly weak (more severe cases)
Infraspinatus atrophy present (more severe cases)
Loss of active motion, particularly abduction. (variable)
Droparm sign present (more severe cases)
Loss of active external rotation (massive tears)

Anterior Instability (Recurrent Subluxation or Dislocation)

Apprehension in response to apprehension test
Reduction of apprehension in response to relocation test
Increased anterior laxity to passive testing (drawer test, load-and-shift test)
Signs of axillary nerve injury (occasionally) (deltoid weakness and numbness over lateral shoulder)
Signs of musculocutaneous nerve injury (rarely) (biceps weakness and numbness over lateral forearm)

Posterior Instability (Recurrent Subluxation or Dislocation)

Increased posterior laxity to passive testing (drawer test, load-and-shift test)
Mildly abnormal sulcus test (variable)
Symptoms reproduced by jerk test or circumduction test (variable)
Voluntary dislocation or subluxation possible (occasionally)

Multidirectional Instability

Abnormal sulcus sign
Increased anterior and/or posterior laxity to passive testing (drawer test, load-and-shift test)
Additional signs of anterior or posterior instability depending on predominant direction of symptomatic episodes
Ability to voluntarily dislocate (occasionally)

Acromioclavicular Joint Injury

Tenderness of acromioclavicular joint
Localized swelling in acromioclavicular joint
Increase in prominence of distal clavicle (variable, depending on severity of injury)
Tenderness of coracoclavicular ligaments (more severe injuries)
Pain with cross-chest adduction
Rarely, distal clavicle displaced posteriorly (Type IV injuries) or inferiorly (Type VI injuries)
O'Brien's test produces pain on top of shoulder (variable)

Biceps Tendinitis

Biceps tendon tender
Speed's test painful
Yergason's test painful (occasionally)
Biceps instability test abnormal (occasionally, if biceps tendon unstable)
Signs of concomitant rotator cuff tear (variable)

Suprascapular Nerve Compression or Injury

Supraspinatus and infraspinatus weakness and atrophy (if compression prior to innervation of supraspinatus)
Infraspinatus weakness and atrophy alone (if compression at the spinoglenoid notch)

Rheumatoid Arthritis

Local warmth and swelling
Muscle atrophy often present
Signs of rheumatoid involvement at other joints

Thoracic Outlet Syndrome

Symptoms reproduced by Roos' test, Wright's maneuver, Adson's test, or hyperabduction test (variable)
Diminution of pulse with Adson's test, Wright's maneuver, Halsted's test, or hyperabduction test (variable)

Adhesive Capsulitis (Frozen Shoulder)

Generalized decrease in both active and passive range of motion, including forward flexion, abduction, internal rotation, and external rotation
Pain elicited by passive range of motion or any passive manipulation that stresses the limits of the patient's reduced motion
Generalized weakness or atrophy (variable)

Stinger Syndrome (Burners)

Tenderness over brachial plexus
Weakness in muscles innervated by involved portion of the plexus (deltoid most commonly involved, elbow flexors second most commonly involved)

Bibliography

American Academy of Orthopaedic Surgeons: Joint Motion: Method of Measuring and Recording. Chicago, American Academy of Orthopaedic Surgeons, 1965.

Beetham WP, Polley HF, Slocum CH, Weaver WF: Physical Examination of the Joints. Philadelphia, WB Saunders 1965, p 41.

Bigliani LU, Perez-Sanz JR, Wolf IN: Treatment of trapezius paralysis. J Bone Joint Surg Am. 1985;67:871–877.

Bigliani LU, Levine WM: Subacromial impingement syndrome. J Bone Joint Surg Am. 1997;79:1854–1868.

Boublik M, Hawkins RJ: Clinical examination of the shoulder complex. J Orthop Sports Phys Ther. 1993;18:379–385.

Burkhead WZ: The biceps tendon. In Rockwood CA, Matsen FA III, eds. The Shoulder. Philadelphia, WB Saunders, 1990, pp 791–836.

Butters KP: The scapula. In Rockwood CA, Matsen FA III, eds. The Shoulder. Philadelphia, WB Saunders, 1990, pp 335–366.

Curran JF, Ellman MH, Brown NL: Rheumatologic aspects of painful conditions affecting the shoulder. Clin Orthop. 1983;173:27–37.

Dameron TB, Rockwood CA: Fractures of the shaft of the clavicle. In Rockwood CA, Wilkins KE, King RE, eds. Fractures in Children. Philadelphia, JB Lippincott, 1984, 608–624.

Fan PT, Blanton, ME: Clinical features and diagnosis of fibromyalgia. J Musculoskeletal Med. 1992;9:24–42.

Gerber C, Hersche O, Farron A: Isolated rupture of the subscapularis tendon: results of operative repair. J Bone Joint Surg Am. 1996;78:1015–1023.

Gerber C, Terrier F, Ganz R: The role of the coracoid process in the chronic impingement syndrome. J Bone Joint Surg Br. 1985;67:703–708.

Gerber C, Ganz R: Clinical assessment of instability of the shoulder. J Bone Joint Surg Br. 1984;66:551–556.

Glockner, SM: Shoulder pain: a diagnostic dilemma. Am Fam Physician. 1995;51:1677–1687.

Gross ML, Distefano MC: Anterior release test. A new test for occult shoulder instability. Clin Orthop. 1997;(339):105–108.

Habermyer P, Kaiser E, Knappe M: Functional anatomy and biomechanics of the long biceps tendon. Unfallchirurgie. 1987;90:319–329.

Hawkins RJ, Neer CS II, Pianta RM, Mendoza FX: Locked posterior dislocation of the shoulder. J Bone Joint Surg Am. 1987;69:9–18.

Hawkins RJ: Cervical spine and the shoulder. Instr Course Lect. 1985;34:191–195.

Hawkins RJ, Boker DJ: Clinical evaluation of shoulder problems. In Rockwood CA, Matsen FA III, eds. The Shoulder. Philadelphia, WB Saunders, 1990, pp 149–177.

Hawkins RJ, Hobeika P: Physical examination of the shoulder. Orthopedics. 1983;6:1270–1278.

Hawkins RJ, Kennedy JC: Impingement syndrome in athletes. Am J Sports Med. 1980;8:151–158.

Hawkins RJ, Mohtadi NGH: Clinical evaluation of shoulder instability. Clin J Sports Med. 1991;1:59–64.

Howard TM, O'Connor FG: The injured shoulder: primary care assessment. Arch Fam Med. 1997;6:376–384.

Inman VT, Saunders DM, Abbot LC: Observations on the function of the shoulder joint. J Bone Joint Surg Am. 1944;24:1–30.

Jobe CM: Superior glenoid impingement. Orthop Clin North Am. 1997;28:137–143.

Jobe FW, Radovich Moynes D: Delineation of diagnostic criteria and a rehabilitation program for rotator cuff injuries. Am J Sports Med. 1982;10:336–339.

Jobe FW, Jobe CM: Painful athletic injuries of the shoulder. Clin Orthop. 1983;(173):117–124.

Kessel L, Watson M: The painful arc syndrome: clinical classification as a guide to management. J Bone Joint Surg Br. 1977;59:166–172.

Kibler WB: Role of the scapula in the overhead scapular motion. Contemp Orthop. 1991;22:525–532.

Kretzler HH, Richardson AB: Rupture of the pectoralis major muscle. Am J Sports Med. 1989;17:453–458.

Kvitne RS, Jobe FW, Jobe CM: Shoulder instability in the overhand or throwing athlete. Clin Sports Med. 1995;14:917–935.

Leffert RD: Thoracic outlet syndrome. J Am Acad Orthop Surg. 1994;2:317–325.

Lerat J-L, Chotel F, Besse JL, et al: Le Ressaut Dynamique Anterieur de l'épaule. Un nouveau test clinique d'instabilité de l'épaule. Étude préliminaire. [The Shoulder Anterior Jerk Test. A New Clinical Examination Test for Shoulder Anterior Instability. Preliminary Report]. Rev Chir Orthop. 1994;80:461–467.

Magee DJ: Orthopedic Physical Assessment. Philadelphia, WB Saunders, 1992, pp 90–142.

Makin GJV, Brown WF, Ebers GC: C7 radiculopathy: importance of scapular winging in clinical diagnosis. J Neurol Neurosurg Psychiatry. 1986;49:640–644.

Matsen FA III, Kirby RM: Office evaluation and management of shoulder pain. Orthop Clin North Am. 1982;13:453–475.

Matsen FA III, Lillitt SB, Sidles JA, Harryman DT: Practical Evaluation and Management of the Shoulder. Philadelphia, WB Saunders, 1994, pp 19–58.

Matsen FA III, Thomas SC, Rockwood CA: Glenohumeral instability. In Rockwood CA, Matsen FA III, eds. The Shoulder. Philadelphia, WB Saunders, 1990, pp 526–622.

Mayfield FH: Neural and vascular compression syndromes of the shoulder girdles and arms. Clin Neurosurg. 1968;15:384–393.

McFarland EG, Torpey BM, Curl LA: Evaluation of shoulder laxity. Sports Med. 1996;4:264–272.

Neer CS: Anterior acromioplasty for the chronic impingement syndrome in the shoulder: a preliminary report. J Bone Joint Surg Am. 1972;54:41–50.

Neer CS, Foster CR: Inferior capsular shift for involuntary inferior and multidirectional instability of the shoulder: a preliminary report. J Bone Joint Surg Am. 1980;62:897–908.

O'Brien SJ, Pagnani MJ, Fealy S, McGlynn SR, Wilson JB: The active compression test: A new and effective test for diagnosing labral tears and acromioclavicular joint injuries. Am J Sports Med. 1998;26:610–613.

Ogino T, Minami A, Kato H, Hara R, Suzuki K: Entrapment neuropathy of the suprascapular nerve by a ganglion, a report of three cases. J Bone Joint Surg Am. 1991;73:141–147.

Pal GP, Bhatt RH, Patel VS: Relationship between the tendon of the long head of the biceps brachii and the glenoid labrum in humans. Anat Rec. 1991;229:278–280.

Pappas AM, Zawacki RM, McCarthy CF: Rehabilitation of the pitching shoulder. Am Journal Sports Med. 1985;13:223–235.

Parsonage MJ, Turner JW: Neuralgic amyotrophy; shoulder-girdle syndrome. Lancet. 1948;1:973–978.

Poppen NK, Walker PS: Normal and abnormal motion of the shoulder. J Bone Joint Surg Am. 1976;58:195–201.

Post M: Physical examination of the shoulder girdle. In Post M, ed. Physical Examination of the Musculoskeletal System. Chicago, Year Book, 1987, pp 13–55.

Post M, Mayer J: Suprascapular nerve entrapment. Diagnosis and treatment. Clin Orthop. 1987;(223):126–136.

Rengachary SS, Burr D, Lucas S, Hassanein K, Mohn MP, Matzke H: Suprascapular entrapment neuropathy: a clinical, anatomical, and comparative study. Neurosurgery. 1979;5:447–451.

Rockwood CA: Disorders of the sternoclavicular joint. In Rockwood CA, Matsen FA III, eds. The Shoulder. Philadelphia, WB Saunders, 1990, pp 477–525.

Rockwood CA, Young CD: Disorders of the acromioclavicular joint. In Rockwood CA, Matsen FA III, eds. Philadelphia WB Saunders, 1990, pp 413–470.

Rowe CR, Zarins B: Recurrent transient subluxation of the shoulder. J Bone Joint Surg Am. 1981;63:863–871.

Shankwiler JA, Burkhead WZ Jr: Evaluation of painful shoulders: entities that may be confused with rotator cuff disease. In Burkhead WZ, ed. Rotator Cuff Disorders. Baltimore, Williams & Wilkins, 1996, pp 59–72.

Silliman JF, Hawkins RJ: Classification and physical diagnosis of instability of the shoulder. Clin. Orthop. 1993;(291):7–19.

Slater RR Jr, Bynum DK: Diagnosis and treatment of carpal tunnel syndrome. Orthop Rev. 1993;22:1095–1105.

Sobel JS, Winters JC, Groenier K, Arendzen JH, de Jong BM: Physical examination of the cervical spine and shoulder girdle in patients with shoulder complaints. J Manipulative Physiol Ther. 1997;20:257–262.

Solheim LF, Roaas A: Compression of the suprascapular nerve after fracture of the scapular notch. Acta Orthop Scand. 1978;49:338–340.

Szalay E, Rockwood CA Jr: Injuries of the shoulder and arm. Emerg Med Clin North Am. 1984;2:279–294.

Turner-Stokes L: Clinical differential diagnosis of shoulder pain. Br J Hosp Med. 1996;56:73–77.

Urschel HC Jr, Paulson DL, McNamara JJ: Thoracic outlet syndrome. Ann Thorac Surg. 1968;6:1–10.

Vangsness CT Jr, Jorgenson SS, Watson T, Johnson DL: The origin of the long head of the biceps from the scapula and glenoid labrum. J Bone Joint Surg Am. 1994;76:951–954.

Wolfe SW, Wickiewicz TL, Cavanaugh JT: Ruptures of the pectoralis major muscle: an anatomical and clinical analysis. Am J Sports Med. 1992;20:587–593.

Wright MH, Jobe C, O'Hara RC, Osborn JM, Alexander G: Cross-sectional anatomy of impingement syndrome [abstract]. J Shoulder Elbow Surg. 1994;3(suppl):573.

Yergason RM: Supination sign. J Bone Joint Surg Am. 1931;13:160.

Roderick Birnie
Bruce Reider

3

Elbow and Forearm

Located in the middle of the upper extremity, the elbow greatly increases the usefulness of the hand. By flexing and extending, the elbow allows an individual to decrease or increase the functional length of the upper limb, producing great flexibility in positioning the hand in space. The major flexor and extensor muscles that cross the elbow joint are powerful motors for lifting, pulling, or pushing.

The rotational capabilities of the forearm complement the elbow's function. The remarkable ability of the forearm to pronate and supinate allows an individual even greater variety in positioning the hand and wrist, while permitting complex rotational tasks that would otherwise be awkward or impossible. In addition, the muscles of the forearm serve as the primary motors of the wrist and hand.

The elbow joint is a complex structure. The principal tasks of flexion and extension are carried out between the distal humerus and the proximal olecranon. The spindle-shaped humeral trochlea fits into the semicircular notch formed by the olecranon and coronoid processes of the proximal ulna, resulting in excellent stability throughout a wide range of motion. Although the head of the proximal radius articulates with the capitellum of the humerus and thus participates in flexion and extension, the modifications in its shape that permit forearm rotation reduce its ability to add stability to the elbow. The round shape of the radial head and the convex nature of the capitellum allow the radius to rotate freely regardless of the degree of elbow flexion, thus permitting forearm rotation in any position of flexion or extension.

Inspection

SURFACE ANATOMY

Anterior Aspect

ANTERIOR FLEXION CREASE. A good landmark for orientation in the anterior elbow is the **anterior flexion crease** (Fig. 3–1). This trans-verse skin line marks the point where the skin folds when the elbow is flexed. The flexion crease occurs at the level of the medial and lateral epicondyles and thus is actually 1 cm to 2 cm proximal to the joint line when the elbow is extended.

SUPERFICIAL VEINS OF THE CUBITAL FOSSA. The superficial veins of the cubital fossa are among the most prominent veins in the body. In lean individuals, especially males, they are easily observed. The **cephalic vein** runs proximally up the lateral border of the anterior forearm, whereas the **basilic vein** runs up the medial side. In between these two lies the prominent **median vein of the forearm.** Just distal to the flexion crease the median vein divides, sending large tributaries to both the cephalic and the basilic veins. This configuration results in a prominent M-shaped pattern. The large basilic vein then continues proximally in the upper arm along the medial border of the biceps brachii muscle, whereas the cephalic vein follows the lateral border of the same muscle. The exact configuration of these veins varies considerably, however, and only the communicating branch, known as the **medial cubital vein,** may be detectable in more obese individuals. This is the vein commonly used for drawing blood. Lymphatic drainage accompanies the superficial and deep veins, terminating in the central and lateral axillary lymph nodes. The **epitrochlear lymph nodes,** located in the basilic system just proximal to the medial epicondyle, may be enlarged in the presence of infection of the hand or the distal forearm.

BONY LANDMARKS AND TENDONS. The prominent musculature of the anterior elbow and forearm obscures most bony prominences when the limb is viewed from this perspective. The **medial epicondyle** is usually visible on the medial border of the elbow at the level of the flexion crease, although it may be obscured by the muscles originating from it. The **lateral epicondyle** is not visible anteriorly. The anterior aspect of the distal upper arm above the elbow is dominated by the oval contour of the **biceps brachii** muscle belly. The distal biceps has a dual insertion. The most prominent portion of the insertion is the **lacertus fibrosus,** a superficial band that inserts into the investing fascia of the proximal

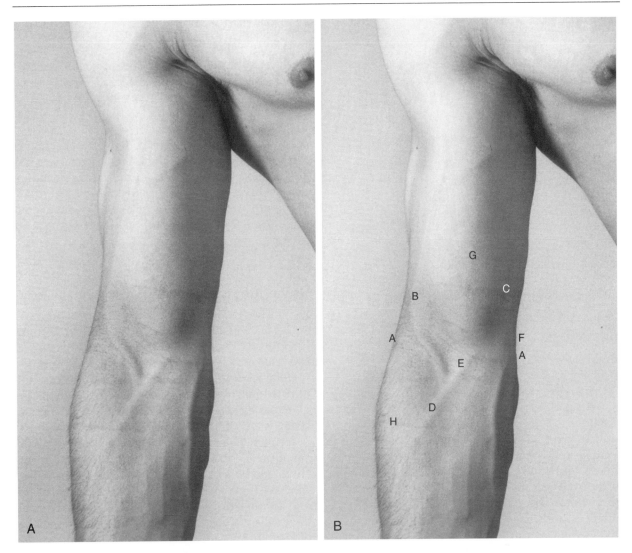

Figure 3–1. *A* and *B,* Anterior aspect of the elbow. A, anterior flexion crease; B, cephalic vein; C, basilic vein; D, median vein of the forearm; E, medial cubital vein; F, medial epicondyle; G, biceps brachii; H, brachioradialis.

medial forearm. This band may be visible even in the relaxed state and becomes quite prominent when the elbow is flexed against resistance (Fig. 3–2). The lacertus fibrosus may obscure the more important insertion of the biceps, the **distal biceps tendon,** which angles laterally to insert into the tuberosity of the proximal radius. This tendon can usually be palpated if the examiner inserts a finger just lateral to the more prominent lacertus fibrosus. It is this insertion into the radius that allows the biceps to function as a powerful supinator of the forearm.

The **brachialis** muscle lies deep to the biceps brachii. It is not distinctly visible, but it contributes to the apparent bulk of the biceps.

If a rupture of the biceps tendon occurs, the biceps retracts proximally, producing considerable deformity of the biceps contour (Fig. 3–3). More rarely, rupture of the biceps muscle can also lead to severe deformity of the biceps.

DEEP VESSELS AND NERVES. The lacertus fibrosus and biceps tendon serve as helpful anatomic landmarks for other structures of the anterior elbow that are not normally visible. The **brachial artery** is just medial to the biceps tendon. The **median nerve,** in turn, lies just medial to the brachial artery. Lateral to the tendon, the **musculocutaneous nerve** emerges from beneath the biceps muscle and continues distally as the **lateral cutaneous nerve of the forearm.**

FOREARM MUSCLES. The proximal portions of the forearm muscles form the inverted triangular depression known as the **cubital fossa (antecubital fossa).** The lateral border of the antecubital fossa is formed by a bulky group of three muscles that originates from the lateral humerus above the elbow: the *brachioradialis,* the *extensor carpi radialis longus,* and the *extensor carpi radialis brevis.* This muscle group was dubbed the

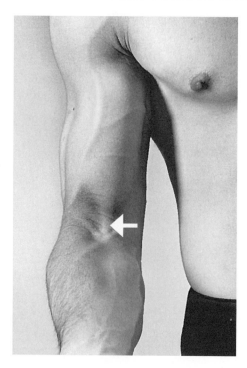

Figure 3–2. Anterior aspect of the elbow during resisted flexion (*arrow* indicates lacertus fibrosus).

mobile wad of three by the anatomist Henry because they can be grasped by the examiner's thumb and index finger and wiggled back and forth if the patient is relaxed. The **brachioradialis,** which arises from the lateral border of the humerus and inserts near the radial styloid, is the only one of these three that is visible anteriorly when the forearm is fully supinated, and it forms the lateral border of the forearm in this position (Fig. 3–4). The muscles that originate from the medial epicondyle are sometimes known as the *flexor-pronator group* because they consist of the pronator teres and the principal flexors of

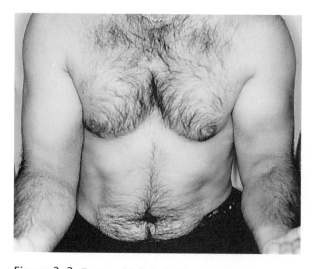

Figure 3–3. Ruptured left distal biceps tendon.

the wrist and fingers. The **pronator teres** is the most centrally situated of these muscles, and it forms the lateral border of the antecubital fossa. The bellies of the wrist flexors (**flexor carpi radialis, palmaris longus,** and **flexor carpi ulnaris**) are located medial to the pronator teres. Together, these four muscles constitute the contour of the medial forearm. Because the finger flexors are located deep to these four muscles, they add to the bulk of the anterior forearm but do not directly influence its contour.

Distally, the forearm muscles taper to tendons, which are discussed in Chapter 4, Hand and Wrist.

Posterior Aspect

OLECRANON PROCESS AND MEDIAL AND LATERAL EPICONDYLES. The posterior aspect of the elbow is dominated by three bony prominences: the **olecranon process** and the **medial** and **lateral epicondyles** (Fig. 3–5). When the elbow is flexed, these three landmarks form a triangle. At 90° of flexion, an equilateral triangle is formed. When the elbow is fully extended, the tip of the olecranon moves proximally, so that the three landmarks lie along a straight line. The relationship of these three bony landmarks to one another can be used to assist in the clinical diagnosis of fractures and dislocations about the elbow. In the presence of a *dislocation of the elbow,* the relationship of the two epicondyles to each other remains normal but their relationship to the olecranon changes. In the case of a *posterior elbow dislocation,* the most common type, the olecranon moves posteriorly with respect to the epicondyles and becomes more prominent. When a *supracondylar fracture* of the humerus occurs, the normal relationship of these three bony landmarks is maintained but the entire triangle is translated or angulated with respect to the humerus, most commonly in the posterior direction. If one of the humeral epicondyles is fractured and displaced or a comminuted supracondylar or intracondylar fracture is present, the normal relationship of the two epicondyles to each other is disrupted.

OLECRANON BURSA. The redundancy of the skin overlying the olecranon process facilitates the extreme amount of flexion possible at the elbow. When the elbow is fully extended, this redundant skin is loose and wrinkled. The **olecranon bursa** lies between the tip of the olecranon and the overlying skin, facilitating the large

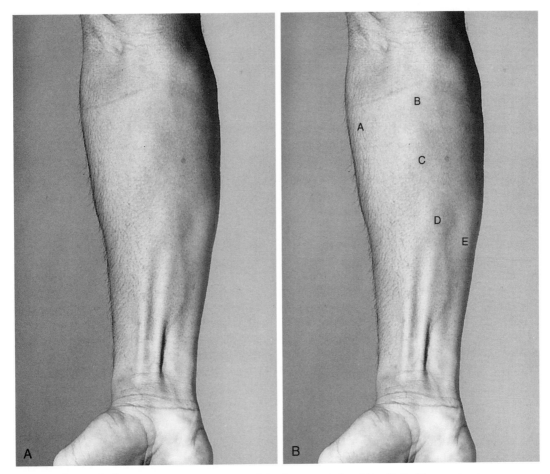

Figure 3–4. *A* and *B,* Anterior aspect of the forearm. A, brachioradialis; B, pronator teres; C, flexor carpi radialis; D, palmaris longus; E, flexor carpi ulnaris.

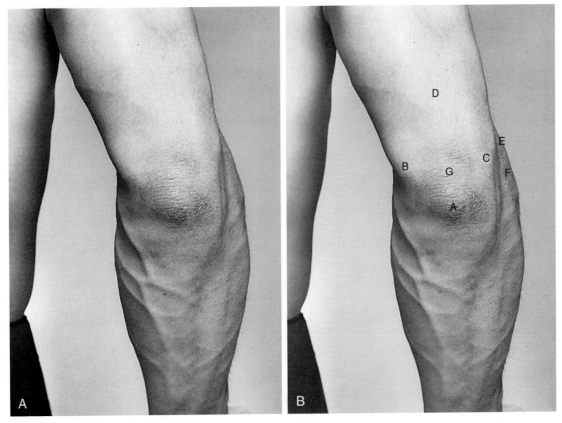

Figure 3–5. *A* and *B,* Posterior aspect of the elbow. A, olecranon process; B, medial epicondyle; C, lateral epicondyle; D, triceps brachii; E, brachioradialis; F, extensor carpi radialis longus; G, olecranon fossa.

amount of sliding motion that takes place between the skin and the bone. Trauma, inflammation, or infection can cause this bursa to fill with blood, synovial fluid, or pus, respectively. The presence of fluid causes the bursa to swell to the size of a Ping-Pong ball or even larger and bulge outward (Fig. 3–6). In the presence of sterile inflammation, the skin overlying the bursa may be slightly warm; in the presence of infection, the skin is normally hot and erythematous.

The tip of the elbow and adjacent subcutaneous border of the proximal ulna is the most common site for formation of **rheumatoid nodules** (Fig. 3–7). When present, these rubbery nodules satisfy one of the criteria for the diagnosis of rheumatoid arthritis.

MUSCULAR CONTOURS. The muscular anatomy of the distal portion of the upper arm is dominated by the **triceps brachii,** the principal extensor of the elbow. The principal insertion of the triceps is into the proximal olecranon, although it also flares into an aponeurosis that covers the small anconeus muscle and blends into the fascia of the posterior forearm. A bulge on the lateral aspect of the posterior elbow marks the proximal portions of the radially innervated **brachioradialis** and **extensor carpi radialis longus** muscles, which originate on the epicondylar ridge above the elbow and course distally to their insertions at the wrist. Together with the **extensor carpi radialis brevis** muscle, these

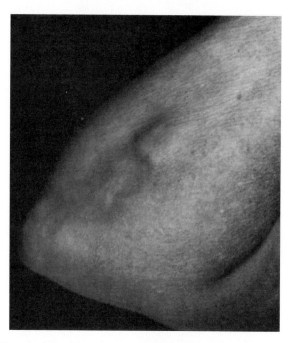

Figure 3–7. Rheumatoid nodules. (From Kelley W, Harris E, Ruddy S, Sledge C: Textbook of Rheumatology, 2nd ed. Philadelphia, WB Saunders, 1985, p 534.)

three constitute the lateral border of the posterior forearm (Fig. 3–8). The central portion of the posterior forearm is occupied by the **extensor digitorum communis** and **extensor carpi ulnaris,** which originate from a common tendon at the lateral epicondyle and course distally across the wrist. In the distal forearm, a group of three muscles, which originates in the midforearm, emerges between the extensor digitorum communis and the extensor carpi radialis brevis muscles and courses obliquely across the radial wrist extensors to the thumb. Owing to the way these muscles emerge obliquely between the other two extensor muscle groups, they are sometimes called the **outcropping muscles of the thumb.** Individually, they are the *abductor pollicis longus, extensor pollicis brevis,* and *extensor pollicis longus.*

ULNA. The muscular contours of the posterior forearm are completed by the ulnar portion of the flexor muscle mass, which bulges out sufficiently to constitute the medial border of the forearm. The subcutaneous border of the **ulna** is often visible as a linear furrow extending distally from the olecranon. In obese patients it may not be visible, but it should be palpable. The subcutaneous border of the ulna constitutes the dividing line between the extensor and the flexor compartments of the forearm.

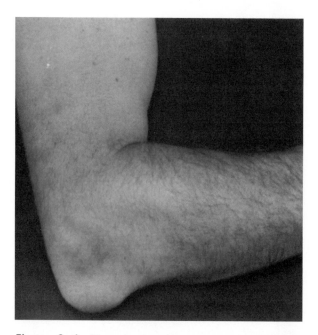

Figure 3–6. Olecranon bursitis. (From Morrey BF: The Elbow and Its Disorders, 2nd ed. Philadelphia, WB Saunders, 1993, p 876.)

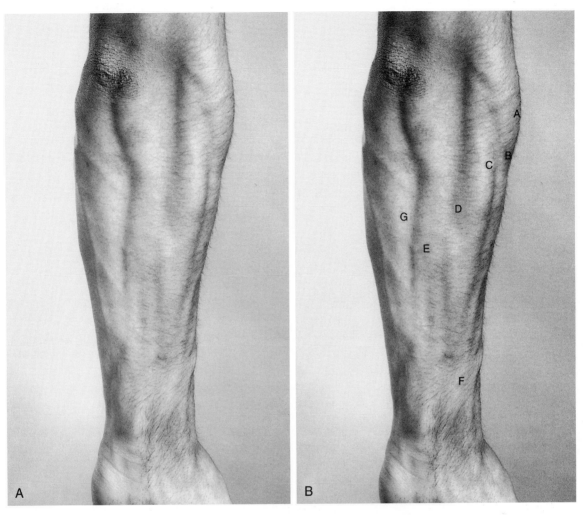

Figure 3–8. *A* and *B,* Posterior aspect of the forearm. A, brachioradialis; B, extensor carpi radialis longus; C, extensor carpi radialis brevis; D, extensor digitorum communis; E, extensor carpi ulnaris; F, outcropping muscles of the thumb; G, subcutaneous border of the ulna.

Lateral Aspect

OLECRANON, LATERAL EPICONDYLE, AND RADIAL HEAD. When the elbow is viewed from the lateral position, the tip of the olecranon, the lateral epicondyle, and the radial head also form an equilateral triangle (Fig. 3–9). The tip of the **olecranon** is a subcutaneous prominence that should be visible in virtually all individuals. The **lateral epicondyle,** the site of origin of the common extensor tendon mass, is visible in most individuals, and in obese patients it may constitute a dimple. In leaner patients, the epicondylar ridge of the distal humerus is visible in continuity with the lateral epicondyle. The **radial head,** however, is not normally visible because it is covered by the extensor muscle mass.

When an *olecranon fracture* occurs, the pull of the triceps muscle usually causes the proximal fragment of the olecranon to retract proximally.

If the patient is examined before much swelling has set in, this displacement is detectable as a disruption in the normal triangular relationship of the three bony landmarks mentioned.

SOFT SPOT. In the center of the triangle created by these three bony landmarks lies a **soft spot** over the lateral elbow capsule. There is relatively little soft tissue overlying the elbow capsule at this point, making it the optimal spot to look for bulging caused by an elbow joint effusion (Fig. 3–10). This soft spot is also generally considered the easiest point at which to aspirate or inject the elbow joint. Distention or fullness at the site of the normal soft spot suggests the presence of intraarticular fluid. The possible causes of such a distention include hemarthrosis due to an intraarticular fracture; synovitis due to arthritis, osteochondritis dissecans, or loose bodies; or infection.

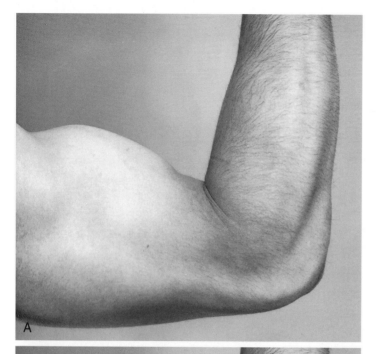

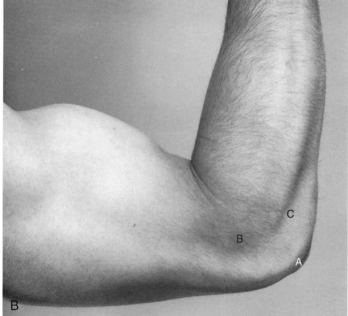

Figure 3–9. *A* and *B,* Lateral aspect of the elbow. A, olecranon; B, lateral epicondyle; C, radial head.

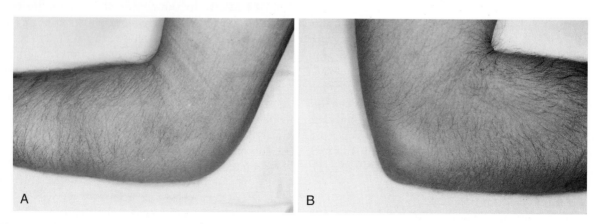

Figure 3–10. *A,* Elbow effusion. *B,* Opposite normal elbow.

Medial Aspect

The medial view of the elbow is dominated by the profile of the **olecranon** process and the prominence of the medial epicondyle (Fig. 3–11). The **medial epicondyle** serves as the origin of the flexor-pronator muscle group. A linear soft tissue ridge may be seen leading down the distal aspect of the upper arm to the medial epicondyle. This represents the medial edge of the **intermuscular septum** of the upper arm. Posterior to this septum lies the **triceps,** and anterior to it lie the **biceps** and **brachialis** muscles.

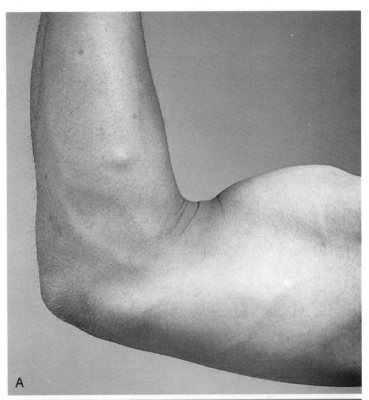

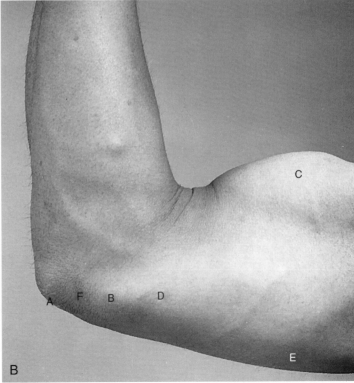

Figure 3–11. *A* and *B,* Medial aspect of the elbow. A, olecranon process; B, medial epicondyle; C, biceps brachii; D, intermuscular septum; E, triceps; F, cubital tunnel.

ULNAR NERVE. The **ulnar nerve** is best identified from the medial aspect. It courses through the posterior compartment of the upper arm just posterior to the intermuscular septum, then passes in the groove between the medial epicondyle and the olecranon before it enters the flexor muscle mass of the forearm between the two heads of the flexor carpi ulnaris. The ulnar nerve is virtually subcutaneous as it passes through the groove between the medial epicondyle and the olecranon; this groove is often called the **cubital tunnel.** In lean individuals, the ulnar nerve may actually be visible in the cubital tunnel as a linear structure about 5 mm to 7 mm in diameter. In patients with more subcutaneous fat, the ulnar nerve is still easily palpable at this location. If ulnar neuropathy is suspected, the examiner should inspect this area very closely as the patient maximally flexes and extends the elbow several times. In some patients, neuropathy is secondary to instability of the ulnar nerve in the cubital tunnel, and the nerve can be seen to pop back and forth across the medial epicondyle as the elbow flexes and extends.

ALIGNMENT

Elbow alignment is normally assessed with the patient standing facing the examiner. The forearms are fully supinated so that the palms face forward and the elbows are fully extended. The shoulders are adducted so that the upper arms

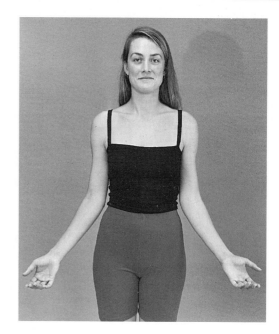

Figure 3–12. Carrying angle in a female.

lie comfortably against the side of the chest. In the normal patient, the examiner observes that the upper extremity is not straight when the elbow is fully extended; instead, the forearm and hand angle away from the body. This normal valgus angulation at the elbow is referred to as the **carrying angle.** Teleologically, this element of design allows humans to place their hands away from the body in more useful positions. There is considerable variation in the carrying angle among individuals, and women as a group

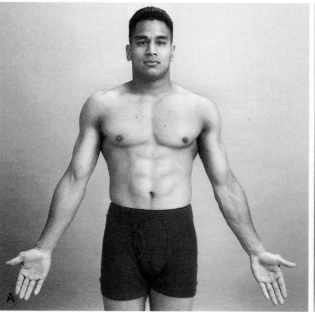
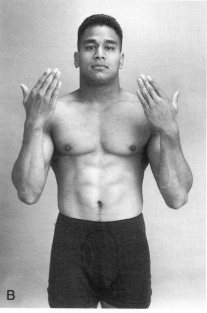

Figure 3–13. *A,* Carrying angle in a male. *B,* Loss of carrying angle in flexion.

have a greater carrying angle than men (Figs. 3–12 and 3–13A). An average of 13° for women and 10° for men is reported. Interestingly, the ulnar-humeral articulation is so engineered that the carrying angle disappears when the elbow is flexed, and the forearm and upper arm overlap perfectly (Fig. 3–13B).

An increase in the carrying angle above the normal range of valgus is called **cubitus valgus** (Fig. 3–14). Pathologic cubitus valgus is usually the result of trauma, such as the nonunion of a fractured lateral condyle of the distal humerus, or any injury that results in the premature closure of the lateral portion of the distal humeral physis. In the case of a growth disturbance, the magnitude of the deformity increases until skeletal growth is completed. This progressive valgus deformity puts abnormal tension on the ulnar nerve, which passes over the medial aspect of the elbow. Ultimately, this can lead to an insidious, progressive deterioration of ulnar nerve function with weakness and atrophy of muscles that are innervated by the ulnar nerve distal to the elbow. This condition is known as a *tardy ulnar nerve palsy* because the neuropathy appears tardily, sometimes years after the fracture has occurred.

Trauma may also lead to a reduction or even reversal of the normal carrying angle. Such a

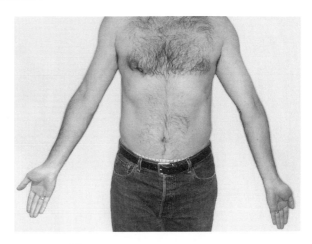

Figure 3–15. Cubitus varus *(left).*

reversal is known as **cubitus varus** and is sometimes called a *gunstock deformity* (Fig. 3–15). The most common cause of cubitus varus is malunion of a supracondylar humerus fracture that occurred in childhood.

Distal to the elbow, the forearm should appear straight regardless of the position of rotation. Unexpected angulation within the forearm suggests malunion of a previous fracture or a developmental abnormality. Such a deformity usually is associated with a diminution or complete loss of normal forearm rotation.

RANGE OF MOTION

Elbow Flexion and Extension

As with the knee, the elbow's freedom of motion is relatively limited in comparison to the shoulder or hip. Although the articular surfaces of the elbow participate in the mechanism that permits forearm rotation, the principal motions of the elbow itself are **flexion** and **extension.** Although the elbow is not a perfect hinge joint, the deviation in the center of rotation is so minimal that, from a practical standpoint, it can be thought to function as a hinge. The center of rotation passes through the midpoint of the capitellum at the anterior inferior aspect of the medial epicondyle. The average arc of motion is from 0° to 140°, although 30° to 130° is thought to be sufficient for most activities of daily living. Many patients exhibit some degree of elbow hyperextension, which may measure as much as 30°. In fact, hyperextension of the elbow is commonly accepted as one of the criteria for generalized joint laxity.

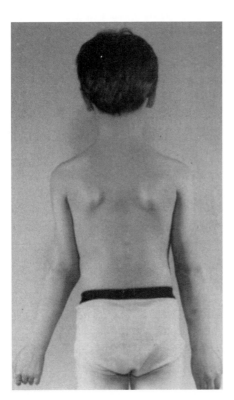

Figure 3–14. Cubitus valgus (left elbow). (From Morrey BF: The Elbow and Its Disorders, 2nd ed. Philadelphia, WB Saunders, 1993, p 255.)

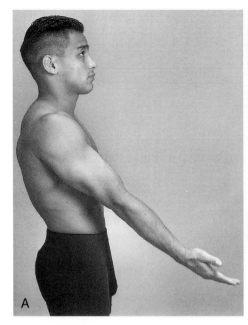

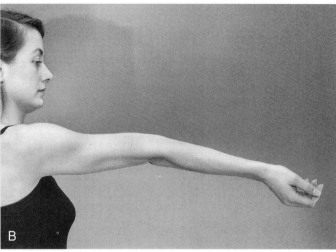

Figure 3–16. *A,* Elbow extension. *B,* Hyperextension.

EXTENSION. In measuring flexion and extension of the elbow, the point at which the forearm is aligned with the upper arm is considered neutral, or 0°. To assess **active elbow extension,** the patient is asked to straighten the elbow as much as possible. A general visual comparison of the two elbows can be done from the anterior perspective, but a lateral view is best for more accurately quantitating the amount of extension present (Fig. 3–16*A*). Extension to at least 0° is considered normal. Hyperextension to 10° is common, and even more hyperextension can be found as an anatomic variant (Fig. 3–16*B*).

If extension to at least 0° is not possible or if the amount of extension differs between the two elbows, the examiner should determine whether further passive extension is possible. To assess **passive elbow extension,** the examiner grasps the upper limb above and below the elbow and gently extends the joint (Fig. 3–17). If this is not painful for the patient, the maneuver can be repeated more swiftly and forcefully to see if pain is elicited. While performing this maneuver, the examiner should note whether the extension stops abruptly, with a hard bony feel, or more softly, with a slight feeling of give to the endpoint. A *hard endpoint* suggests a bony block, such as might be caused by the accretion of osteophytes on the olecranon process or large loose bodies in the posterior compartment of the elbow. A *softer endpoint* suggests that an anterior soft tissue contracture is responsible for the loss of extension. A mild loss of extension due to such a

contracture is common in the dominant elbow of athletes who throw.

Posterior elbow pain produced by **forceful passive extension** suggests either bony or soft tissue impingement in the olecranon fossa. Athletes who throw are subject to a condition called *valgus extension overload,* in which the recurrent valgus stresses that occur during throwing cause impingement of the proximal and medial olecranon, eventually leading to the development of osteophytes in these areas. Such patients normally feel posterior elbow pain when their elbows are forcefully extended.

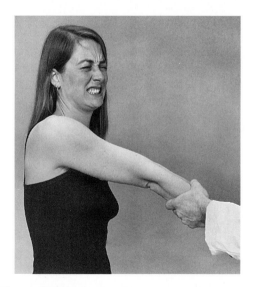

Figure 3–17. Passive elbow extension.

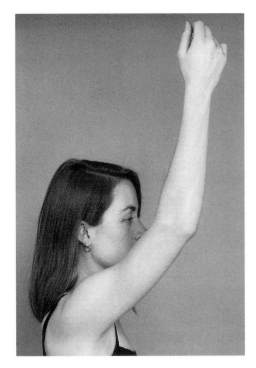

Figure 3–18. Elbow extension against gravity.

Weakness or paralysis of the triceps due to tendon rupture or radial nerve injury should cause a dramatic difference between active and passive extension of the elbow, just as quadriceps weakness can result in an extension lag at the

knee. However, this extension lag can easily be overlooked at the elbow because the normal upright body position causes the elbow to fall into extension with the force of gravity. If such a condition is suspected, the patient should be asked to extend the elbow with the arm in the overhead position to see whether full **elbow extension against gravity** is possible (Fig. 3–18).

FLEXION. To assess active elbow flexion, the examiner should ask the patient to bend both elbows as far as possible (Fig. 3–19A). Normal patients should be able to flex to 130° or 140°. If active flexion appears deficient or asymmetric, the examiner should grasp the patient's limb above and below the elbow joint and gently attempt further passive flexion (Fig. 3–19B). The normal flexion endpoint of the elbow is softer than the normal extension endpoint because flexion is usually limited by the impingement of the flexor muscle groups of the upper arm and forearm. In patients with unusually well-developed biceps, the loss of flexion can be considerable. Loss of flexion in the presence of a firmer, bony endpoint suggests an anterior impingement due to osteophytes on the coronoid process of the ulna, ectopic calcification, or large loose bodies. Limitation of flexion owing to posterior soft tissue contracture is unlikely.

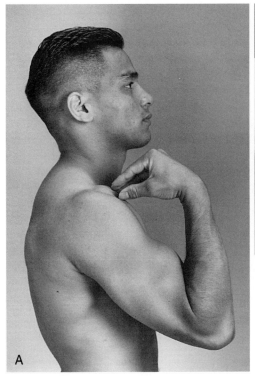

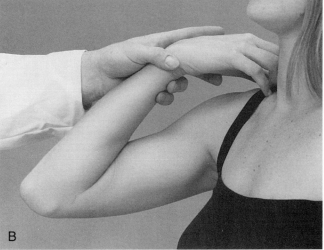

Figure 3–19. *A,* Active elbow flexion. *B,* Passive elbow flexion.

Forearm Rotation

Rotation of the forearm is a complex process that involves both the elbow and the wrist. To produce forearm rotation, the curved radius rotates around the straight ulna. At its proximal end, the circular, slightly concave radial head rotates in place against the convex capitellum. The configuration of the capitellum allows this rotation to occur in virtually any position of flexion or extension. This movement also occurs at the distal radial-ulnar joint and is guided by the triangular fibrocartilage and associated ligaments. When the forearm is fully supinated, the radius and ulna are roughly parallel to each other; when the forearm is fully pronated, the radius crosses over the ulna. Abnormalities of any of the structures involved in this complex mechanism can lead to significant loss of forearm rotation.

The average amount of rotation is 70° to 80° of pronation and 85° of supination, although 50° of pronation and 50° of supination are considered sufficient to perform most activities of daily living. Because patients often unconsciously make up for loss of forearm rotation with compensatory shoulder motion (Fig. 3–20), such compensatory motion should be carefully prevented when assessing forearm rotation.

SUPINATION. To measure forearm rotation, the patient stands facing the examiner with elbows tucked snugly against the sides. The patient should be instructed to keep the elbows at the sides during the testing procedure. The elbows are flexed 90°. When the thumb is facing upward, the forearm is considered to be in the neutral position (Fig. 3–21A). To test **supination,** the patient is then instructed to rotate the forearms until the palms are facing up (Fig. 3–21B). The angle of rotation with respect to a vertical line is considered the amount of supination present. In a patient with 85° of supination, the plane of the palm would be almost parallel to the floor.

PRONATION. To test **pronation,** the patient is then instructed to rotate both forearms until the palms are facing down (see Fig. 3–21C). The examiner should verify that the elbows' positions against the sides of the body remain unchanged. Again, the amount of pronation is estimated as the angle between the plane of the palms and a vertical line.

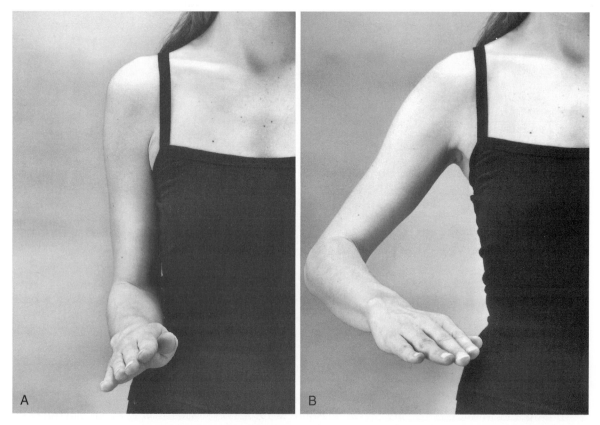

Figure 3–20. *A* and *B*, Compensating for deficient forearm rotation with shoulder motion.

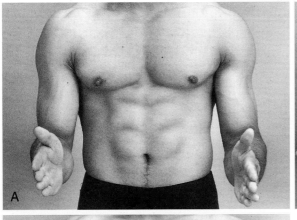

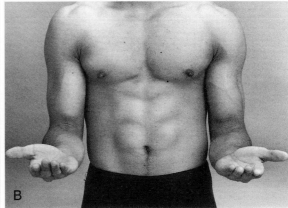

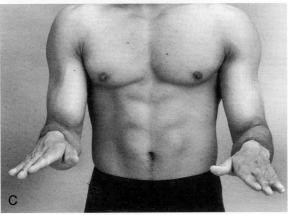

Figure 3–21. Forearm rotation. *A*, Neutral position. *B*, Supination. *C*, Pronation.

Palpation

Anterior Aspect

BICEPS TENDON AND LACERTUS FIBROSUS.
As previously noted, the distal biceps tendon and the associated lacertus fibrosus are the dominant features of the anterior elbow. The prominence of both these structures is increased by resisted supination or resisted elbow flexion in the supinated position. The **lacertus fibrosus** is more superficial and usually obscures the main portion of the tendon. If biceps tendinitis is suspected, the **biceps tendon** should be palpated carefully down toward its insertion on the radius. To do so, the examiner curves a finger around the lateral border of the lacertus fibrosus at the level of the elbow flexion crease (Fig. 3–22). The tendon should be palpable as a taut cord diving deep toward the radius. Tenderness of the distal tendon, especially when exacerbated by resisted elbow flexion or forearm supination, is suggestive of *biceps tendinitis.* In the presence of a distal *biceps tendon rupture,* the tendon would be difficult to palpate and would not feel taut.

BRACHIAL ARTERY AND MEDIAN NERVE. The **brachial artery** lies just medial to the biceps tendon and passes beneath the lacertus fibrosus. The brachial artery pulse can usually be palpated just medial to these structures, slightly above the flexion crease of the elbow (Fig. 3–23). Supporting the patient's limb so that it is relaxed with the elbow slightly flexed often facilitates palpation of the brachial pulse. The artery in turn can be used as a landmark for the **median nerve,** which is located just medial to it. The nerve itself, however, cannot be distinctly identified by palpation.

The most common site of median nerve compression is the point at which the median nerve passes between the two heads of the pronator teres muscle, a condition therefore referred to as *pronator syndrome.* This relatively uncommon nerve compression syndrome presents with a vague aching pain in the proximal flexor mass of the forearm that is made worse by repetitive strenuous motions such as heavy lifting. Paresthesias in the sensory distribution of the median nerve in the hand may be an associated symptom. To **screen for pronator syndrome,** the examiner positions the patient to test for pronation strength. With one hand, the examiner re-

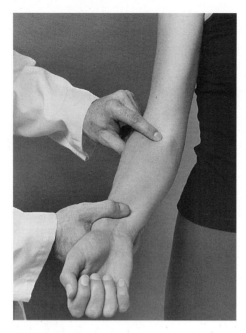

Figure 3–22. Palpation of the biceps tendon.

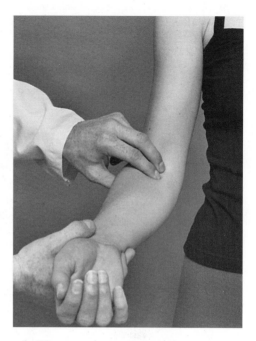

Figure 3–23. Palpation of the brachial artery.

sists the patient's attempt to pronate the forearm, while with his or her opposite thumb, the examiner applies firm pressure to the pronator mass 3 fingerbreadths distal to the elbow crease (Fig. 3–24).

Posterior Aspect

OLECRANON PROCESS. Palpation of the posterior elbow begins with the olecranon process (see Fig. 3–5). In the setting of acute trauma, tenderness of the olecranon, especially when accompanied by swelling and ecchymosis, suggests an olecranon fracture. The olecranon also has a separate apophyseal growth plate, which may be injured in the adolescent athlete by weightlifting or throwing. This overuse *olecranon apophysitis* is usually associated with localized bony tenderness but very little, if any, edema.

OLECRANON FOSSA. Firm palpation of the flexed elbow just superior to the olecranon process reveals a soft depression corresponding to the **olecranon fossa** of the posterior humerus. The examiner is actually palpating the olecranon fossa through the overlying triceps tendon. Tenderness of the distal **triceps tendon** suggests the possibility of *triceps tendinitis,* especially if the tenderness is exacerbated by resisted elbow extension. Loose bodies in the posterior compartment of the elbow can cause tenderness in the olecranon fossa. Tenderness along the superior

and medial margins of the olecranon process in an athlete who throws suggests the possibility of *valgus extension overload,* a process in which the valgus force imparted by throwing causes the medial border of the olecranon to impinge on the adjacent surface of the olecranon fossa in extension.

OLECRANON BURSA. As already noted, fluid distention of the olecranon bursa is usually quite visible. Chronic or previous inflammation of the

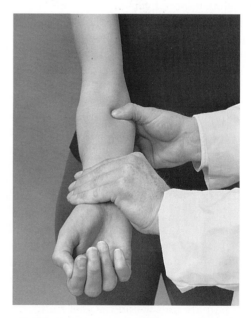

Figure 3–24. Palpation to screen for pronator syndrome.

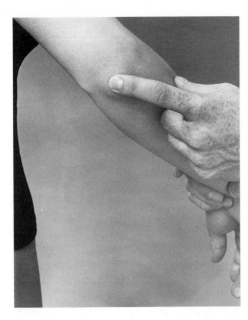

Figure 3–25. Palpation of the olecranon bursa.

bursa can be associated with subtler findings that may be detected by gentle palpation. By gently rubbing one or two fingers over such an olecranon bursa, the examiner often detects ridges corresponding to the thickened walls of the bursa (Fig. 3–25). In some cases, firm nodules about the size of a grain of rice are palpable.

ULNA. Proceeding distally from the olecranon, the examiner should gently palpate the entire subcutaneous border of the **ulna** (see Fig. 3–8). This usually is readily apparent as a firm narrow bony ridge. Although fractures of both bones of the forearm are usually accompanied by obvious instability and deformity, isolated fractures of the ulna may have a more subtle presentation. Isolated fracture of the ulna is usually due to a direct blow and is sometimes called a *nightstick fracture*. In the presence of such a fracture, careful palpation of the subcutaneous border of the ulna usually reveals localized tenderness and sometimes a palpable discontinuity of the bony contour.

POSTERIOR INTEROSSEOUS NERVE. The most common entrapment neuropathy of the radial nerve or its branches involves the **posterior interosseous nerve** as it passes between the two heads of the supinator muscle under a thick ligamentous band known as the *arcade of Frohse*. Entrapment of the posterior interosseous nerve at this location is also known as *radial tunnel syndrome*. Patients with this syndrome usually present with an aching pain in the extensor muscle mass of the proximal forearm that commonly radiates further distally in the forearm and even

proximally above the elbow. As there is no sensory nerve involved, paresthesias are not a feature.

The most common site of compression is best palpated with the patient's forearm relaxed and pronated. Because the arcade of Frohse is located about 4 fingerbreadths distal to the lateral epicondyle, four fingers of the examiner's hand are placed over the extensor muscle mass in a line extending distally from the lateral epicondyle. The examiner's index finger should now be located over the arcade of Frohse. In a patient with radial tunnel syndrome, pressure from the examiner's index finger at this site usually reproduces or exacerbates the patient's familiar pain (Fig. 3–26). This should help to differentiate the condition from the more common *lateral epicondylitis,* in which the maximal tenderness is usually located within 1 fingerbreadth of the lateral epicondyle. Other provocative tests to distinguish these two conditions are described in the Manipulation section.

INTERSECTION SYNDROME. Another uncommon condition that affects the extensor side of the forearm is intersection syndrome. Intersection syndrome is a condition characterized by inflammation at the location where two of the outcropping muscles, the abductor pollicis longus and extensor pollicis brevis, cross the extensor carpi radialis longus and brevis. To **screen for intersection syndrome,** the examiner should palpate the dorsum of the patient's distal forearm with the forearm fully pronated. Because the intersection point is located about 4 fingerbreadths proximal to the wrist, the four fingers of the examiner's hand are placed in a line along the dorsum of the patient's distal radius with the little finger adjacent to Lister's tubercle (Fig. 3–27A). The examiner's index finger should now

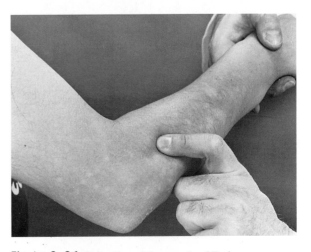

Figure 3–26. Palpation of the arcade of Frohse.

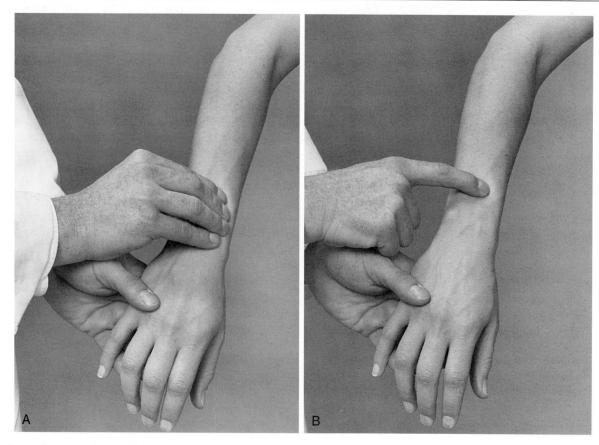

Figure 3–27. *A and B*, Palpation for intersection syndrome.

be over the intersection point (Fig. 3–27*B*). In a patient with intersection syndrome, digital pressure at this site may reproduce or exacerbate the patient's pain. Having the patient dorsiflex the wrist against resistance during palpation of the

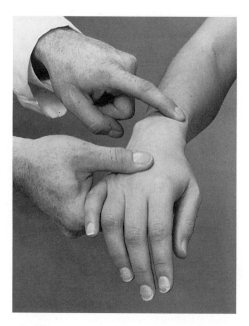

Figure 3–28. Pronated forearm, palpating the distal radius.

intersection point may further intensify the discomfort.

RADIUS. Unlike the ulna, the **radius** is not easily palpable throughout its length. Distal to the radial head, the rest of the proximal radius is covered by the bellies of the brachioradialis and other extensor muscles; therefore, the proximal radius is only vaguely palpable. Further distally, however, the muscles become tendinous. The dorsum of the distal half of the radius is therefore easy to palpate in the pronated forearm because it is covered only by the tendons of the mobile wad and of the three outcropping muscles of the thumb. Firm palpation of the pronated forearm should allow the examiner to delineate the outlines of the distal radius (Fig. 3–28).

Lateral Aspect

RADIAL HEAD AND CAPITELLUM. The tip of the olecranon and lateral epicondyle are clearly visible landmarks of the lateral elbow, but the **radial head** must be palpated for identification. If the examiner remembers that these three landmarks form a roughly equilateral triangle, the

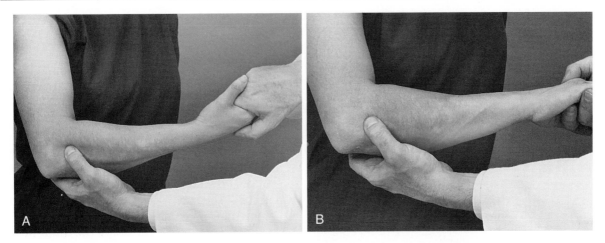

Figure 3–29. *A* and *B,* Palpating the radial head while rotating the forearm.

approximate location of the radial head deep to the extensor muscle mass can be estimated (see Fig. 3–9). Firm palpation at this site with the elbow flexed 90° and the forearm relaxed reveals a firm bony resistance corresponding to the radial head. The examiner can verify that the correct structure has been identified by passively rotating the patient's forearm during palpation (Fig. 3–29). If the examiner is palpating the correct spot, the rotational movement of the radius can be felt beneath the palpating digit. Tenderness over the radial head following a fall on the outstretched hand suggests a *radial head fracture,* especially when forearm rotation reproduces or exacerbates the pain. The **capitellum,** which articulates with the radial head, is the usual site of osteochondritis dissecans in the elbow. Thus, tenderness in the same area in an adolescent, especially an athlete who throws or a gymnast, suggests a diagnosis of osteochondritis dissecans of the capitellum, also known as *Panner's disease.*

LATERAL EPICONDYLE. A common painful condition of the lateral elbow is *lateral epicondylitis,*

commonly known as *tennis elbow.* This condition might more properly be called *extensor origin tendinitis,* because it is not the epicondyle itself, but the tendons that originate there, that are involved in this disorder. The condition consists of degeneration of the affected tendon related to overuse and most commonly involves the *extensor carpi radialis brevis* with the rest of the *common extensor tendon* variably involved. Maximal tenderness is usually detected just distal to the *lateral epicondyle* within the tendons themselves. To pinpoint this tenderness, the examiner should palpate very carefully with one finger while the patient's elbow is flexed to 90° and the forearm muscles are relaxed (Fig. 3–30). Resisted wrist extension may exacerbate the pain of palpation.

Medial Aspect

MEDIAL EPICONDYLE. The most prominent structure of the medial elbow is the medial epicondyle, the site of origin of the flexor-pronator muscle group. The medial epicondyle has a separate apophyseal growth center and may be avulsed in children or adolescents, either in association with an elbow dislocation or as an isolated injury. In preadolescent or adolescent athletes who throw, repeated traction from the flexor pronator muscle group can cause an overuse injury known as *medial epicondyle apophysitis* or *Little Leaguer's elbow.* In the presence of this condition, firm palpation of the medial epicondyle is painful. Because the epicondyle is so prominent, the examiner can actually grasp it between the thumb and the index finger and attempt to move it back and forth. Although no motion with respect to the rest of the humerus is detectable, this manipulation is usually quite painful if Little Leaguer's elbow is present (Fig. 3–31).

In older patients, the flexor-pronator tendon origin is subject to a tendinitis similar to that

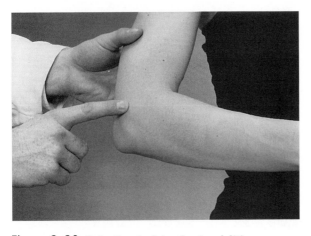

Figure 3–30. Palpation for lateral epicondylitis.

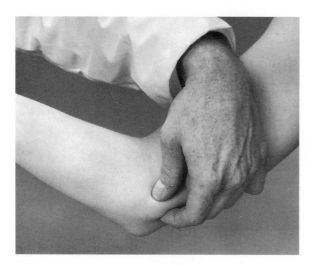

Figure 3–31. Stressing the medial epicondyle.

seen on the lateral side of the elbow. This *flexor-pronator origin tendinitis* is referred to by many names: *medial epicondylitis, golfer's elbow, reverse tennis elbow, medial tennis elbow.* To **screen for flexor pronator origin tendinitis,** the examiner firmly palpates with one index finger just distal to the medial epicondyle with the patient's elbow flexed and forearm relaxed (Fig. 3–32). If the patient's response is equivocal, the tenderness may be accentuated by palpating the tendon while the patient pronates the forearm against resistance.

ULNAR NERVE. The **ulnar nerve** can usually be palpated as a fairly soft longitudinal structure slightly thicker than a sneaker shoelace. Palpation of the ulnar nerve should be very gentle because it can be quite sensitive. Sensitivity of the nerve is reflected in its common names: *crazy bone* or *funny bone.* If an ulnar neuropathy is suspected, the examiner should attempt to elicit **Tinel's sign** by tapping gently on the exposed portion of the nerve with the tip of the long finger (Fig. 3–33). In a normal patient, such tapping may be mildly uncomfortable. If the tapping produces a feeling of paresthesias or dysesthesias radiating distally from the point of impact into the forearm, Tinel's sign is said to be present. Tinel's sign reflects irritation of the ulnar nerve. Common causes of ulnar nerve irritation at the elbow include compression where the ulnar nerve enters the flexor carpi ulnaris muscle, external compression from leaning on the elbow, irritation owing to habitual subluxation of the nerve over the medial epicondyle, and traction due to cubitus valgus or valgus instability of the elbow.

To **screen for ulnar nerve instability,** the examiner should gently palpate the nerve between the medial epicondyle and the olecranon while passively flexing and extending the patient's elbow (Fig. 3–34). If nerve instability is present, the examiner feels the nerve pass anteriorly over the epicondyle when the elbow is flexed, usually with a soft palpable snap. When ulnar nerve injury at the elbow is detected in an athlete who throws, the elbow should be examined carefully for valgus instability as the underlying cause of the neuropathy.

MEDIAL (ULNAR) COLLATERAL LIGAMENT. The most important ligamentous stabilizer of the elbow is the **medial collateral ligament (ulnar collateral ligament).** This ligament is triangular with two main limbs. The more important

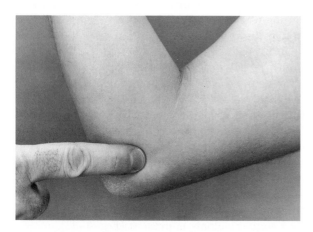

Figure 3–32. Palpation for medial epicondylitis.

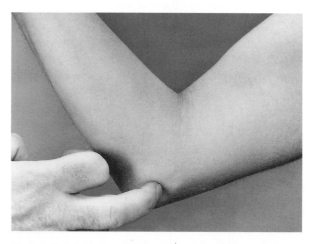

Figure 3–33. Tinel's test of the ulnar nerve.

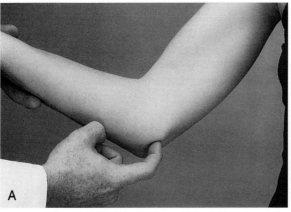 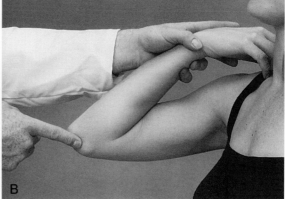

Figure 3–34. *A and B,* Palpation for ulnar nerve instability.

anterior limb arises from the medial epicondyle deep to the flexor pronator origin and inserts on a small tubercle on the medial border of the coronoid process of the ulna. The posterior limb arises from the medial epicondyle behind the anterior limb and inserts into the medial border of the olecranon, forming the floor of the cubital tunnel. The posterior portion of the ligament is thus covered by the ulnar nerve, but the anterior portion is more exposed and can be palpated just anterior to the nerve with the elbow flexed from 30° to 60° (Fig. 3–35). The goal of palpation is to elicit tenderness because the outlines of the ligament cannot be clearly discerned. Because the act of throwing places a valgus stress on the elbow, this ligament is subject to overuse injury in athletes who throw. Such an injury is manifested by tenderness of the medial collateral ligament and, in more severe cases, abnormal valgus laxity of the elbow.

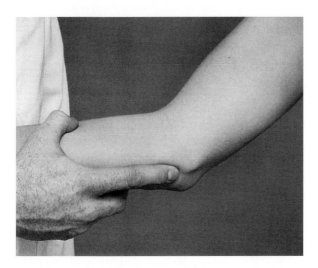

Figure 3–35. Palpation of the ulnar collateral ligament.

Manipulation

MUSCLE TESTING

Elbow Flexors

The **biceps brachii** is the principal elbow flexor and an important supinator of the forearm. The biceps is innervated by the *musculocutaneous nerve.* To test for biceps strength in elbow flexion, the examiner faces the patient and asks him or her to flex the elbow. The examiner stabilizes the patient's arm by grasping it at the posterior elbow and holds the patient's forearm just proximal to the wrist. The examiner then attempts to passively extend the elbow while the patient resists maximally (Fig. 3–36). In a normal patient, the examiner is able to extend the elbow only with difficulty; a strong patient may be able to overcome the examiner's resistance and flex the elbow further. Because there is wide variation in biceps strength, it is important to compare both arms. The **brachialis** muscle also assists in elbow flexion. It is not easy to isolate from the biceps brachii and is tested along with it.

The **brachioradialis** is a unique elbow flexor. Unlike the other flexor muscles, it arises close to the elbow from the lateral epicondylar ridge and inserts close to the wrist in the distal radius. Although brachioradialis strength cannot be isolated from that of the other elbow flexors, the muscle can be demonstrated to its best advantage by testing with the forearm in the position of neutral rotation. The patient is instructed to flex the elbow to 90°. The examiner then pushes downward on the patient's wrist while the patient provides maximal upward resistance. The

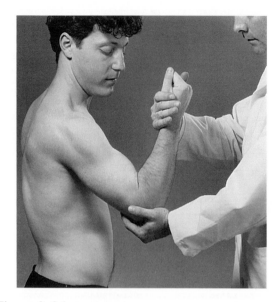

Figure 3–36. Assessing biceps strength (elbow flexion).

brachioradialis stands out distinctively from the other forearm muscles and its function, thus, is easily confirmed (Fig. 3–37).

The brachioradialis is innervated by the *radial nerve.* Injury to the radial nerve in the upper arm, such as might occur in association with a fracture of the humerus, denervates the brachioradialis along with the other wrist and finger extensors that are innervated further distally.

Elbow Extenders

The **triceps brachii** is the principal extender of the elbow and is innervated by the radial nerve. It is tested in a manner analogous to that of testing elbow flexion. The examiner stabilizes the patient's arm at the elbow in the same manner as used to test the biceps but this time provides

resistance against the ulna as the patient is instructed to extend the elbow as forcefully as possible (Fig. 3–38). As with the biceps, triceps strength varies considerably and should always be compared with the opposite side. The examiner should be able to overcome the normal triceps only with difficulty and may indeed be unable to resist the force of extension in a strong patient.

Forearm Rotators

SUPINATION STRENGTH. Supination strength is provided primarily by the **biceps brachii,** innervated by the *musculocutaneous nerve,* and the **supinator** muscle, innervated by the *radial nerve.* To test supination strength, the patient sits or stands with the elbow flexed 90° and the upper arm held snugly against the body. This ensures that the shoulder muscles are not being used to supplement the strength of forearm supination. The test begins with the patient's forearm fully pronated. Both of the examiner's hands then firmly grasp the patient's hand. The patient is instructed to attempt to turn the hand over with as much force as possible (Fig. 3–39). Normally, the examiner's two hands should be able to prevent this motion, although strong patients may be able to overcome the examiner. Rupture of the long head biceps tendon at the shoulder, a common occurrence, normally produces only a mild decrease in supination strength. Rupture of the distal biceps tendon at the elbow, however, produces a dramatic loss of supination strength. Denervation of the biceps owing to cervical radic-

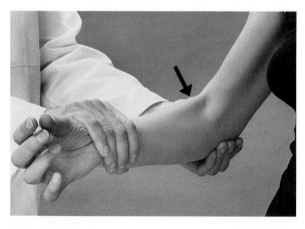

Figure 3–37. Showing brachioradialis contraction *(arrow).*

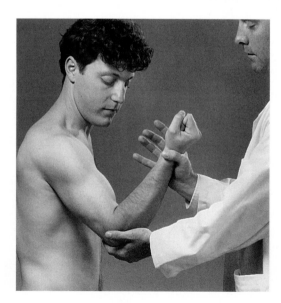

Figure 3–38. Assessing triceps strength.

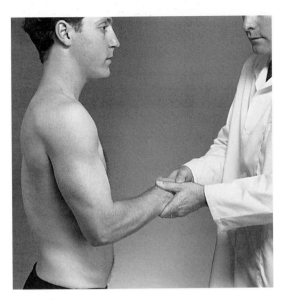

Figure 3–39. Assessing supination strength.

ulopathy or musculocutaneous nerve injury or of the supinator due to radial nerve injury also produce a diminution of supination strength.

Supination strength is normally about 15% greater than pronation strength. The dominant extremity is normally about 5% to 10% stronger than the nondominant side, but this difference may be more marked in certain individuals, such as manual laborers.

PRONATION STRENGTH. Pronation strength is provided by the **pronator teres** and **pronator quadratus,** both innervated by the *median nerve.* To test the strength of pronation, the patient is asked to assume the same general position as that used for testing supination strength. This time, the test is begun with the patient's forearm fully supinated. The examiner grasps

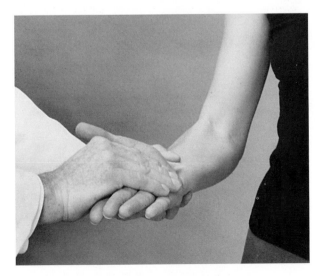

Figure 3–40. Assessing pronation strength.

the patient's hand in this position and instructs the patient to attempt to turn the hand over as forcefully as possible (Fig. 3–40). In most cases, the strength of the examiner's two hands is sufficient to prevent the patient's forearm from pronating. Testing with the elbow fully flexed puts the pronator teres at a disadvantage and thus is a way of relatively isolating the pronator quadratus.

Other Forearm Muscles

The other forearm muscles are primarily motors of the wrist and hand. Strength testing of these muscles is described in Chapter 4, Hand and Wrist.

SENSATION TESTING

Nerve injuries at the elbow and forearm can result in sensory deficits in the hand and wrist. Sensation of the fingertips is best evaluated by testing for two-point discrimination. In other parts of the hand, light touch or pinprick testing may be used.

With any **median nerve** injury, there is potential for loss of sensation in the median nerve distribution, which includes the palmar surface of the thumb, the index finger, the long finger, and the radial aspect of the ring finger. If the injury takes place in the proximal portion of the forearm, sensation to the palmar aspect of the base of the thumb is also affected. If a more distal injury occurs, such as a carpal tunnel syndrome, sensation is preserved on the palmar aspect of the base of the thumb because the palmar cutaneous branch of the median nerve is given off before the median nerve enters the carpal tunnel (Fig. 3–41).

Anterior interosseous nerve syndrome has no associated sensory deficit.

The **ulnar nerve** supplies sensation to the little finger and the ulnar aspect of the ring finger. Any injury to the ulnar nerve at the level of the wrist or more proximally results in the loss of sensation in this distribution. Injuries that occur more proximally, such as at the elbow, also affect sensation over the dorsal ulnar part of the hand (Fig. 3–42).

The **radial nerve** supplies sensation to the dorsum of the hand, particularly over the first web space. An injury to the radial nerve at the level of the elbow or above affects sensation in this area (Fig. 3–43).

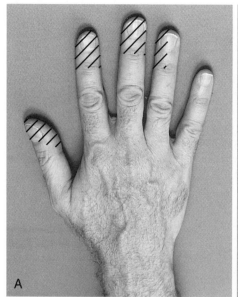
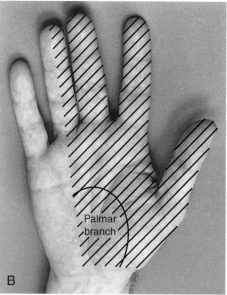

Figure 3–41. *A* and *B*, Sensory distribution of the median nerve in the hand.

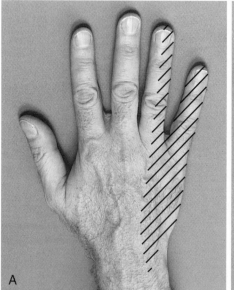
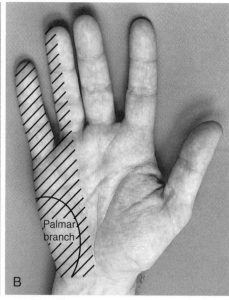

Figure 3–42. *A* and *B*, Sensory distribution of the ulnar nerve in the hand.

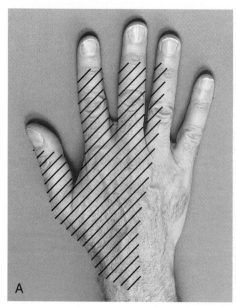
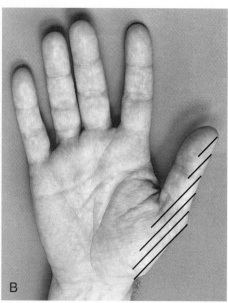

Figure 3–43. *A* and *B*, Sensory distribution of the radial nerve in the hand.

SPECIAL TESTS

Nerve Compression Syndromes

CUBITAL TUNNEL SYNDROME. The most common nerve compression syndrome occurring about the elbow is the cubital tunnel syndrome involving the ulnar nerve. This syndrome can occur spontaneously or in association with many other factors, such as activities requiring repetitive elbow movements, osteoarthritis, rheumatoid arthritis, fractures and dislocations, cubitus valgus, and instability of the ulnar nerve. Rarely, an anomalous muscle known as the *anconeus epitrochlearus* crosses the ulnar nerve in the region of the medial epicondyle and may also cause this syndrome. Typical symptoms of cubital tunnel syndrome include achy pain in the medial forearm and paresthesias in the sensory distribution of the ulnar nerve in the hand.

The most common screening test for cubital tunnel syndrome is described in the Palpation section, under Medial Aspect, Ulnar Nerve: percussion of the ulnar nerve between the medial epicondyle and the olecranon process to elicit **Tinel's sign.** The **elbow flexion test** is another provocative test for ulnar nerve compression at the elbow. To perform the elbow flexion test, the examiner passively flexes the patient's elbow to the maximal degree possible and holds it in this position for a minute or more (Fig. 3–44). In the presence of cubital tunnel syndrome, the patient often reports the gradual development of paresthesias in the small finger and the ring finger. These symptoms may be further accentuated by applying digital pressure directly over the ulnar nerve as it runs through the cubital tunnel. This combination of prolonged passive elbow flexion

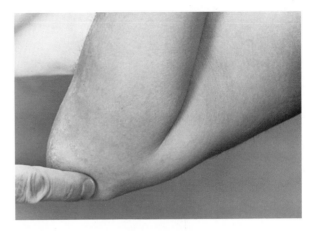

Figure 3–45. Ulnar nerve compression test.

and digital pressure over the cubital tunnel is known as the **ulnar nerve compression test** (Fig. 3–45).

In more advanced cases of ulnar nerve compression, weakness and eventually atrophy of muscles innervated by the ulnar nerve are noted. The pattern of muscle weakness can be used to differentiate between ulnar nerve compression at the elbow and the less common ulnar nerve compression at the wrist. Compression at either location can produce weakness of the intrinsic muscles of the hand innervated by the ulnar nerve. This would result in weakness of finger abduction and adduction. In addition to this intrinsic weakness, however, compression of the ulnar nerve at the elbow may produce weakness of the flexor digitorum profundus to the small finger and the ring finger and of the flexor carpi ulnaris, which are innervated below the elbow but above the wrist. The documentation of weakness in the flexor digitorum profundus to the little finger and the ring finger and weakness of wrist flexion in ulnar deviation thus confirms that the site of compression must be proximal to the wrist. A high ulnar nerve palsy can produce a deformity called **benediction hand,** in which the little finger and the ring finger are clawed (flexed at the interphalangeal joints and hyperextended at the metacarpophalangeal joints) (Fig. 3–46).

LESS COMMON NERVE COMPRESSION SYNDROMES. Less common nerve compression syndromes in the elbow and the forearm may involve the radial or median nerves. The **radial nerve** and its major branches, the **posterior interosseous nerve** and the **superficial sensory branch,** can be compressed anywhere from the level of the lateral head of the triceps to the region of the elbow, the proximal forearm, and

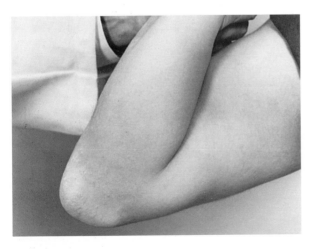

Figure 3–44. Elbow flexion test for cubital tunnel syndrome.

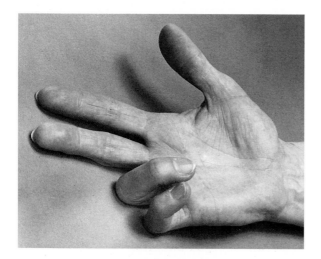

Figure 3–46. Benediction hand deformity.

even into the distal forearm. Possible causes include adhesions, muscular anomalies, vascular aberrations, fibrotic bands, inflammatory conditions, tumors, and fractures. The presentation depends on which branch of the nerve is involved and at what level.

RADIAL TUNNEL SYNDROME. As previously noted, the most common entrapment neuropathy of the radial nerve occurs in the radial tunnel at the arcade of Frohse. In addition to the finding of tenderness at this site, the **long finger extension test** can also suggest the presence of a radial tunnel syndrome. To perform the long finger extension test, the examiner instructs the patient to fully extend the fingers with the wrist also extended about 30°. The patient is instructed to maintain extension of the fingers while the examiner presses down on the dorsum of the long finger, attempting to passively flex the metacarpophalangeal joint (Fig. 3–47). If this maneuver reproduces the patient's familiar pain in the region of the radial tunnel, the diagnosis of radial tunnel syndrome is further strengthened. The long finger extension test can sometimes be painful in the presence of extensor origin tendinitis (lateral epicondylitis). The site of maximal tenderness can usually be used to distinguish these two conditions, however, because in extensor origin tendinitis the point of maximal tenderness is just distal to the lateral epicondyle whereas in radial tunnel syndrome, the point of maximal tenderness is about 4 fingerbreadths distal to this same landmark.

Muscular weakness is unusual in radial tunnel syndrome. When weakness is encountered in the presence of an apparent radial neuropathy, care-

ful documentation of the muscles involved often delineates the site of compression. Vital to this differentiation is the knowledge that the brachioradialis, extensor carpi radialis brevis, and extensor carpi radialis longus are innervated proximal to the radial tunnel, whereas the extensor carpi ulnaris, extensor digitorum communis, extensor pollicis longus, and extensor pollicis brevis are all innervated distal to it by the posterior interosseous nerve. Strength testing of these muscles is described in Chapter 4, Hand and Wrist. In the presence of an apparent radial nerve palsy, therefore, documentation of weakness of the brachioradialis, extensor carpi radialis longus, and extensor carpi radialis brevis indicates that the site of compression is proximal to the radial tunnel. Severe compression of the **posterior interosseous nerve** at the radial tunnel leaves those three muscles unaffected but may produce weakness of the extensor digitorum communis, the extensors pollicis longus and brevis, and the extensor carpi ulnaris. In such a patient, the wrist deviates to the radial side when the patient is instructed to actively extend it because the radial wrist extensors are functioning but the extensor carpi ulnaris is not.

PRONATOR SYNDROME. As already mentioned, the most common site of **median nerve** compression in the forearm is the point at which the nerve passes between the two heads of the pronator teres. Pronator syndrome is much less common than compression of the medial nerve at the carpal tunnel and is difficult to diagnose. As noted in the Palpation section, the reproduction of the patient's symptoms by direct pressure over the pronator teres during resisted forearm pronation is the most reliable screening test for prona-

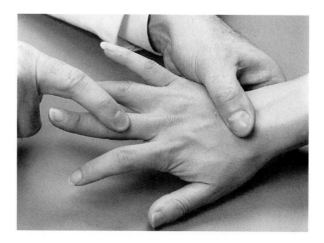

Figure 3–47. Long finger extension test.

tor syndrome. If pronator syndrome is suspected, the effect of **prolonged resisted pronation** should also be investigated. This test is performed in the same manner described for testing pronation strength (see Fig. 3–40). In this case, however, the examiner resists the patient's attempts at pronation for 60 seconds or more. Reproduction of the patient's symptoms by this maneuver further reinforces the possibility of pronator syndrome.

OTHER SITES OF MEDIAN NERVE COMPRESSION. Several other less common sites of median nerve compression about the elbow and in the forearm are possible. At the elbow, the median nerve may be compressed by the lacertus fibrosus. If this is the case, the patient's symptoms may usually be reproduced by **prolonged resisted elbow flexion** and **resisted forearm supination.**

The median nerve may also be compressed by the origin of the flexor digitorum superficialis. In this case, the resisted **long finger PIP flexion test** will sometimes reproduce the patient's symptoms. In this test, which is analogous to the long finger extension test, the patient is asked to flex the fingers of the involved hand with the forearm supinated. The examiner's finger is then hooked under the middle phalanx of the patient's long finger, and the examiner attempts to extend the PIP joint while the patient resists as strongly as possible (Fig. 3–48). Reproduction of the patient's symptoms by this maneuver suggests median nerve compression by the flexor digitorum superficialis.

The site of a median nerve injury can usually be defined by the muscles that are affected. An injury proximal to the elbow affects all median-

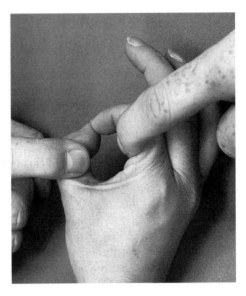

Figure 3–49. Testing flexor pollicis longus and flexor digitorum profundus strength for anterior interosseous nerve syndrome.

innervated functions, including wrist flexion, finger flexion, thumb flexion, and thumb opposition. If the nerve is injured in the proximal forearm, wrist flexion may be unaffected. Finally, if the injury is at the wrist, only the muscles of the thenar eminence, most easily tested by evaluating thumb opposition, are affected.

ANTERIOR INTEROSSEOUS NERVE SYNDROME. Anterior interosseous nerve syndrome may occur spontaneously or secondary to a number of causes including trauma, forearm masses, or anomalous muscles. Its presentation is quite similar to that of pronator syndrome, with aching pain in the proximal forearm. In more severe cases of anterior interosseous nerve syndrome, weakness of the flexor pollicis longus and flexor digitorum profundus to the index finger may be present. To test the strength of these muscles, the patient is instructed to make a tight O by opposing the tips of the thumb and index finger. The examiner then hooks each of his or her own index fingers within the O and attempts to separate the patient's thumb and index finger (Fig. 3–49). Comparison with the patient's opposite hand should be used to assess whether weakness of the muscles innervated by the anterior interosseous nerve may be present. Weakness of the pronator quadratus, which is also innervated by the anterior interosseous nerve, may be looked for by testing pronator strength with the elbow fully flexed. As noted, there is no sensory deficit associated with anterior interosseous nerve syndrome.

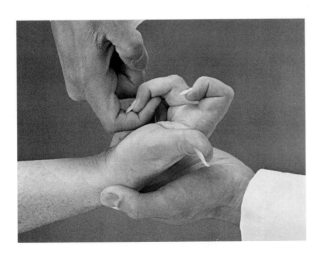

Figure 3–48. Long finger flexion test.

ence of abnormal valgus laxity, the examiner feels the bones separate slightly when this stress is applied and clunk back together when the stress is relaxed.

The position of forearm rotation can affect the results of the valgus stress test. Valgus laxity with the forearm pronated reflects injury to the anterior portion of the medial collateral ligament, whereas valgus laxity in supination may be due to laxity of the anterior portion of the medial collateral ligament or the ulnar part of the lateral collateral ligament (see under Posterolateral Rotatory Instability Test, later).

VARUS STRESS TEST. Chronic varus laxity of the elbow is assessed using the **varus stress test.** The details of the varus stress test are analogous to those of the valgus stress test, but the direction of force application is reversed. This time, the limb is positioned with the shoulder more internally rotated. The examiner grasps the patient's limb above the elbow with one hand and below the elbow with the other hand and applies a controlled varus stress (Fig. 3–54). Again, care must be taken to avoid rotating the entire limb when the varus stress is applied.

In the presence of abnormal laxity of the lateral ligament complex, the examiner feels the bones separate at the elbow when the varus

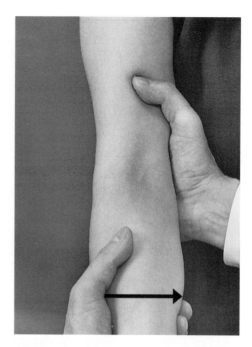

Figure 3–54. Varus stress test (*arrow* indicates direction of force applied to forearm).

stress is applied and come back together with a clunk when the stress is relaxed. As in the valgus test, comparison with the other side is helpful in determining whether a perceived increase in laxity is truly pathologic.

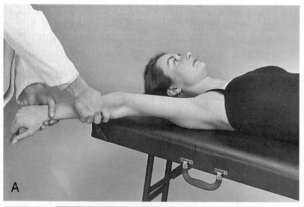

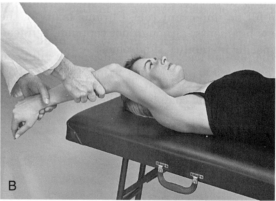

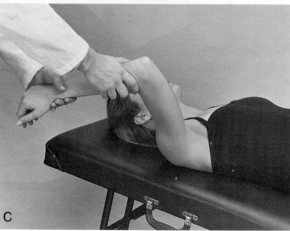

Figure 3–55. *A–C,* Posterolateral rotatory instability test.

POSTEROLATERAL ROTATORY INSTABILITY TEST (PIVOT SHIFT TEST).

The **posterolateral rotatory instability test,** or **pivot shift test,** is designed to detect posterolateral instability of the elbow, a condition that occurs owing to insufficiency of the portion of the lateral ligamentous complex known as the *lateral ulnar collateral ligament.* This syndrome is manifested by episodes suggestive of subluxation or dislocation. The posterolateral rotatory instability test may be performed with the upper limb at the patient's side or with the shoulder flexed so that the limb lies above the patient's head. O'Driscoll and colleagues, who first described this test, preferred the latter position. The test is performed with the patient supine and the shoulder flexed overhead. The examiner grasps the patient's forearm, externally rotating the shoulder to its limit to prevent humeral rotation and placing the forearm in a supinated position. The test begins with the patient's elbow in full extension. The examiner applies valgus and axial compression forces to the elbow and a supination torque to the forearm. This produces a rotatory subluxation of the ulnohumeral joint with a coupled posterolateral dislocation of the radial head from the humerus (Fig. 3–55A). As the elbow is flexed to about 40°, the posterolateral rotatory subluxation increases to its maximum (Fig. 3–55B). The radial head creates a posterolateral prominence with an obvious dimple in the skin located just proximal to it. Additional flexion results in sudden reduction of the radiohumeral and ulnohumeral joints (Fig. 3–55C). The dimple disappears, and the radius and ulna can be felt and seen to snap back into place on the humerus. The palpable subluxation and reduction just described are usually appreciated only when the test is performed with the patient under general anesthesia. If the test is performed with the patient awake, an abnormal result is signified by the patient's apprehension; only occasionally can a sudden reduction of the radiohumeral and ulnohumeral joints be elicited.

The physical findings in common conditions of the elbow and forearm are summarized in Table 3–1.

TABLE 3–1.
PHYSICAL FINDINGS IN COMMON CONDITIONS OF THE ELBOW AND FOREARM

Cubital Tunnel Syndrome

Tenderness over the course of the ulnar nerve
Abnormal Tinel's sign over the ulnar nerve as it passes through the cubital tunnel
Ulnar nerve compression test abnormal
Elbow flexion text abnormal (variable)
Abnormal sensation (two-point discrimination or light touch), little finger, ulnar aspect of ring finger; ulnar aspect of hand (variable)
Weakness and atrophy of the ulnar-innervated intrinsic muscles of the hand (variable)
Weakness of the flexor digitorum profundus to the little finger (variable)
Signs of concomitant ulnar nerve instability, elbow instability, or elbow deformity (occasionally)

Lateral Epicondylitis (Extensor Origin Tendinitis)

Tenderness at the lateral epicondyle and at the origin of the involved tendons
Pain produced by resisted wrist extension
Pain with passive flexion of the fingers and the wrist with the elbow fully extended (variable)

Radial Tunnel Syndrome

Tenderness in the extensor muscle mass of the forearm at the arcade of Frohse
Long finger extension test reproduces familiar pain
Weakness of finger and thumb extensors and extensor carpi ulnaris (unusual)

Pronator Syndrome

Tenderness in the proximal forearm over pronator teres
Abnormal sensation (two-point discrimination or light touch) in the thumb, the index finger, the long finger, and the radial side of the ring finger (variable)
Prolonged resisted pronation reproduces symptoms
Weakness of median innervated muscles (variable)

Other Median Nerve Compression Syndromes

Resisted elbow flexion and forearm supination reproduces symptoms (compression at the lacertus fibrosus)
Resisted long finger proximal interphalangeal joint flexion reproduces symptoms (compression by the flexor digitorum superficialis)
Weakness of median innervated muscles (variable)

Anterior Interosseous Nerve Syndrome

Weakness of flexor pollicis longus and flexor digitorum profundus to index finger (O sign)
Weakness of pronator quadratus (variable)

Medial Epicondylitis (Flexor-Pronator Tendinitis)

Tenderness over the common flexor origin
Resisted wrist flexion test reproduces pain
Resisted forearm pronation reproduces pain

Distal Biceps Tendon Rupture

Swelling
Ecchymosis
Palpable gap in the biceps tendon
Weak supination and elbow flexion

Valgus Extension Overload Syndrome

Tenderness around the tip of the olecranon
Pain with forced passive elbow extension
Increased valgus laxity (variable)

Osteoarthritis

Restricted flexion or extension
Effusion (variable)

Bibliography

Askew LJ, An KN, Morrey BF, Chao EY: Functional evaluation of the elbow: normal motion requirements and strength determination. Orthop Trans. 1981; 5:304.

Beals RK: The normal carrying angle of the elbow. A radiographic study of 422 patients. Clin Orthop. 1976; 119:194–196.

Buehler MJ, Thayer DT: The elbow flexion test. A clinical test for the cubital tunnel syndrome. Clin Orthop. 1988; 233:213–216.

Callaway GH, Field LD, Deng XH, et al: Biomechanical evaluation of the medial collateral ligament of the elbow. J Bone Joint Surg Am. 1997; 79:1223–1231.

Childress HM: Recurrent ulnar nerve dislocation at the elbow. Clin Orthop. 1975; 108:168–173.

Henry AK: Extensile Exposure, 2nd ed. Edinburgh, Churchill Livingstone, 1973, p 90.

Huss CD, Puhl JJ: Myositis ossificans of the upper arm. Am J Sports Med. 1980; 8:419–424.

Jobe FW, Stark H, Lombardo SJ: Reconstruction of the ulnar collateral ligament in athletes. J Bone Joint Surg Am. 1986; 68:1158–1163.

Morrey BF, Askew LJ, Chao EY: A biomechanical study of normal functional elbow motion. J Bone Joint Surg Am. 1981; 63:872–877.

Morrey BF, An KN: Articular and ligamentous contributions to the stability of the elbow joint. Am J Sports Med. 1983; 11:315–319.

Morrey BF: The Elbow and its Disorders, 2nd ed. Philadelphia, WB Saunders, 1993, p 1876.

Moss SH, Switzer HE: Radial tunnel syndrome: a spectrum of clinical presentations. J Hand Surg [Am]. 1983; 8:414–420.

Nirschl RP: Tennis elbow. Orthop Clin North Am. 1973; 3:787–800.

Novak CB, Lee GW, Mackinnon SE, et al: Provocative testing for cubital tunnel syndrome. J Hand Surg [Am]. 1994; 19:817–820.

O'Driscoll SW, Bell DF, Morrey BF: Posterolateral rotatory instability of the elbow. J Bone Joint Surg Am. 1991; 73:440–446.

Pappas AM, Zawacki RM, Sullivan JI: Biomechanics of baseball pitching: a preliminary report. Am J Sports Med. 1985; 13:216–222.

Pavlov H, Torg JS, Jacobs B, Vigorita V: Nonunion of olecranon epiphysis: two cases in adolescent baseball pitchers. AJR. 1981; 136:819–820.

Regan WD, Korinek SL, Morrey BF, An KN: Biomechanical study of ligaments about the elbow joint. Clin Orthop. 1991; 271:170–179.

Schwab GH, Bennett JB, Woods GW, Tullos HS: Biomechanics of elbow instability: the role of the medial collateral ligament. Clin Orthop. 1980; 146:42–52.

Spinner M: Injuries to the Major Branches of the Nerves in the Forearm, 2nd ed. Philadelphia, WB Saunders, 1978.

Wilson FD, Andrews JR, Blackburn TA, McCluskey G: Valgus extension overload in the pitching elbow. Am J Sports Med. 1983; 11:83–88.

Daniel P. Mass
Bruce Reider

4

Hand and Wrist

Without the human hand, the most refined creations of the human mind would be mere theoretical concepts. The hand is the focal point of human beings' interactions with the environment; it is the instrument used to deliver a knockout punch or to perform brain surgery. The hand is an organ of such complexity that many devote their lives to studying it and curing its ills.

The varied functions of the hand include grasping, pinching, and acting as a hook or paperweight. About 45% of the work of the hand utilizes *grasp,* a power function that requires coordinated action of both the intrinsic hand muscles and the extrinsic thumb and finger flexors. Variations of the grasp mechanism allow a person to make a tight fist or to securely hold an object such as a ball or glass (Fig. 4–1A). Another 45% of hand function utilizes *pinch.* Varieties of pinch include *side pinch (key pinch),* between the tip of the thumb and the side of the index finger (Fig. 4–1B); *tip pinch,* between the tip of the fully opposed thumb and the tip of one of the remaining fingers (Fig. 4–1C); and *chuck pinch,* in which less rotation is required to allow the tip of the thumb to form a triangular chuck with the tips of the index and long fingers (Fig. 4–1D). About 5% of the hand's activities require functioning as a *hook.* This more primitive function allows the curved fingers to span handles or support thin objects (Fig. 4–1E). In the remaining 5% of tasks, the hand functions as a *paperweight* (Fig. 4–1F). This most primitive of hand functions does not require the intrinsic strength or fine manipulative abilities necessary for more delicate tasks.

The hand functions well because it is suspended at the end of the arm. The shoulder and elbow serve to position the hand in space, allowing it to perform the precise functions required. Before commencing a detailed examination of the hand and the wrist, the examiner must perform a general assessment of the shoulder, elbow, and forearm. This may be done rapidly by asking the patient to raise the hands overhead until the arms touch the ears, to bring the arms down by the sides, to place the hands behind the head, to place the hands behind the back, to place the arms at the sides with the elbows flexed to 90°, then to fully pronate and supinate the forearms, to flex the elbows fully, and to extend the elbows fully. This sequence gives the examiner a brief overview of the range of motion of the other joints of the upper extremity and allows the examiner to screen for any gross abnormality that might secondarily affect hand and wrist function.

Inspection

SURFACE ANATOMY

For comfort and convenience, the hand and wrist are usually inspected with the patient seated. The hands may be rested on a small table or desk, on a pillow resting on the patient's lap, or on the lap itself. With the hands extended in front of the patient and the forearms pronated, the forearm, hand, and extended fingers should form a straight line. Any break in that line is abnormal and requires further investigation.

Orientation

When describing locations in the hand and wrist, the traditional terms *anterior, posterior, medial,* and *lateral* are usually replaced by the terms **volar (palmar), dorsal, ulnar,** and **radial.** The ability of the forearm to rotate changes the position of structures in the distal forearm and hand in relation to the rest of the human body; it is thus less confusing to describe them in relationship to surfaces within the hand and wrist. Thus, *dorsal* refers to the back of the hand and wrist, *volar* or *palmar* refer to the anterior, or palm, surface of the hand and wrist, *radial* refers to the side of the hand and wrist on which the thumb and radius are located, and *ulnar* refers to the side of the hand and wrist on which the little finger and ulna are located.

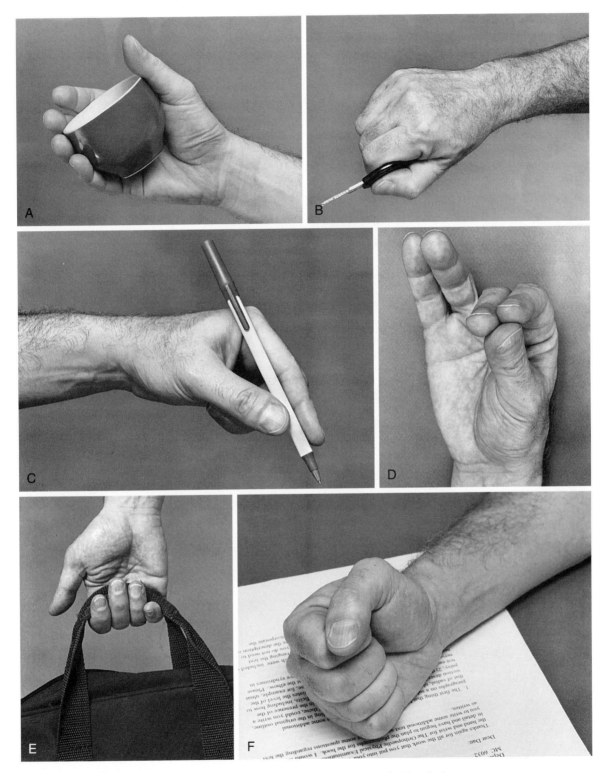

Figure 4–1. Functions of the hand. *A,* Grasp. *B,* Side pinch (key pinch). *C,* Tip pinch. *D,* Chuck pinch. *E,* Hook. *F,* Paperweight.

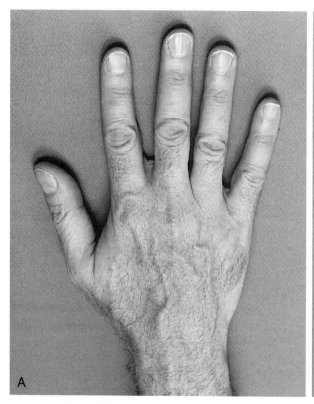
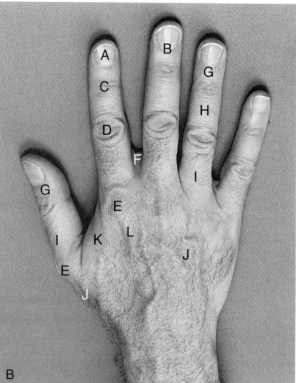

Figure 4–2. *A* and *B*, Dorsal aspect of the hand. A, fingernail; B, cuticle; C, distal interphalangeal joint; D, proximal interphalangeal joint; E, metacarpophalangeal joint; F, web space; G, distal phalanx; H, middle phalanx; I, proximal phalanx; J, metacarpal; K, first dorsal interosseous; L, extensor tendon (index finger).

Dorsal Aspect

The dorsal aspect of the hand and wrist is inspected with the patient's forearm pronated.

FINGERNAILS. Closest to the examiner are the **fingernails,** which protect the dorsal tips of the digits (Fig. 4–2). A smooth **eponychium,** or cuticle, surrounds the base of the nail. Ideally, the nail itself should be smooth and oval. The **nailbed** itself, visible through the nail, should be a healthy pink, with the exception of a small white crescent or **lunula** at the base of some nails. The color of a nail reflects the circulatory status of that particular digit; the color of the nails as a whole may reflect the circulatory status of the hand and the cardiovascular function of the patient.

Deformities of the nail are legion and may reflect injury to the nailbed or systemic disease. Common nail deformities include splitting owing to a previously lacerated nailbed and pitting owing to psoriatic arthritis. Fungal nail infections, more common in the foot, may also leave the fingernails thickened and deformed. The appear-

ance of the nails may reflect not only the patient's health status but his or her occupation and personality as well. Swelling around the base of the fingernail, often asymmetric and accompanied by erythema, many times reflects an infection known as a *paronychia* (Fig. 4–3). Maroon discoloration at the base of the nail usually reflects a *subungual hematoma*, which often results from a

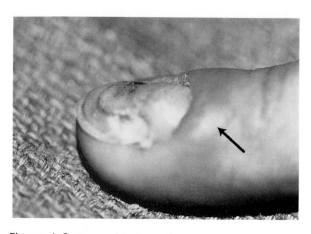

Figure 4–3. Paronychia (*arrow*).

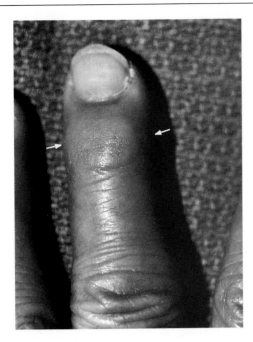

Figure 4–4. Heberden's nodes *(arrows).*

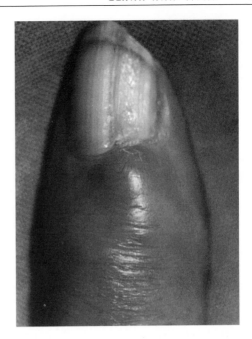

Figure 4–5. Mucous cyst.

direct blow to the fingertip. Subungual hematoma may be associated with an underlying fracture of the distal phalanx.

DIGITS. The digits themselves should appear straight, with transverse wrinkles marking the locations of the interphalangeal joints. The thumb is composed of proximal and distal phalanges linked by an interphalangeal joint. Localized swelling may reflect a specific injury or a more systemic disease process. Multiple bony swellings around the **distal interphalangeal (DIP) joints** are known as **Heberden's nodes**

(Fig. 4–4) and are typical of osteoarthritis. A *mucous cyst* is a cystic lesion on the dorsum of the finger near the DIP joint and the fingernail (Fig. 4–5). It is associated with degenerative arthritis of the DIP joint and arises from the joint itself.

Degenerative swollen **proximal interphalangeal (PIP) joints** may also occur in osteoarthritis. These firm, bony swellings are known as **Bouchard's nodes** (Fig. 4–6). When these joints are involved with rheumatoid arthritis, the swelling is soft and puffy. The PIP joints are also common sites of dislocations and collateral liga-

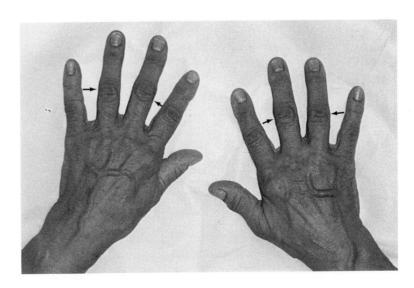

Figure 4–6. Bouchard's nodes *(arrows).*

ment sprains. These injuries produce localized swelling and a visible step-off if a nonreduced dislocation is present.

Fractures may occur in any of the **phalanges.** They are marked by localized ecchymosis and fusiform swelling. Angular or rotational deformities may also be present. More complex deformities of the fingers are discussed under Alignment.

The webbing at the base of the finger slants distally from the dorsal toward the volar side of the hand. The distal limit of the **web spaces** between the fingers actually marks the midpoint of the **proximal phalanges.** The **metacarpophalangeal (MCP) joints** are usually subtly visible as a series of bumps in line with the fingers. Swelling around one of these joints following trauma usually reflects a fracture, sprain, or dislocation. Inflammatory swelling of the metacarpophalangeal joints is commonly found in rheumatoid arthritis.

HAND. The dorsal skin of the hand is normally loose and redundant (Fig. 4–7). The **extensor tendons** to the four fingers are usually visible as they cross the metacarpophalangeal joints. Asking the patient to forcefully hyperextend the fingers usually increases the prominence of the extensor tendons (Fig. 4–8). Common causes of swelling over the dorsum of the hand include metacarpal fracture, hematoma, and inflammatory tenosynovitis. Because the **metacarpals** are

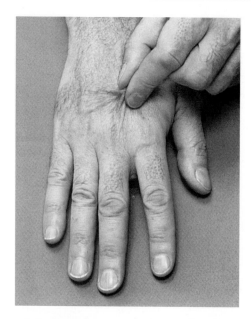

Figure 4–7. Looseness of dorsal skin.

subcutaneous, angulation associated with fractures of their shafts is usually visible once the initial swelling has declined. In the presence of severe ulnar neuropathy, the consequent atrophy of the ulnar-innervated interosseous muscles makes the metacarpal shafts more visible. Fracture of the metacarpal shaft just proximal to the metacarpophalangeal joint is particularly com-

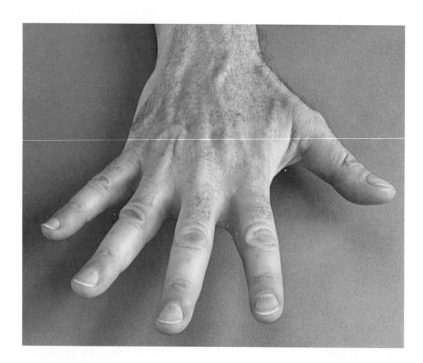

Figure 4–8. Active extension increases the prominence of the finger extensor tendons.

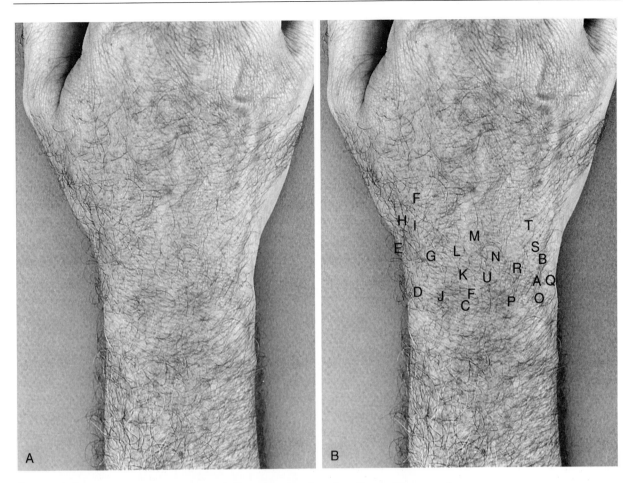

Figure 4–9. *A* and *B,* Dorsal aspect of the wrist. A, triangular fibrocartilage complex (TFCC); B, extensor carpi ulnaris tendon; C, Lister's tubercle; D, radial styloid; E, abductor pollicis longus and extensor pollicis brevis; F, extensor pollicis longus; G, scaphoid; H, trapezium; I, scapho-trapezio-trapezoid (STT) joint; J, extensor carpi radialis brevis and longus tendons; K, scapholunate ligament; L, scapholunate capitate joint; M, head of the capitate; N, extensor digitorum communis tendons; O, ulnar head; P, distal radioulnar joint; Q, ulnar styloid; R, lunotriquetral ligament; S, triquetrum; T, hamate; U, lunate.

mon in the fifth metacarpal, where it is known as a *boxer's fracture.* Such fractures often produce a **dropped knuckle;** the metacarpal head is depressed and its normal prominence disappears. **Carpal bossing** is the term for benign bony prominences that can form on the dorsum of the proximal ends of the second and third metacarpals.

The **first dorsal interosseous** is the most prominent muscle mass of the dorsum of the hand. Located along the radial border of the second metacarpal, the first dorsal interosseous creates a large fleshy prominence between this metacarpal and the thumb. Visible atrophy of the first dorsal interosseous is associated with severe degrees of ulnar neuropathy.

WRIST. The bump caused by the **head of the distal ulna** is the most prominent bony landmark of the dorsal wrist (Fig. 4–9). Just distal to the head of the ulna is a small hollow marking the location of the **triangular fibrocartilage complex (TFCC).** The **extensor carpi ulnaris** tendon passes over the ulnar aspect of the pronated ulna and may occasionally be visible just distal to it, especially if the wrist is actively extended and ulnar-deviated. The tendons of the **extensors carpi radialis longus** and **brevis** are more apt to be visible as they cross the wrist to insert at the base of the second and third metacarpals. Again, asking the patient to dorsiflex the wrist actively increases the prominence of these tendons. Active extension of the thumb

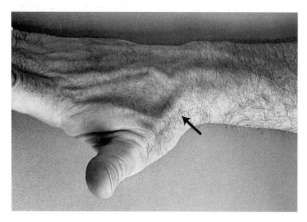

Figure 4–10. Active extension to demonstrate extensor pollicis longus tendon (*arrow*).

also makes the tendon of the **extensor pollicis longus** quite visible (Fig. 4–10). This tendon enters the wrist from the distal forearm, where it makes a sharply angled turn at the prominence of the radius known as **Lister's tubercle,** en route to its insertion at the base of the thumb. This is a common site for rupture of the tendon following fracture of the distal radius or rheumatoid synovitis. In the case of such a rupture, the normal prominence of the tendon disappears.

Diffuse swelling over the dorsum of the wrist is common in *rheumatoid arthritis* or from hemorrhage following fracture of one of the carpal bones or injury to the intercarpal ligaments (Fig. 4–11A). The swelling due to synovitis is more

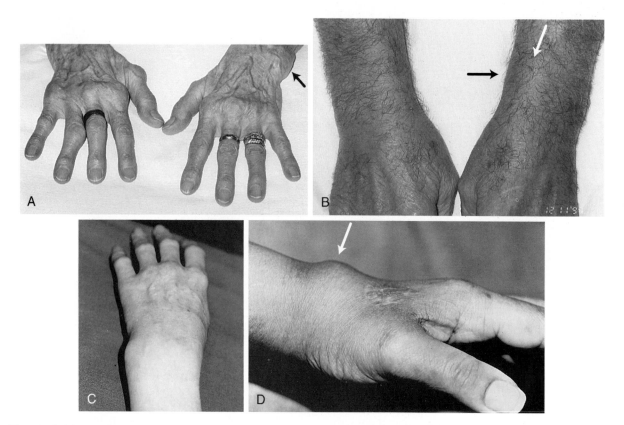

Figure 4–11. *A,* Wrist swelling in rheumatoid arthritis (*arrow*). *B,* Swelling from nondisplaced fracture of the distal radius (*arrows*). *C,* Silver fork deformity. *D,* Dorsal wrist ganglion (*arrow*).

diffuse and extends further distally over the dorsum of the hand compared with the hematoma associated with a fracture or a ligament injury. Fracture of the distal radius is extremely common and causes swelling that is slightly more proximal (Fig. 4–11*B*). When such fractures occur, the distal fragment most commonly displaces dorsally. This produces the so-called **silver fork deformity,** in which the distal radius and hand appear dorsally displaced with respect to the rest of the forearm (Fig. 4–11*C*).

A localized spherical mass on the dorsum of the wrist is most commonly due to a *ganglion cyst*. These cysts can range from just barely palpable to golf ball-sized. They most commonly appear immediately adjacent to the radial wrist extensors, but they may dissect more proximally and distally as they enlarge (see Fig. 4–11*D*). Ganglia become more prominent with wrist flexion. The transillumination test can confirm

the diagnosis of a ganglion cyst (see the Manipulation section).

Radial (Lateral) Aspect

THUMB. Rotating the patient's forearm into the neutral position allows the examiner to study the radial aspect of the hand and wrist directly (Fig. 4–12). This position allows a more direct view of the dorsum of the **thumb.** As in the fingers, in the thumb the examiner looks for abnormalities about the fingernail or areas of swelling or ecchymosis that might signify a fracture or joint injury. The metacarpophalangeal joint of the thumb, the **first metacarpophalangeal joint,** is normally quite prominent and easily visualized. Injuries to the ulnar collateral ligament of the first metacarpophalangeal joint, often

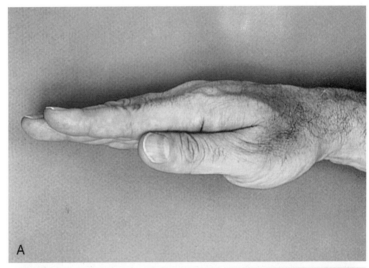

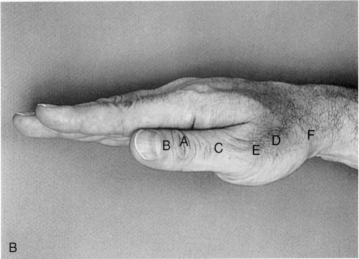

Figure 4–12. *A* and *B*, Radial aspect of the hand. A, interphalangeal joint of the thumb; B, distal phalanx; C, proximal phalanx; D, first metacarpal; E, first metacarpophalangeal joint; F, basilar joint.

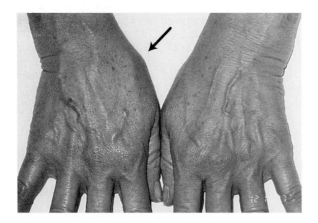

Figure 4–13. Swollen basilar joint (*arrow*).

the **anatomic snuffbox** (Fig. 4–14). The anatomic snuffbox is bordered dorsally by the tendon of the **extensor pollicis longus** and volarly by the adjacent tendons of the **extensor pollicis brevis** and **abductor pollicis longus.** The visibility of these tendons may be accentuated by asking the patient to extend the thumb forcefully.

The waist of the **scaphoid** bone, a common site of fracture, lies deep to the anatomic snuffbox. Thus, puffy swelling in the anatomic snuffbox following trauma suggests the possibility of a scaphoid fracture.

Volar (Palmar) Aspect

called *skier's thumb* or *gamekeeper's thumb,* are a common cause of swelling at that location.

Although the thumb has only two phalanges, its metacarpal is much more mobile than the metacarpals of the other fingers and thus assumes some of the functions of a third phalanx. The proximal end or base of the **first metacarpal,** which serves as the insertion site of the abductor pollicis longus tendon, produces a visible step-off in the contour of the hand. Abnormal enlargement of this prominence is a common sign of arthritis of the **basilar joint** (Fig. 4–13) between the base of the first metacarpal and the trapezium.

WRIST. Looking proximally from the base of the first metacarpal, the examiner encounters a hollow depression and then a slight prominence produced by the styloid process of the distal radius. The hollow marks an area often known as

FINGERS AND PALM. Further rotating the patient's forearm into the fully supinated position allows inspection of the palmar aspect of the hand and volar wrist. The palmar aspect of the normal hand is not flat but marked by a number of curves and contours (Fig. 4–15). A **longitudinal arch** begins with a prominence at the base of the hand, curves away from the examiner in the middle of the palm, and then curves back toward the examiner at the distal palm and fingers. This arch is formed by the natural resting tension that exists in the finger flexors when the wrist is extended. A **transverse arch,** oriented perpendicular to the longitudinal arch, traverses the hand from one side to the other. Flexing the metacarpophalangeal joints of the fingers and flexing and adducting the thumb accentuates these arches, producing the cupped configuration helpful for swimming or scooping water

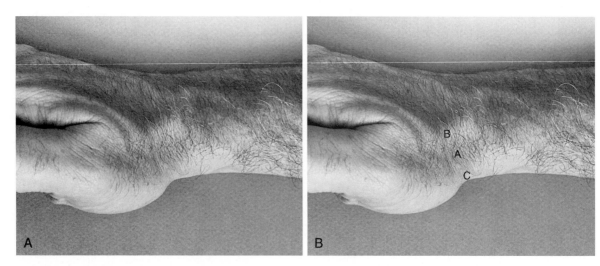

Figure 4–14. *A* and *B,* Radial aspect of the wrist. A, anatomic snuffbox; B, extensor pollicis longus; C, extensor pollicis brevis and abductor pollicis longus.

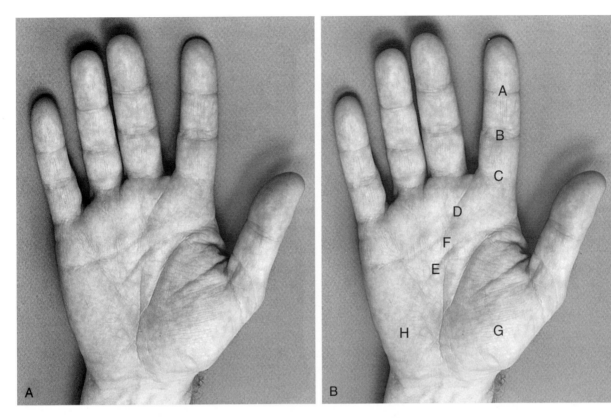

Figure 4–15. *A* and *B*, Palmar aspect of the hand. A, distal flexion crease of index finger; B, proximal flexion crease of index finger; C, web flexion crease of index finger; D, distal palmar crease; E, proximal palmar crease; F, level of metacarpophalangeal joints; G, thenar eminence; H, hypothenar eminence.

(Fig. 4–16). A break in either of these arches reflects a serious injury to the hand.

The examiner should carefully note the normal resting position of the fingers. When the wrist is extended, the normal resting tension on the flexor tendons of the fingers causes them to lie in an **arcade of flexion,** which progresses from slight flexion of the index finger to marked flexion of the little finger (Fig. 4–17). A break in this normal arcade usually signifies a flexor tendon injury or restricted joint motion in the involved finger.

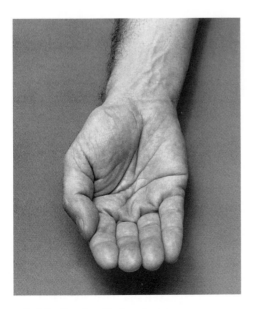

Figure 4–16. Cupping the hand.

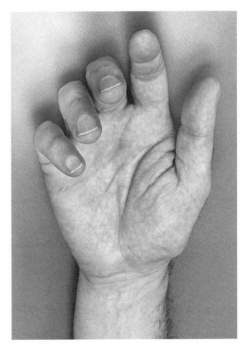

Figure 4–17. Normal resting arcade of finger flexion.

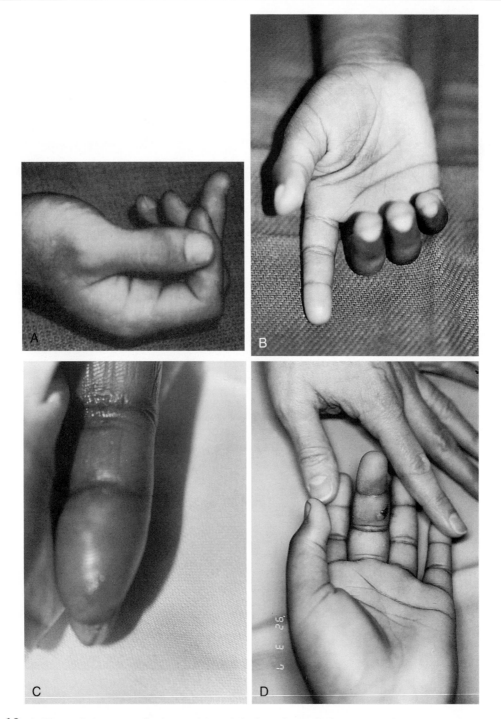

Figure 4–18. *A*, Flexor digitorum profundus avulsion of the long finger. *B*, Laceration of both flexor profundus and superficialis tendons to the index finger. *C*, Felon. *D*, Flexor tendon sheath infection. (*A*, From Reider B: Sports Medicine: The School-Age Athlete, 2nd ed. Philadelphia, WB Saunders, 1996, p 252.)

Disruption of the flexor tendons may be due to laceration or a closed rupture. The most common example of a closed rupture is avulsion of the **flexor digitorum profundus** insertion from the base of the distal phalanx. This condition is sometimes called *jersey finger* because it can occur when the fingers of a football player are pulled into extension as he attempts to grasp the jersey of an opponent. This usually occurs in the ring finger, whose profundus tendon is tethered to those of the little finger and the long finger. *Flexor profundus avulsion* causes disruption of the normal resting arcade of the fingers because the DIP joint of the involved finger comes to lie in a relatively extended position (Fig. 4–18*A*). Deformities caused by flexor tendon laceration

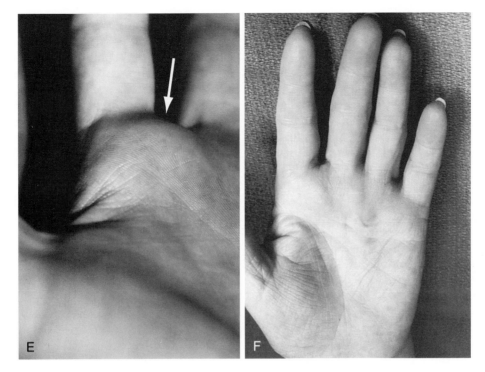

Figure 4–18 *Continued. E,* Flexor tendon sheath ganglion *(arrow). F,* Dupuytren's disease of the ring finger.

vary depending on the tendons involved. *Laceration of the profundus tendon* alone would produce isolated loss of DIP joint flexion similar to that produced by jersey finger. *Laceration of the superficialis tendon* alone would produce only a slight break in the arcade of flexion, because the profundus tendon would still be able to flex both interphalangeal joints of the involved finger. *Laceration of both tendons,* however, results in loss of ability to flex both the PIP and the DIP joints of the involved finger. This causes the affected finger to lie with both interphalangeal joints extended while the other fingers form the normal resting arcade (Fig. 4–18*B*).

The skin of the palmar surface of the hand is dramatically different from that of the dorsum. The **palmar skin** is thickened, hairless, and marked with discrete creases that identify the sites of motion. Localized calluses may give clues about the person's occupation or avocations. Unlike the dorsal skin, the palmar skin is tightly bound down through fascial tetherings that allow the palm to transmit shear forces to objects being manipulated.

The **distal** and **proximal flexion creases of the fingers** mark the approximate locations of the DIP and the PIP joints, respectively (Fig. 4–15). The **web flexion creases** at the level of the web spaces are misleading because they mark the midpoint of the proximal phalanges. The true location of the metacarpophalangeal joints is signified by the **palmar creases.**

Because the palmar skin is the common site of interface between human beings and the surrounding environment, it is frequently subject to lacerations and penetrating injuries. These injuries, in turn, may lead to closed-space infections of the fingers and hand. Localized swelling and erythema of the fingertip, for example, may reflect a *felon,* the common term for a closed-space infection of the **fingertip** (see Fig. 4–18*C*). The presence of vesicles suggests a *herpetic felon* or *herpetic whitlow.* Fusiform swelling extending along the middle and proximal phalanges into the distal palm may signify a closed infection of the flexor tendon sheath (see Fig. 4–18*D*). This fusiform swelling is one of the four classic signs of flexor tendon sheath infection, often called the four **cardinal signs of Kanavel.** The other three are the volar surface of the involved finger is tender, the finger is held in a flexed position at rest, and passive extension of the finger exacerbates the patient's pain. Other closed-space infections may occur in the **thenar** or **midpalmar spaces.** These would result in localized painful swelling over the thenar eminence or center of the palm, respectively.

Epidermal inclusion cysts, the result of old penetrating injuries, may cause nodular swellings of the fingertips or other areas of the volar surface of the fingers. A nodular swelling at the level of the proximal flexion crease of the fingers is most commonly due to a *ganglion of the flexor tendon sheath* (see Fig. 4–18*E*). These ganglia are normally only a few millimeters and thus only palpable, although large ones may occasionally be visible.

In most individuals two creases, known as the **distal palmar flexion crease** and the **proximal palmar flexion crease,** cross the hand. The more transverse portions of these two palmar flexion creases combine to identify the level of the metacarpophalangeal joints of the fingers **(transverse palmar crease).**

Just deep to the palmar skin lies a layer of fascia known as the **palmar aponeurosis.** In its normal state, this tissue is not directly visible. However, a visible nodule in line with the ring or little fingers may be the first sign of *Dupuytren's disease* (see Fig. 4–18*F*). This condition, which is often familial and tends to occur in older men, can progress to the formation of longitudinal fibrous bands that gradually pull the involved finger or fingers into a progressively flexed, contracted position.

Proximal to the palmar flexion creases, the fleshy mounds of the thenar and hypothenar eminences are the predominant contours. The **thenar eminence** is created by the muscle bellies of the major intrinsic muscles of the thumb including the adductor pollicis, the flexor pollicis brevis, the abductor pollicis brevis, and the opponens pollicis. The *ulnar nerve* supplies the adductor pollicis and the deep head of the flexor pollicis brevis, whereas the rest of the thenar eminence is innervated by the *median nerve*. The **hypothenar eminence** is composed of the intrinsic muscles to the little finger. The smaller size of the hypothenar eminence reflects the reduced strength and opposability of this digit compared with the thumb. The hypothenar muscles include the abductor digiti minimi (quinti), which forms the medial border of the hand; the flexor digiti minimi (quinti); and the opponens digiti minimi (quinti), all innervated by the *ulnar nerve*.

WRIST. Where the hand joins the forearm at the wrist, a series of flexion creases is usually

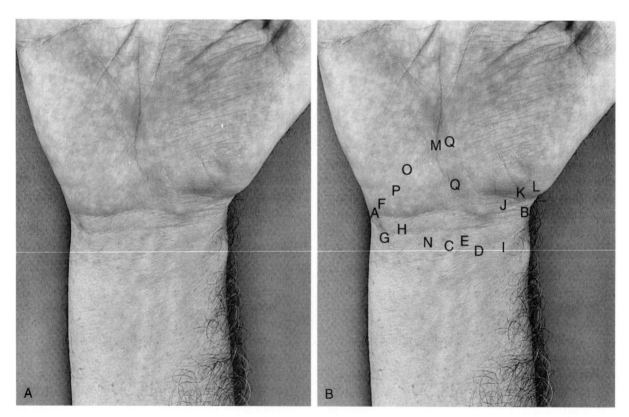

Figure 4–19. *A* and *B,* Volar aspect of the wrist. A, distal flexion crease; B, abductor pollicis longus; C, palmaris longus; D, flexor carpi radialis; E, median nerve; F, pisiform; G, flexor carpi ulnaris; H, ulnar artery and nerve; I, radial artery; J, scaphoid tubercle; K, trapezium; L, basilar joint; M, longitudinal interthenar crease; N, flexor digitorum tendons; O, hook of the hamate; P, Guyon's canal; Q, proximal and distal margins of the transverse carpal ligament.

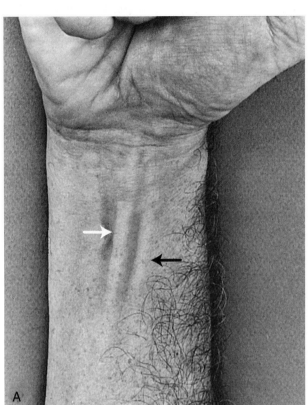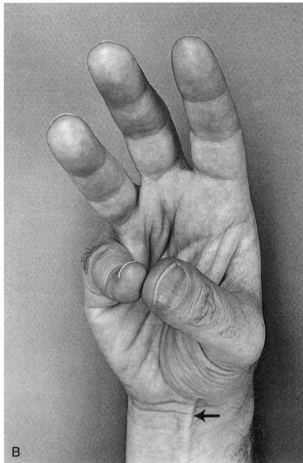

Figure 4–20. *A*, Prominence of flexor carpi radialis (*solid arrow*) and palmaris longus (*open arrow*) increased by active wrist flexion. *B*, Demonstration of palmaris longus tendon by pinching (*arrow*).

visible (Fig. 4–19). The **distal flexion crease of the wrist** marks the proximal limit of the **flexor retinaculum (transverse carpal ligament),** the tough fascial tissue that forms the roof of the carpal tunnel. On the lateral border of the wrist, the prominence of the base of the first metacarpal is again visible along the lateral border of the thenar eminence. The tendon of the **abductor pollicis longus** forms the border of the contour of the wrist as it courses distally to insert on the base of the first metacarpal. Moving medially, the next tendon that is usually visible through the skin is that of the **flexor carpi radialis** (Fig. 4–20*A*). Between the abductor pollicis longus and the flexor carpi radialis lies the distal portion of the **radial artery.** Its pulsations are often visible on careful inspection.

Running just lateral and parallel to the flexor carpi radialis tendon is the **palmaris longus** tendon. This structure, present in about 80% of

individuals, can be brought out by asking the patient to pinch the tips of the opposed thumb and little finger firmly together with the wrist in slight flexion (see Fig. 4–20*B*). The depression between the flexor carpi radialis and the palmaris longus tendons overlies the **median nerve,** which is not itself visible.

At the lateral side of the wrist, the **pisiform** bone creates a bony prominence at the base of the hypothenar eminence. The pisiform is a sesamoid bone within the **flexor carpi ulnaris** tendon, a structure that is usually visible and defines the medial border of the wrist. The prominence of both the flexor carpi ulnaris and the flexor carpi radialis tendons may be increased by having the patient flex the wrist against resistance. The **ulnar artery** and **nerve** lie just radial to the flexor carpi ulnaris tendon. The pulsations of the ulnar artery are not normally visible but can be palpated.

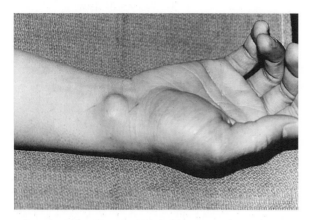

Figure 4–21. Volar wrist ganglion.

The most common mass of the volar wrist is a *volar wrist ganglion* (Fig. 4–21). These ganglia may vary in size from small ones, which are only palpable, to larger, visible ones of 1 cm or more. When visible, they usually appear at the radial side of the wrist. More diffuse swelling over the carpus may be due to *inflammatory synovitis* or *hemorrhage* from a fracture or ligamentous injury.

Ulnar (Medial) Aspect

The ulnar aspect of the hand and wrist may be most easily inspected by having the patient flex the elbow until the ulnar border of the hand is facing the examiner. This perspective furnishes fewer distinguishing landmarks than the other aspects (Fig. 4–22). The superior border of the dorsum of the hand is delineated by the straight contour of the shaft of the **fifth metacarpal.** Flexion deformities due to acute or malunited boxer's fractures of the neck of the fifth metacarpal should be most clearly appreciated from this perspective. Volar to the metacarpal, the fleshy prominence of the **hypothenar eminence** bulges toward the examiner. More proximally, the bony prominence of the **head of the distal ulna** is usually visible on the dorsum of the wrist. An increase in this normal prominence may be due to degenerative arthritis of the distal radioulnar joint, rheumatoid synovitis, or a tear of the TFCC. In severe cases of rheumatoid arthritis, the carpal bones may sublux volarly with respect to the distal ulna and radius. This subluxation occurs more on the ulnar side than on the radial side, thus accentuating the prominence of the distal ulna. This condition is known as *capita ulna syndrome.*

ALIGNMENT

Alignment may be first assessed with the fingers and the thumb fully extended and the wrist in a neutral position. Whether viewed from their dorsal or volar aspects, the fingers and the thumb should appear straight and in alignment with their respective metacarpals (Fig. 4–23A). Acute

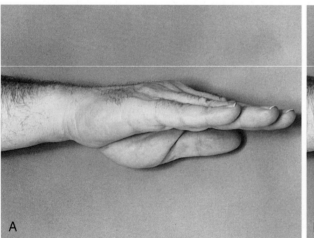
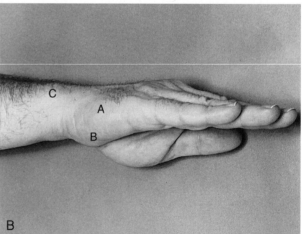

Figure 4–22. *A* and *B,* Ulnar aspect of the hand and wrist. A, Fifth metacarpal; B, hypothenar eminence; C, head of the ulna.

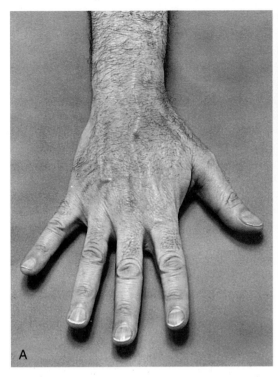

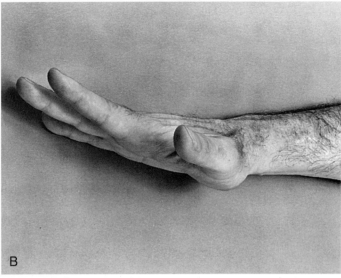

A

B

Figure 4–23. *A,* Normal alignment, dorsal view. *B,* Normal alignment, sagittal view.

or malunited fractures of the phalanges are the most common cause of angular deviations from normal straight alignment. **Ulnar deviation of the MCP joints** of the fingers is a common deformity in rheumatoid arthritis (Fig. 4–24). In this case, the rheumatoid synovitis disrupts the extensor hoods over the heads of the digital metacarpals, allowing the extensor tendons to slide to the ulnar aspect of each metacarpal and thus pull the fingers into flexion and ulnar deviation.

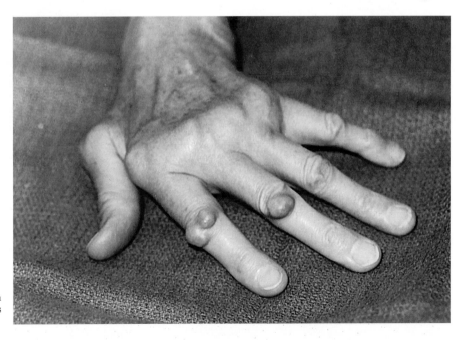

Figure 4–24. Ulnar deviation of metacarpophalangeal joints in rheumatoid arthritis.

FINGER DEFORMITIES. Sagittal alignment may be assessed by inspecting the fingers and thumb from either side while the patient holds the digits in full extension. When fully extended, the normal fingers and thumb should hyperextend slightly, exhibiting a smooth, gentle curve (see Fig. 4–23B). A number of common deformities are visible from this perspective. Avulsion of the insertion of the extensor digitorum communis from the dorsal base of the distal phalanx of one of the fingers is called a **mallet finger.** When a mallet finger deformity is present, the DIP joint of the involved finger remains in slight flexion when the patient attempts to extend all fingers (Fig. 4–25A).

Damage to the insertion of the central slip of the extensor digitorum communis tendon at the dorsal base of the middle phalanx can cause a **boutonnière deformity,** a combination of flexion contracture of the PIP joint and extension deformity of the DIP joint (see Fig. 4–25B). This insertion may rupture acutely owing to a jamming injury of the finger or attenuate gradually owing to rheumatoid synovitis. Initially, this damage results in a flexion deformity at the PIP joint when the patient attempts to extend the involved finger. Overpull of the extensor tendon, which is still attached to the distal phalanx, results in hyperextension of the DIP joint. With time, the lateral bands of the extensor tendon sublux volarly past the center of rotation of the PIP joint, causing the boutonnière deformity to become more rigid.

A **swan neck deformity** may follow an untreated mallet injury, follow an untreated PIP joint dislocation, or occur within the context of rheumatoid arthritis (see Fig. 4–25C). It is a combination of flexion deformity of the DIP joint and hyperextension of the PIP joint. The insertion of the extensor digitorum communis tendon at the base of the distal phalanx is avulsed or the volar plate of the PIP joint is attenuated by rheumatoid synovitis or trauma. This allows the extensor tendon to retract and overpull, resulting in a hyperextension deformity of the PIP joint. Initially, the hyperextension of the PIP joint is reversible by active flexion, but ultimately the joint can become stiff and fixed.

NERVE PALSIES. Two classic deformities that are due to peripheral nerve injuries are benedic-

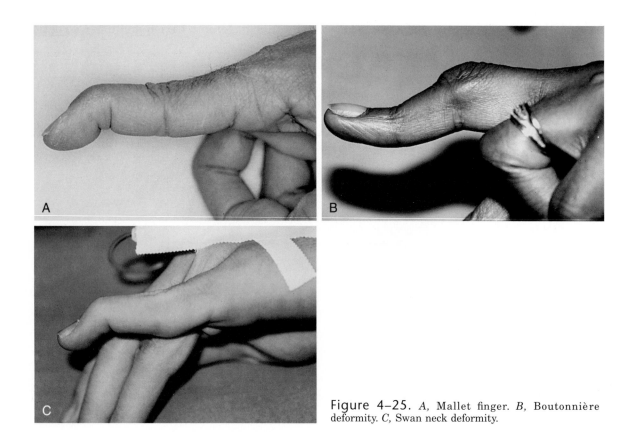

Figure 4–25. *A,* Mallet finger. *B,* Boutonnière deformity. *C,* Swan neck deformity.

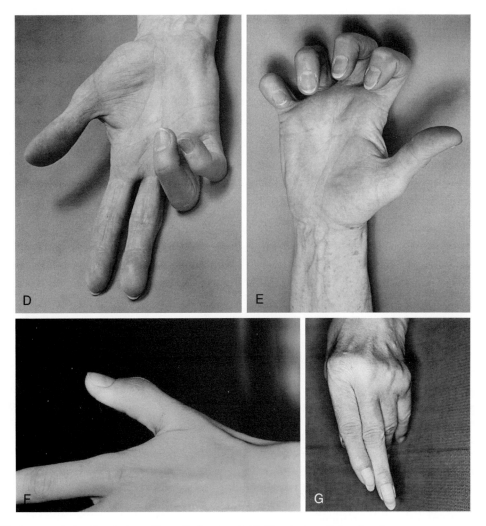

Figure 4–25 *Continued. D,* Simulation of benediction hand. *E,* Simulation of claw hand. *F,* Extensor pollicis longus rupture. *G,* Extensor digitorum communis rupture (ring and little fingers).

tion hand and claw hand. A severe ulnar nerve palsy produces the **benediction hand** deformity, in which the little finger and the ring finger are claw-shaped (hyperextended at the MCP joints but flexed at the interphalangeal joints) owing to denervation of the interossei muscles, hypothenar muscles, and ulnar two lumbricals (see Fig. 4–25*D*). Combined median and ulnar nerve palsy can produce a **claw hand,** in which all fingers are claw-shaped owing to overpull of the finger extensors (see Fig. 4–25*E*).

JOINT DISLOCATIONS. *Dislocations of the PIP joint* are common and disrupt normal sagittal alignment. Most commonly, the middle phalanx displaces dorsally, producing a visible step-off at

the PIP joint. *Dislocations of the MCP joints* are more unusual. In this case, the proximal phalanx usually dislocates dorsally on the head of the corresponding metacarpal. In addition to the dorsal swelling created by the displacement of the proximal phalanx, a volar bulge may also be visible due to the prominence of the metacarpal head in the palm. Dislocation of the metacarpophalangeal joint of the thumb produces a similar deformity, although additional rotation and angulation of the proximal phalanx is often present.

TENDON RUPTURES. Flexion deformities of the thumb and fingers may also be due to rupture of the relevant extensor tendon. *Rupture of the extensor pollicis longus tendon* at the wrist, the most common of these injuries, may occur following a fracture of the distal radius or may be due to rheumatoid synovitis. In the presence of extensor pollicis longus rupture, the patient has particular difficulty extending the interphalangeal joint of the thumb (see Fig. 4–25F).

Rheumatoid arthritis may also produce *ruptures of the extensor digitorum communis tendons.* These ruptures produce a flexion deformity of the involved metacarpophalangeal joints because the patient is still able to extend the interphalangeal joints using the intrinsic muscles of the hand (see Fig. 4–25G). The extensor slip to the little finger is usually the first to rupture, followed progressively by the tendons to the ring, long, and index fingers over a variable period of time. This progressive series of extensor tendon ruptures is known as the *Vaughan-Jackson lesion.*

ROTATIONAL MALALIGNMENT. Finger alignment can be further assessed by asking the patient to supinate the hand and flex the fingers together. The examiner begins by inspecting the fingertips end-on while the fingers are partly flexed. When viewed from this perspective, the nail of the index finger faces slightly away from that of the long finger while the nails of the ring finger and the little finger are slightly rotated in the opposite direction (Fig. 4–26). Deviations from this alignment are most commonly due to

rotational deformity following the malunion of a phalangeal fracture.

The examiner can further test the rotational alignment of the fingers and metacarpals by asking the patient to individually flex each of the four fingers toward the palm. When flexed individually, each finger should face the scaphoid tubercle at the base of the thumb (Fig. 4–27A–D). When flexed as a group, they should stay in parallel alignment with each other (Fig. 4–27E). Rotational malalignment following an acute or malunited fracture of one of the metacarpals or phalanges causes the associated finger to deviate from the normal flexion alignment, possibly causing the adjacent fingers to cross when they are flexed simultaneously (Fig. 4–27F).

WRIST. The wrist may also be the site of posttraumatic or rheumatoid deformities. When fractures of the distal radius occur, the hand and distal radius are most commonly pushed dorsally. If this is incompletely reduced, the distal radius and hand remain dorsally displaced, resulting in a permanent step-off (see Fig. 4–11C). Dislocations or fracture-dislocations at the radiocarpal or midcarpal joints can also produce step-off deformities, although the details may be quickly obscured by the dramatic swelling that can accompany such injuries.

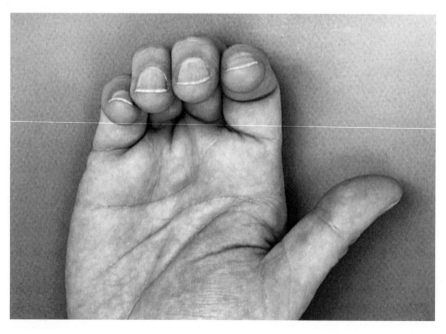

Figure 4–26. Normal fingertip alignment.

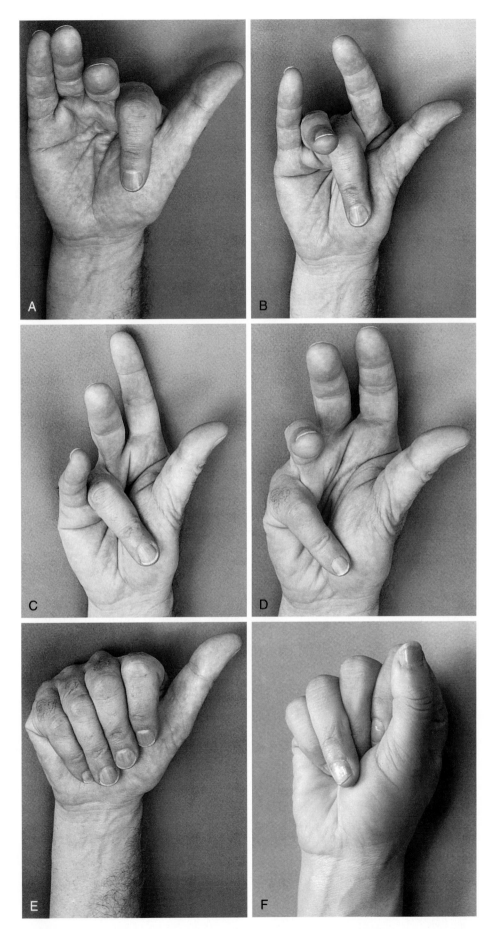

Figure 4–27. Normal flexion alignment of fingers. *A,* Index. *B,* Long. *C,* Ring. *D,* Little. *E,* All four together. *F,* Simulated rotational malalignment following a metacarpal fracture.

RANGE OF MOTION

A thorough assessment of the range of motion (ROM) of the joints of the hand and wrist should include an evaluation of **forearm rotation** as described in Chapter 3, Elbow and Forearm, because forearm rotation requires proper functioning of the distal radioulnar joint of the wrist. Conditions of the wrist that can lead to reduced forearm rotation include fractures of the distal radius involving the distal radioulnar joint, Galeazzi's fractures (fractures of the shaft of the distal radius associated with subluxation or dislocation of the distal radioulnar joint), and injuries of the triangular fibrocartilage complex.

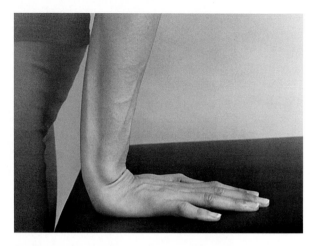

Figure 4–29. Passive wrist extension.

Wrist Motion

Wrist motion is a complex process involving coordinated movements at the *radiocarpal* and *intercarpal joints*. Loss of wrist motion is a common sequela of fractures or ligamentous injuries of or near the wrist. For measurement purposes, wrist motion is usually documented in four directions: flexion, extension, radial deviation, and ulnar deviation. During actual function, these motions can be combined in differing proportions, so that complete circumduction is possible. Wrist range of motion is usually evaluated with the elbow flexed to 90° and the forearm pronated. When measuring flexion and extension of the wrist, the neutral, or 0°, position is the point at which the dorsum of the wrist forms a straight line with the dorsum of the distal forearm.

EXTENSION AND FLEXION. To evaluate wrist **extension (dorsiflexion),** ask the patient to pull the hand upward as far as possible (Fig. 4–28). In most normal wrists, active extension is possible to 60° or 70°. When a passive force is added to the wrist, such as when an individual performs a pushup, extension may increase to 90° (Fig. 4–29). **Flexion (palmar flexion)** is then evaluated by asking the patient to bend the wrist downward as far as possible (Fig. 4–30). Normal flexion ranges from about 60° to 80°.

If the patient's hand is relaxed while demonstrating extension and flexion of the wrist, the **tenodesis effect** of the normal resting tension in the flexors and extensors of the fingers and thumb is demonstrated. When the wrist is passively extended, the flexor tendons are passively tightened, causing the fingers and thumb to flex

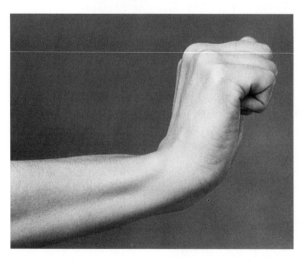

Figure 4–28. Active wrist extension.

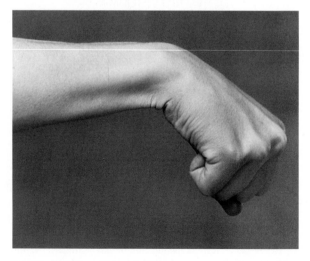

Figure 4–30. Active wrist flexion.

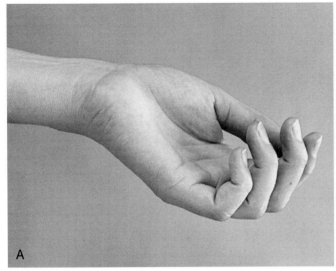

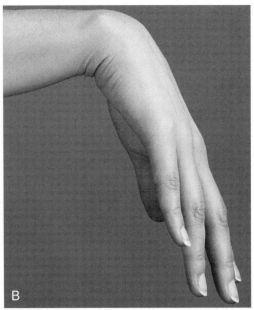

Figure 4–31. Tenodesis effect. *A*, Wrist extension with finger flexion. *B*, Wrist flexion with finger extension.

(Fig. 4–31*A*). Differential tension in the flexor tendons of the fingers causes them to assume the progressive arcade of flexion previously described. When the wrist is passively flexed, the extensor tendons are passively tightened and the flexor tendons relaxed, causing the fingers and thumb to passively extend (Fig. 4–31*B*). Either portion of the tenodesis effect can be overcome by active movement of the fingers.

RADIAL AND ULNAR DEVIATION. The two remaining movements of the wrist are radial and ulnar deviation. The neutral, or 0°, position for the measurement of deviation is the point at which an imaginary line through the long finger and third metacarpal aligns with the axis of the forearm. To assess **radial deviation,** the patient is asked to bend the wrist toward the radial side of the forearm (Fig. 4–32). The average amount

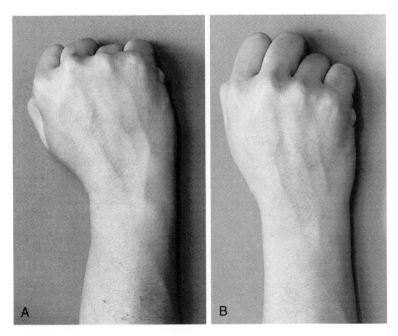

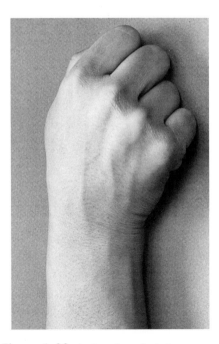

Figure 4–32. *A*, Active radial deviation. *B*, Neutral.

Figure 4–33. Active ulnar deviation.

of normal radial deviation is about 20°. **Ulnar deviation** is assessed by asking the patient to bend the wrist toward the ulnar side of the forearm (Fig. 4–33). Normal ulnar deviation averages about 30° to 40°. If the examiner assesses ulnar deviation with the patient's forearm supinated, a mild increase in motion is noted.

Finger Motion

Evaluation of the range of motion of the fingers and thumb involves the assessment of many individual joints and movements. A good screening test for thumb and finger motion is to ask the patient first to make a tight fist and then to fully extend the fingers and thumb. This brief procedure allows the examiner to pinpoint an area of potential abnormality and to focus on it in the detailed examination.

All joints of the fingers are capable of flexion and extension. In the assessment of flexion and extension, the neutral position is usually considered the point at which the dorsum of the extended finger is parallel with the dorsum of the hand.

EXTENSION AND FLEXION. Extension of the DIP, the PIP, and the MCP joints is usually assessed simultaneously. With the forearm pronated, the patient is asked to straighten the fingers as far as possible (Fig. 4–34). It is best to have the patient extend all four fingers together because tethering among the flexor tendons limits extension to a varying degree if the patient attempts to extend the fingers one at a time while

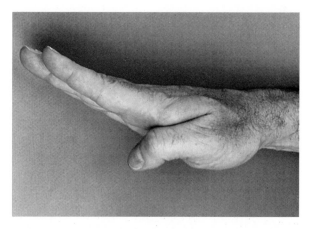

Figure 4–34. Active finger extension.

keeping the others flexed. **Active extension** of the DIP, the PIP, and the MCP joints should be possible to at least a neutral position. Mild hyperextension is common, especially in the MCP joints. Some loose-jointed patients exhibit hyperextension at the MCP joints measuring 30° or more. **Passive extension** of the fingers can be measured by gently pushing the finger upward with the examiner's own finger or thumb (Fig. 4–35). In most individuals, this leads to minimal increases in extension of the interphalangeal joints but a marked increase in extension of the MCP joint. Passive hyperextension of the MCP joint of the index finger to 70° or 80° is not unusual. The ability to passively hyperextend the index MCP joint to 90° or more is considered by many to be a sign of generalized ligamentous laxity.

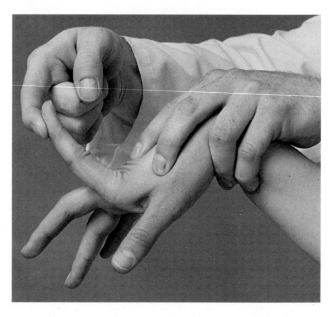

Figure 4–35. Passive finger extension.

Active flexion of the finger joints is assessed by asking the patient to bend the fingers downward into a tight fist. Flexing the fingers so that the tips are pressed against the **midpalmar crease** allows assessment of flexion of the DIP, the PIP, and the MCP joints (Fig. 4–36*A*). If the fingertips are pressed against the **web flexion crease** of the fingers, flexion of the interphalangeal joints can be assessed independent of MCP joint motion (Fig. 4–36*B*). Normal DIP joint flexion ranges from 70° to 90°. Normal PIP joint flexion is greater, averaging about 110°. Normal active MCP joint flexion also ranges from about 80° to 90°.

In addition to recording the individual flexion angles of the finger joints, an overall assessment of finger flexion can be made by measuring the **distance between the fingertips and the transverse palmar crease.** Normally, the fingertips should be able to touch the transverse palmar crease when a tight fist is made. If they cannot reach it, the distance may be measured in millimeters (see Fig. 4–36*C*). This method is helpful for serial assessment of improvement following treatment of hand injuries.

If flexion of the interphalangeal joints of the fingers is limited, the most common causes are posttraumatic scarring of the extensor tendons with secondary contracture of the capsule of the involved interphalangeal joint or contracture of the intrinsic muscles resulting in excessive tension on the finger extensor tendons. The **Bunnell-Littler test** for intrinsic tightness can be used to differentiate between these two possibilities. To perform this test, the examiner stabilizes the MCP joint of an individual finger in the ex-

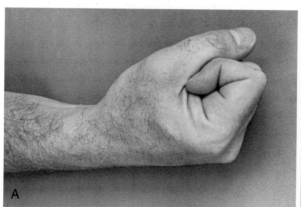
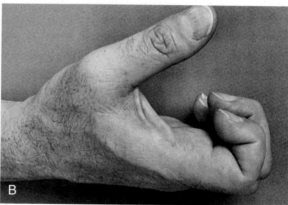
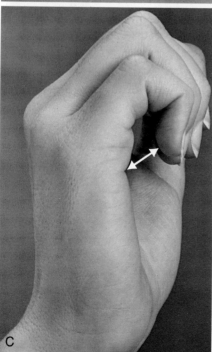

Figure 4–36. *A*, Active finger flexion. *B*, Active flexion of the interphalangeal joints only. *C*, Limited finger flexion may be assessed by measuring the distance between the fingertips and the midpalmar crease *(arrow)*.

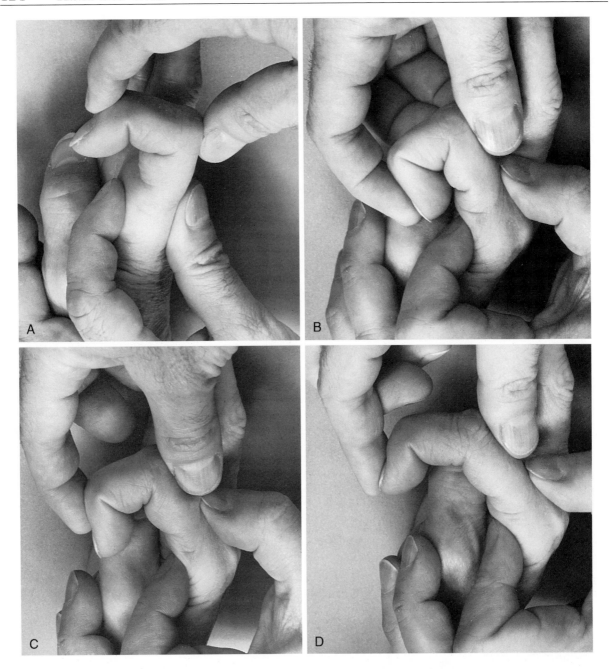

Figure 4–37. Bunnell-Littler test. *A*, Metacarpophalangeal joint extended. *B*, Metacarpophalangeal joint flexed, interphalangeal joint flexion increased. *C*, Metacarpophalangeal joint flexed, interphalangeal joint flexion unchanged. *D*, Metacarpophalangeal joint flexed, interphalangeal joint flexion decreased.

tended position and attempts to passively flex the finger (Fig. 4–37*A*). The amount of finger flexion is noted. The examiner then passively flexes the MCP joint and again assesses the passive flexion of the finger. If passive interphalangeal joint flexion increases with flexion of the MCP joint, this is evidence for tightness of the intrinsic muscles because flexion of the MCP joint relaxes the intrinsics (Fig. 4–37*B*). If, on the other hand, passive flexion of the MCP joint does not increase the limited flexion of the involved

interphalangeal joint, the limitation is primarily a result of a contracture or deformity within the interphalangeal joint itself (Fig. 4–37*C*). Extrinsic contracture of the long finger extensors can also limit interphalangeal joint flexion through a tenodesis effect. In this case, passively flexing the MCP joint actually produces a decrease in interphalangeal joint flexion because MCP joint flexion further tightens the contracted long finger extensor and thus passively reduces flexion of the interphalangeal joints (Fig. 4–37*D*).

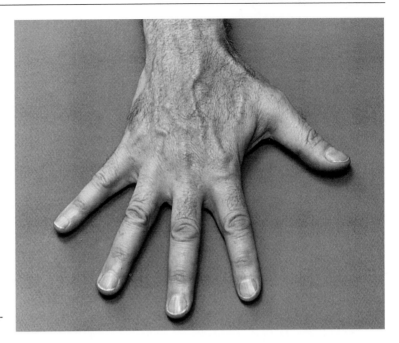

Figure 4–38. Abduction of metacarpophalangeal joints.

ABDUCTION AND ADDUCTION. The MCP joints are capable of an additional plane of motion not possible in the interphalangeal joints: **abduction** and **adduction.** The cam shape of the metacarpal heads allows the collateral ligaments of the MCP joints to be lax when the joints are extended, thus permitting abduction-adduction. When the metacarpophalangeal joints are flexed to 90°, the collateral ligaments are fully taut and abduction-adduction is not possible. At positions of flexion between 0° and 90°, abduction-adduction of the metacarpophalangeal joints is proportionally limited according to the amount of flexion present. Because the collateral ligaments of the interphalangeal joints are taut in all positions of flexion, abduction-adduction at these joints is not possible.

Abduction-adduction of the MCP joints is usually tested with the elbow flexed to 90°, the forearm pronated, and the fingers fully extended. The neutral position is that in which the fingers are held side by side. To measure **abduction** at the MCP joints, the patient is asked to spread the fingers as wide as possible (Fig. 4–38). A line drawn through the long finger and the third metacarpal is considered the neutral axis for measurement of abduction. Abduction can be quantitated by measuring the angle that each fully abducted finger makes with this neutral axis. The overall amount of abduction can also be quantitated by measuring the span between the tips of the index and the little fingers. Finger abduction is often assessed simply on a qualita-tive basis. Abnormalities of the *ulnar nerve,* which innervates the intrinsic muscles, weaken or prevent active abduction. To assess **adduction,** the patient is asked to return the fingers to the neutral position (Fig. 4–39).

When abduction is measured in this fashion, the long finger remains in the neutral position. Abduction of the long finger can be measured, if desired, by asking the patient to abduct the other

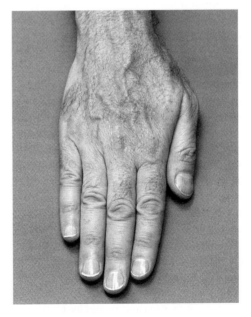

Figure 4–39. Adduction of metacarpophalangeal joints.

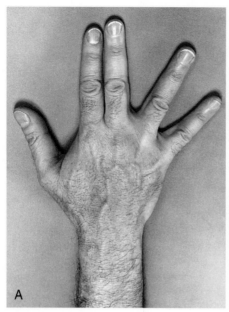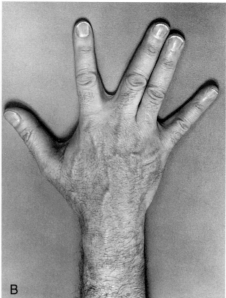

Figure 4–40. *A* and *B,* Long finger abduction.

fingers and then abduct the long finger to each side in turn until it touches the index and the ring fingers, respectively (Fig. 4–40).

Thumb Motion

The thumb is capable of complex combinations of motion. Many believe that it is the versatility of the thumb that has permitted the advancement of human technology. The complexity of these motions has also made for some confusion in descriptive nomenclature.

FLEXION AND EXTENSION. The motions of the **interphalangeal and MCP joints** of the thumb are fairly straightforward. Movement at these two joints is limited primarily to flexion and extension and is usually assessed simultaneously. The neutral position is considered to be that point at which the dorsum of the distal phalanx, proximal phalanx, and first metacarpal all form a straight line. To assess **flexion** of the interphalangeal and MCP joints of the thumb, the patient is asked to bend the thumb across the palm as far as possible (Fig. 4–41). Flexion of the interphalangeal joint is normally possible to 80° or 90° degrees. Flexion at the MCP joint varies more widely; it may be as little as 20° degrees or as great as 90° degrees. Comparison with the opposite side is important to establish the normal amount for each particular patient. To measure **extension** of the interphalangeal and MCP

joints of the thumb, the patient is asked to extend the thumb as fully as possible, as if hitchhiking (Fig. 4–42). Hyperextension of about 10° degrees is usually possible in the interphalangeal joint, and hyperextension of 10° degrees in the MCP joint is not unusual. Reduced motion in these two joints is most commonly the result of stiffness following a soft tissue injury or posttraumatic arthritis.

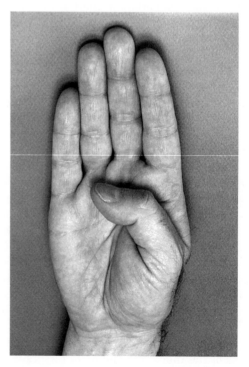

Figure 4–41. Flexion of the thumb.

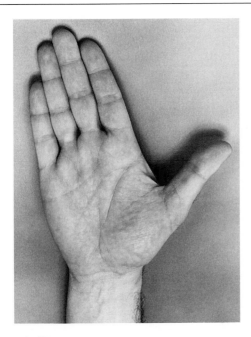

Figure 4–42. Extension of the thumb.

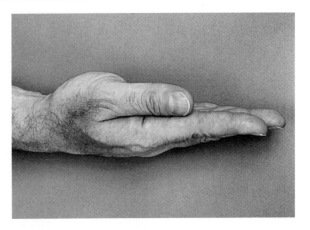

Figure 4–44. Palmar adduction of the thumb.

ABDUCTION AND ADDUCTION. The greater freedom of movement at the **trapeziometacarpal** or **basilar joint** of the thumb makes assessment much more complex. Abduction and adduction are most commonly assessed in the plane perpendicular to the palm, and this is described as palmar abduction and adduction.

To assess **palmar abduction,** the elbow is positioned in 90° of flexion with the forearm fully supinated. With the interphalangeal and MCP joints in extension, the patient is asked to move the thumb as far away from the palm and the rest of the hand as possible in a plane perpendicular to the palm (Fig. 4–43). Although this movement occurs primarily at the basilar joint, some concomitant motion at the MCP joint also takes

place. The angle between the axis of the thumb and the plane of the hand is considered the amount of palmar abduction present. In the normal patient, this motion averages about 60°. To assess **palmar adduction,** the patient is asked to return the side of the thumb to the palm and index finger (Fig. 4–44). Full approximation to this neutral position should be possible.

Radial abduction can also be measured in the plane of the palm. To assess radial abduction, the patient is asked to bring the extended thumb as far away from the index finger as possible while keeping it in the plane of the palm (Fig. 4–45). Radial abduction may be assessed with the forearm either pronated or supinated. It is

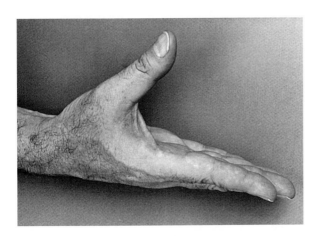

Figure 4–43. Palmar abduction of the thumb.

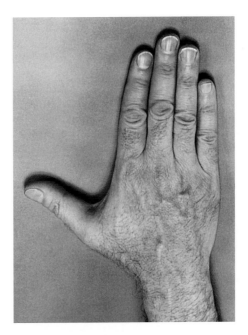

Figure 4–45. Radial abduction of the thumb.

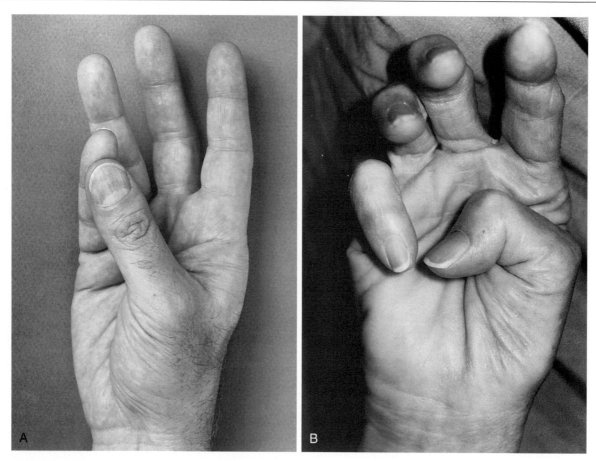

Figure 4–46. *A,* Opposition of the thumb. *B,* Lack of normal opposition in median nerve palsy.

quantitated by measuring the angle between the axis of the thumb and the axis of the index finger. In the normal individual, this measures about 70° to 80°.

OPPOSITION. The most distinctive motion of the basilar joint is **opposition.** True opposition involves palmar abduction and rotation of the entire thumb at the basilar joint so that the volar surface of the tip of the thumb touches that of the tip of the little finger. To test opposition of the thumb, the patient is asked to bring the tips of the thumb and little finger together so that the palmar surfaces of the two digits meet (Fig. 4–46). Opposition is usually assessed qualitatively rather than quantitatively. When normal opposition is present, the patient should be able to oppose the tips of the thumb and little finger so that the fingernails are almost parallel to each other.

Palpation

Dorsal Aspect

Palpation of the dorsal aspect of the fingers and hand is fairly straightforward because most of the anatomic structures are fairly superficial (see Fig. 4–2). Palpation should be directed at structures that appeared swollen, discolored, or deformed during inspection. When diffuse swelling of a finger is present, careful palpation may allow the examiner to pinpoint the probable site of injury. For example, maximal tenderness over the midshaft of the phalanx suggests a diaphyseal fracture, whereas maximal tenderness around a joint suggests a periarticular fracture, a ligamentous injury, or a tendon insertion injury.

Digits

DISTAL INTERPHALANGEAL JOINTS. When a particular joint is swollen, careful palpation around the joint helps identify the specific structures involved. When the **DIP joint** is swollen, for example, tenderness on the dorsum at the base of the distal phalanx suggests a *mallet injury* to the insertion of the **extensor digitorum communis** tendon, in the case of the finger, or the **extensor pollicis longus** tendon, in the case of the interphalangeal joint of the thumb. Maximal tenderness on either side of the DIP joints of the fingers or the interphalangeal joint of the thumb suggests injury to the corresponding **collateral ligament.** Such a finding should be followed by the appropriate stability test as described in the Manipulation section.

PROXIMAL INTERPHALANGEAL JOINTS. If a **PIP joint** of one of the fingers is swollen following trauma, a similar method may be used to pinpoint the injured structure. For example, tenderness on the dorsum of the PIP joint at the base of the middle phalanx suggests a potential *boutonnière injury* to the insertion of the **central slip of the extensor digitorum communis** tendon at the base of the middle phalanx. This is an important finding to detect because partial injury to the extensor insertion can later develop into a boutonnière deformity if the joint is not properly protected. As in the DIP joints, the finding of maximal tenderness on one side of the joint or the other suggests injury to the corresponding **collateral ligament.** Maximal tenderness on the volar aspect of the joint suggests injury to the thick volar portion of the joint capsule known as the *volar plate*. It is important to remember that the area of tenderness in any of these ligament or tendon injuries can be mimicked by a periarticular fracture.

METACARPOPHALANGEAL JOINTS. Despite the greater play available in the MCP joints, injury to the collateral ligaments of these joints can occur. On palpating for tenderness of the **collateral ligaments** of the MCP joints of the fingers, it is important to remember that the joints are located at the level of the knuckles and not at the level of the web space. The examiner gently inserts a fingertip between the metacarpal heads and gently palpates the side of the MCP joint to detect the tenderness of these collateral ligament injuries (Fig. 4–47A).

Injuries to the collateral ligaments of the MCP joint of the thumb are common. Of these, sprains of the **ulnar collateral ligament,** often called *skier's thumb* or *gamekeeper's thumb,* are particularly frequent. The finding of tenderness on the appropriate side of the thumb's MCP joint suggests such an injury. Stability testing of the MCP joints of the thumb and fingers is described in the Manipulation section.

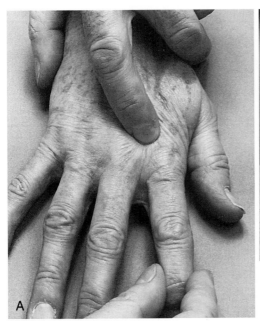

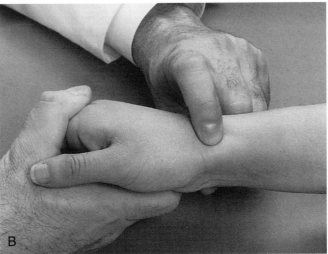

Figure 4–47. *A,* Palpation of the ulnar collateral ligament of the metacarpophalangeal joint of the index finger. *B,* Palpation of the scaphoid.

Metacarpals

Fractures of the **metacarpals** of the fingers are common, especially in the fourth and fifth metacarpals. These fractures may occur just proximal to the metacarpal head or within the metacarpal shaft. Point tenderness of a particular metacarpal suggests the possibility of fracture at that location; palpation may also allow the examiner to detect the deformity caused by a displaced fracture of one of these subcutaneous bones.

Fractures of the **first metacarpal** of the thumb may occur in the shaft or at the base, where the most common type is called *Bennett's fracture.* Tenderness at the base of the first metacarpal following trauma should lead the examiner to suspect such a fracture.

Wrist

Palpation of the dorsal wrist begins on the radial side (see Fig. 4–9). The firm bony resistance of the **radial styloid** is a reliable landmark for orientation at the radial side of the wrist. Continuing distally from the radial styloid, the examiner can identify the tendons of the *first dorsal compartment,* the **abductor pollicis longus** and the **extensor pollicis brevis.** This is the first of six synovial compartments into which the tendons of the dorsal wrist are grouped. These tendons form the volar border of the **anatomic snuffbox.** Tenderness or palpable synovial thickening of the first dorsal compartment over the radial styloid suggests a diagnosis of *de Quervain's disease.*

About 2 cm to the ulnar side of the radial styloid, the examiner can palpate a small bump on the dorsum of the distal radius known as **Lister's tubercle.** Lister's tubercle is an important landmark for palpating the bones and ligaments of the dorsal wrist. Running past the ulnar side of Lister's tubercle to its insertion on the dorsum of the distal phalanx of the thumb is the **extensor pollicis longus** tendon. The extensor pollicis longus makes up the *third dorsal compartment* and forms the dorsal border of the anatomic snuffbox.

Palpable just distal to the radial styloid, within the confines of the anatomic snuffbox, is an area of bony resistance corresponding to the waist of the **scaphoid** bone (see Fig. 4–47*B*). Slight ulnar deviation of the wrist may make the scaphoid more easily palpable. Tenderness over the waist of the scaphoid is an important finding because fractures at this location are common and notoriously difficult to diagnose radiographically.

Gentle palpation further distal in the anatomic snuffbox reveals a pulsating structure that is the **dorsal branch of the radial artery.** Firmer palpation just distal to this pulse reveals the bony resistance that corresponds to the **trapezium.** Another 3 mm or 4 mm more distal, the examiner should be able to palpate the outlines of the **trapeziometacarpal joint,** or **basilar joint,** of the thumb. Tenderness here suggests degenerative arthritis, which is particularly common in women over 50 years. If arthritis is present, palpable osteophytes may be noted. Other tests for arthritis or instability of the basilar joint are described in the Manipulation section.

Just to the ulnar side of the junction between the scaphoid and the trapezium, the examiner should be able to palpate a deep indentation that corresponds to the **scaphotrapeziotrapezoid (STT) joint.**

The tendons of the **extensors carpi radialis longus and brevis** pass beneath the extensor pollicis longus before they insert on the dorsum of the second and third metacarpals. Nevertheless, they should be palpable, particularly if the patient is asked to extend the wrist against resistance. These tendons constitute the *second dorsal compartment.* This is the site where a *dorsal wrist ganglion* is most likely to appear. A large ganglion presents as an obvious mass, but careful palpation may be necessary to detect a small one, which feels like a firm spherical mass only a few millimeters in diameter.

Palpating just distal to Lister's tubercle with the wrist in slight flexion, the examiner's finger falls from the distal edge of the radius into the radiocarpal joint at the site of the **scapholunate ligament.** This ligament links the scaphoid, which is located to the radial side of Lister's tubercle, and the **lunate,** which extends from that point to about the middle of the ulnar head.

As the palpating finger passes distally, a second indentation can be felt about 1 cm more distal from Lister's tubercle. This indentation corresponds to the **midcarpal joint** or, more specifically, the **scapholunate capitate joint.** A position of slight flexion of the wrist may make the midcarpal joint more palpable. Tenderness, swelling, or bogginess at this site suggests injury to the ligaments connecting the scaphoid, the lunate, and the capitate. As the examiner continues palpating in the ulnar direction, an area of firm resistance corresponding to the **head of the capitate** is felt just distally.

The **extensor digitorum communis** tendons occupy the *fourth dorsal compartment* of the wrist. These tendons can be palpated as a group at the point where they traverse the wrist by asking the patient to actively extend the fingers (see Fig. 4–8). Lumpy synovial thickening around these tendons as well as the other dorsal tendons is a common finding in *rheumatoid arthritis.*

The little finger has the distinction of having its own individual extensor tendon, the **extensor digiti minimi (quinti).** This tendon occupies the *fifth dorsal compartment* and traverses the wrist over the distal radioulnar joint. It can be palpated at the level of the wrist by asking the patient to extend the little finger by itself (see Fig. 4–8).

The most prominent bony landmark of the ulnar side of the dorsal wrist is the **head of the ulna.** The head of the ulna is a round bump about 1 cm or more across that is clearly visible in most individuals. The depression on the radial side of this bump marks the location of the **distal radioulnar joint,** one of the articulations through which rotation of the forearm occurs. Arthritis of the distal radioulnar joint, a fairly common condition, is associated with tenderness and sometimes palpable osteophytes at this location.

If the examiner palpates along the ulnar border of the ulnar head, a bony projection a few millimeters in length is detected. This is the **ulnar styloid,** a small protruberance of the distal ulna that serves as the anchoring point for the **triangular fibrocartilage complex (TFCC).** The TFCC connects the ulnar styloid to the distal radius and functions as an important component of the mechanism of forearm rotation at the wrist. Injuries of the TFCC are common and may produce pain and popping sensations. To directly palpate the TFCC, the examiner identifies the ulnar head and palpates distally until the tip of the palpating finger falls into a small depression. This depression overlies the TFCC. Tenderness here highly suggests a TFCC injury. Palpating the TFCC, the examiner may ask the patient to

alternately radial-deviate and ulnar-deviate the wrist. In the presence of a TFCC tear, the examiner may feel popping emanating from the TFCC as the patient executes this maneuver.

The tendon of the **extensor carpi ulnaris** passes through a groove on the ulnar side of the ulnar head just distal to the styloid and traverses the wrist en route to its insertion at the base of the fifth metacarpal. The extensor carpi ulnaris tendon, which constitutes the *sixth dorsal compartment,* can be felt as a distinct longitudinal prominence in this location. Asking the patient to ulnarly deviate the wrist and then extend it against resistance increases the prominence of the extensor carpi ulnaris tendon. Tenderness of the tendon, particularly if increased by resistance, usually indicates the presence of *extensor carpi ulnaris tendinitis.* Sometimes the restraining sheath of the extensor carpi ulnaris tendon can tear, resulting in recurrent subluxation of the tendon from its groove on the distal ulna. **Subluxation of the extensor carpi ulnaris tendon** can be looked for by palpating the tendon during active forearm rotation. The examiner begins by palpating the tendon while the patient's forearm is supinated with the wrist in a radially deviated and extended position (Fig. 4–48*A*). The patient is instructed to then pronate the forearm while flexing the ulnarly deviated wrist in one smooth motion (Fig. 4–48*B*). The examiner usually is able to feel the extensor carpi ulnaris tendon pop from its groove during this maneuver if instability is present.

Distal to the triangular fibrocartilage, but in line with the middle of the ulnar head, the examiner may feel another subtle indentation, which corresponds to the **lunotriquetral ligament.** Positioning the wrist in flexion and radial deviation makes this indentation easier to detect. Just distal to this indentation, the palpating finger

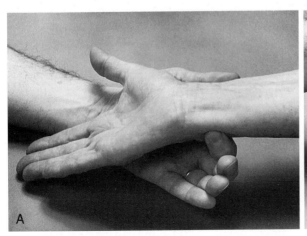
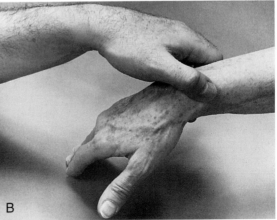

Figure 4–48. *A* and *B,* Testing for instability of the extensor carpi ulnaris tendon.

encounters the bony resistance of the **triquetrum** itself. Proceeding further distally, the examiner should be able to identify the dorsum of the **hamate** and finally the mobile **carpometacarpal joints** with the fourth and fifth metacarpals.

Volar (Palmar) Aspect

Fingers and Palm

As in dorsal palpation, palpation of the volar aspect of the fingers and hand should include areas of obvious swelling or deformity (see Fig. 4–15). Palpation of suspected fractures or joint injuries is described under Dorsal Aspect in the Palpation section.

INFECTIONS. As already mentioned, **closed-space infections** tend to occur on the volar surface of the fingers and palm. If swelling or erythema is noted in any of the following locations, the surface should be palpated very gently for associated tenderness: the volar fingertip (*felon*), the volar surface over the middle and proximal phalanges (*flexor tendon sheath infection*), the middle and distal portions of the palm (*midpalmar space infection*), and the thenar eminence (*thenar space infection*). These closed-space infections can be extremely tender, so initial palpation should be very gentle.

SWEATING. While palpating the volar surfaces of the hand, the examiner should note that the skin is slightly moist. This **moisture** increases function and improves grip. In the presence of a nerve injury such as a median, ulnar, or digital nerve laceration, the skin in the sensory distribution of the injured nerve should feel dry, hence slick, owing to loss of normal neuroregulation of sweating.

MASSES. Ganglia of the flexor tendon sheath usually occur at the level of the web flexion creases of the fingers. The examiner should remember that these creases are located at about the midpoint of the proximal phalanx. A **flexor sheath ganglion** is rarely visible, but it can usually be palpated as a firm round nodule 3 mm to 5 mm in diameter located centrally or to one side of the flexor tendon of a finger. A **giant cell tumor** is a less common cause of a mass in the finger. It tends to occur between the joints and is firmer and larger than a ganglion.

Further proximally, at the level of the transverse flexion crease of the palm or the proximal flexion crease of the thumb, the examiner can palpate the nodular swelling usually associated with **trigger finger.** In trigger finger, the flexor digitorum superficialis tendon tends to catch in a constriction caused by thickening of one of the pulleys that normally prevents the flexor tendons from bowstringing. To palpate a trigger finger, the examiner presses gently over the volar aspect of the involved flexor tendon at the level of the MCP joint. The patient is asked to make a tight fist, then extend the fingers fully (Fig. 4–49). In the presence of trigger finger, the examiner feels the tendon tend to catch at the constricted pulley. Flexor sheath ganglia may also occur in this location and be palpable near or over the tendon.

EMINENCES. In the palm of the hand, the **thenar and hypothenar eminences** can also be palpated for muscle tone and bulk. If the thenar eminence is palpated while the patient is pressing the tips of the thumb and the little finger firmly together, the muscle should feel rock hard. A softened thenar eminence is usually caused by median nerve neuropathy or basilar joint arthritis. The thenar eminence appears wasted and flaccid in advanced cases of *median nerve neuropathy,* whereas *ulnar nerve neuropathy* can lead to atrophy of the hypothenar eminence.

Wrist

The volar aspect of the wrist is palpated with the patient's elbow flexed and forearm supinated. The tendons of the *first dorsal compartment* are actually situated quite volarly and form the radial border of the volar aspect of the wrist (see Fig. 4–19). Just to the ulnar side of these tendons is a soft spot. Gentle palpation in this soft spot allows the examiner to detect the pulsations of the **radial artery** (Fig. 4–50A). Just distal to the distal flexion crease of the wrist, in line with the radial pulse, the examiner feels a firm resistance corresponding to the **tubercle of the scaphoid.** Continuing distally in line with the scaphoid, the examiner can palpate the volar aspect of the **trapezium** and then the **basilar joint.** This area provides another site at which the tenderness associated with basilar joint arthritis can be sought.

As the examiner continues to palpate in the ulnar direction, the next distinct structure is the linear mass of the **flexor carpi radialis** tendon. This tendon is often visible and can be made even more prominent by asking the patient to flex the wrist against resistance (see Fig. 4–20). The flexor carpi radialis inserts at the base of the second metacarpal. Continuing in the ulnar di-

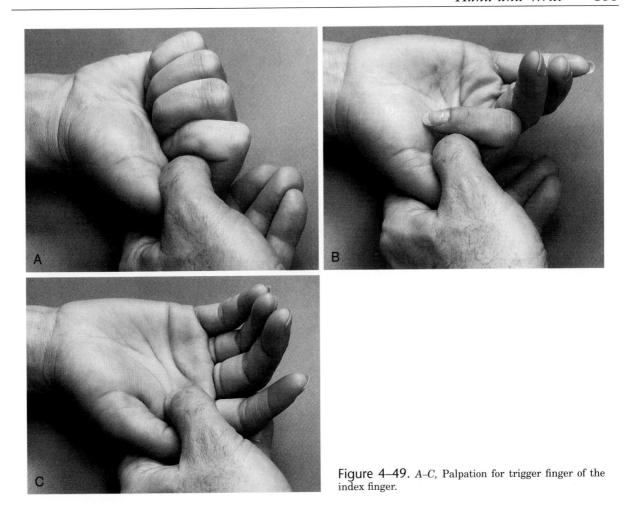

Figure 4–49. *A–C,* Palpation for trigger finger of the index finger.

rection, the examiner next encounters the most superficial tendon of the volar wrist, the **palmaris longus.** The prominence of the palmaris longus can be increased by asking the patient to pinch the tips of the thumb and the little finger together with the wrist slightly flexed (see Fig. 4–20). The palmaris longus, which inserts into the palmar fascia at the base of the palm, exists in only about 80% of individuals.

The narrow depression between the flexor carpi radialis and the palmaris longus tendons indicates the location of the **median nerve.** The

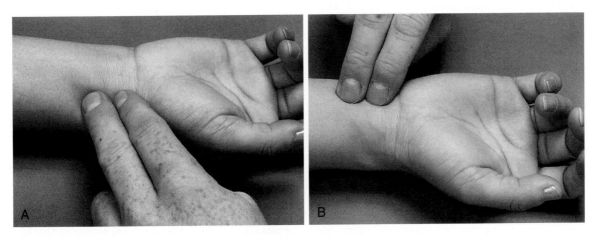

Figure 4–50. *A,* Palpation of the radial artery. *B,* Palpation of the ulnar artery.

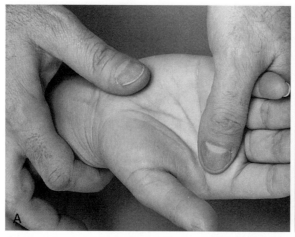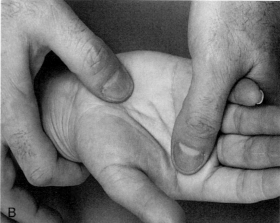

Figure 4–51. *A* and *B,* Palpation of the hook of the hamate.

nerve itself cannot be distinguished by palpation. Specific tests to identify median nerve compression at the wrist, a condition known as *carpal tunnel syndrome,* are described later in this chapter.

If the examiner palpates distally along the palmaris longus tendon, the soft tissues of the wrist are felt to grow firmer as the palpating finger reaches the distal wrist crease. This corresponds to the proximal edge of the **transverse carpal ligament** or **flexor retinaculum,** the tough fascial tissue that forms the roof of the carpal tunnel. If the examiner continues to palpate distally along the longitudinal interthenar skin crease, the tissues are noted to soften again when the palpating finger reaches the distal edge of the transverse carpal ligament. The distance between the proximal and the distal edges of the palmar aponeurosis is usually about 3 cm.

To the ulnar side of the palmaris longus tendons, the **flexor digitorum profundus** and the **flexor digitorum superficialis** tendons traverse the carpal tunnel. Although the outlines of the individual tendons cannot be palpated, they can be felt to glide beneath the examiner's fingertips if this area is palpated while the patient flexes and extends his or her fingers. Palpable synovial thickening around these tendons is a common occurrence in *rheumatoid arthritis.*

Continuing in the ulnar direction, moderately firm palpation allows the examiner to detect the pulsations of the **ulnar artery** (see Fig. 4–50*B*). The **flexor carpi ulnaris** tendon, a thick tendon along the ulnar border of the volar wrist, can be used as a landmark to locate the ulnar pulse. The ulnar artery lies just to the radial side of the flexor carpi ulnaris. The prominence of the flexor carpi ulnaris can be further increased by asking the patient to ulnar-deviate the wrist and then flex it against resistance. The **ulnar nerve** travels deep to the ulnar artery and cannot be distinctly palpated.

As the flexor carpi ulnaris tendon is followed distally, it can be noted to insert into an oval bony prominence, the **pisiform** bone, at the base of the hypothenar eminence. The pisiform can be used as a landmark to locate the **hook of the hamate** bone. If the examiner's own thumb is placed over the pisiform, so that the interphalangeal flexion crease of the examiner's thumb lies at the proximal end of the pisiform and the tip of the examiner's thumb is aimed toward the base of the patient's index finger, firm palpation with the tip of the examiner's thumb compresses a hard bony prominence corresponding to the *hook of the hamate* (Fig. 4–51). The hook of the hamate is distal and radial to the pisiform, in line with the ring finger. The fascial structure connecting these two landmarks, the *pisohamate ligament,* forms the roof of the **ulnar tunnel (Guyon's canal).** The ulnar nerve and artery run through this tunnel and may become compressed there.

Manipulation

MUSCLE TESTING

Wrist and Finger Extensors

The primary extensors of the wrist are the **extensor carpi ulnaris** and the **extensors carpi radialis longus and brevis.** Because the finger extensors cross the wrist, they also can assist in wrist extension. Wrist extensor strength is usually tested with the patient's elbow flexed and forearm pronated. The patient is asked to make a fist and extend the wrist. The examiner then supports the patient's forearm while pressing downward on the dorsum of the patient's hand. The patient is instructed to resist this pressure as strongly as possible (Fig. 4–52*A*). If normal strength is present, the examiner is unable to break the strength of the extensors or is able to break the strength only with considerable difficulty.

The method just described tests the extensor carpi ulnaris, the extensor carpi radialis brevis, and the extensor carpi radialis longus as a group. If the examiner wishes to focus the test on the **extensor carpi ulnaris,** the patient is asked to extend the wrist in an ulnar-deviated position (see Fig. 4–52*B*). Similarly, if the examiner wishes to focus on the **extensors carpi radialis longus and brevis,** the patient is asked to extend the wrist in the radial-deviated position (see Fig. 4–52*C*). Palpation of the individual tendon

in question provides supplementary verification that the tendon is indeed under tension.

The extensors carpi radialis longus and brevis are innervated by the *radial nerve* itself, whereas the extensor carpi ulnaris is innervated by the *posterior interosseous branch* of the radial nerve. A *posterior interosseous nerve palsy,* therefore, denervates the extensor carpi ulnaris but leaves the radial wrist extensors unaffected. In this case, the patient's wrist tends to deviate to the radial side whenever the patient attempts to perform active wrist extension.

The primary extensor of the four fingers is the **extensor digitorum communis.** In addition, the index finger and the little finger have their own supplementary extensors, the *extensor indicis proprius* and the *extensor digiti minimi (extensor digiti quinti),* respectively. All of these muscles are innervated by the *posterior interosseous branch* of the radial nerve. Complicating the evaluation of the finger extensors is the role of the **intrinsic muscles** of the hand, the *lumbricals* and *interossei.* Owing to their insertions at

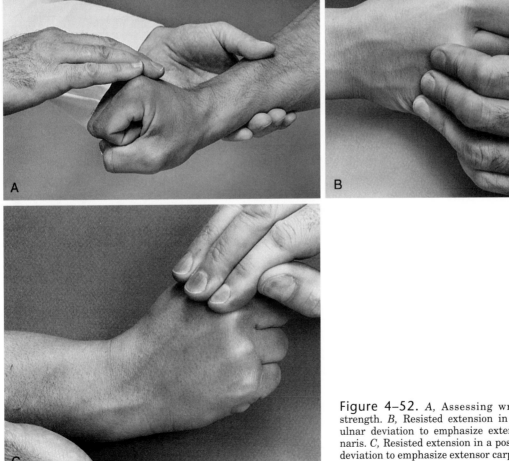

Figure 4–52. *A,* Assessing wrist extensor strength. *B,* Resisted extension in a position of ulnar deviation to emphasize extensor carpi ulnaris. *C,* Resisted extension in a position of radial deviation to emphasize extensor carpi radialis longus and brevis.

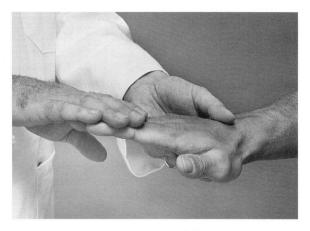

Figure 4–53. Assessing finger extension strength.

the base of the proximal phalanx and into the dorsal hood of the extensor tendon, the intrinsic muscles tend to act as flexors of the MCP joints but extensors of the interphalangeal joints of the fingers. For this reason, testing the patient's ability to extend the MCP joints against resistance is the best way to evaluate the long finger extensors by themselves.

Extension of the four fingers is usually tested together because tethering among the extensor tendons by the *junctura tendinae* makes it difficult to extend the long finger and the ring finger if the others are held in flexion. The index finger and the little finger are less tethered because they have independent extensors, and they may be tested independently, if desired. To test the **extensor digitorum communis** strength, the patient's elbow is flexed and the forearm fully pronated. The patient is instructed to extend the fingers fully at all joints and to retain that position against the examiner's attempt to passively

flex the fingers. One of the examiner's hands then supports the patient's hand while the examiner's other hand presses downward on the patient's fingers in an attempt to flex the MCP joints (Fig. 4–53). The examiner should be careful to position this hand proximal to the patient's PIP joints so that extension of the MCP joints is isolated. The average examiner should be able to break the finger extensor strength of most patients, but moderate resistance should be noted.

Wrist and Finger Flexors

The principal wrist flexors are the **flexor carpi radialis** and **flexor carpi ulnaris.** They are assisted by the long finger flexors and the palmaris longus. To test the strength of wrist flexion, the patient's elbow is flexed and the forearm is fully supinated. The patient is instructed to make a fist and to flex the wrist. The examiner positions one hand to support the patient's forearm and the other to press downward on the patient's hand. The patient is instructed to resist the examiner's attempt to passively extend the wrist (Fig. 4–54A). The examiner should be able to overcome the patient's flexors with considerable difficulty, and in some cases he or she will not be able to break them. As in the testing of the wrist extensors, performing the test with the wrist in an ulnar-deviated position tends to isolate the **flexor carpi ulnaris** (Fig. 4–54B), whereas performing the test with the wrist in a radial-deviated position tends to isolate the **flexor carpi radialis.** The flexor carpi radialis is innervated by the *median nerve,* whereas the flexor carpi ulnaris is innervated by the *ulnar*

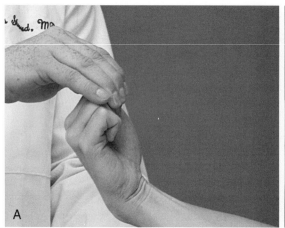
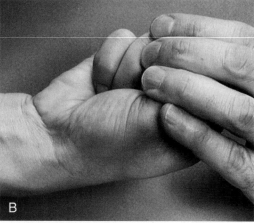

Figure 4–54. *A,* Assessing wrist flexion strength. *B,* Emphasizing flexor carpi ulnaris.

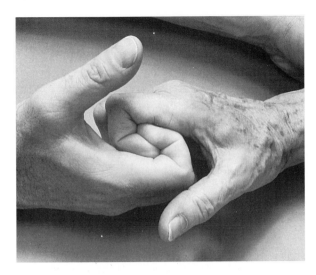

Figure 4–55. Assessing overall finger flexor strength.

nerve. Thus, in the presence of a *median nerve palsy,* attempted active wrist flexion tends to deviate the wrist to the ulnar side. Conversely, in the presence of an *ulnar nerve palsy,* attempted active wrist flexion tends to deviate the wrist to the radial side.

The principal finger flexors are the **flexor digitorum superficialis** and **flexor digitorum profundus.** As already noted, the **intrinsic muscles** of the hand assist with flexion of the MCP joints. Because the flexor digitorum profundus tendons insert at the base of the distal phalanges, the flexor digitorum profundus acts to flex all three joints of the fingers. Because the flexor digitorum superficialis tendons insert at the base of the middle phalanges, the flexor digitorum superficialis tendons have no effect on the DIP joints. This anatomic fact can be used to

differentiate function of the flexor digitorum profundus from the flexor digitorum superficialis.

Overall finger flexor strength is usually tested with the patient's elbow flexed and forearm pronated. The examiner's fingers are hooked beneath the patient's fingers and the patient is instructed to make a tight fist. The patient is then told to resist as strongly as possible the examiner's attempt to pull the patient's fingers into extension (Fig. 4–55). The examiner should be able to overcome the strength of most normal patients but with considerable difficulty.

Independent function of the **flexor digitorum profundus** tendons is verified by testing each finger separately. The examiner stabilizes the PIP joint in extension of the finger being tested, and he or she asks the patient to flex the DIP joint (Fig. 4–56). The patient should be able to flex the DIP joint about 45° when thus restrained. The examiner's index finger may be used to provide a resistive force, if desired. The innervation of the flexor digitorum profundus is unusual; it is split between the median and the ulnar nerves. The *anterior interosseous branch* of the *median nerve* usually innervates the flexor profundus to the index finger and the long finger, whereas the *ulnar nerve* innervates the flexor profundus to the ring finger and the little finger. An isolated *ulnar nerve palsy,* therefore, can result in diminution of flexor profundus strength in the ring finger and the little finger, while flexor profundus function of the index finger and the long finger remains intact. Isolated loss of flexor profundus function to the ring finger alone, on the other hand, may be due to avulsion of the flexor profundus slip to that digit, the condition known as *jersey finger.*

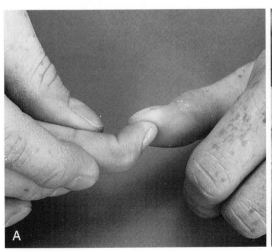
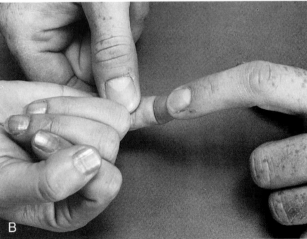

Figure 4–56. Assessing flexor digitorum profundus. *A,* To the index finger. *B,* To the little finger.

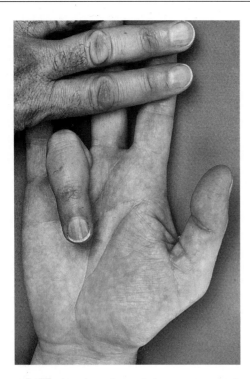

Figure 4–57. Assessing flexor digitorum superficialis function to the ring finger.

To test the **flexor digitorum superficialis** function in isolation, the patient is instructed to flex the fingers one at a time while the examiner holds the other three fingers in full extension at all joints (Fig. 4–57). Because the flexor profundus tendons are tethered together proximally, holding the other three fingers in extension incapacitates the flexor profundus of the finger being tested. The flexor superficialis acts alone, thus only the PIP joint and the MCP joint of the tested finger are flexed. If the flexor digitorum superficialis tendon of a given finger has been lacerated, the patient is unable to flex that finger when the other three are held in extension. Because the flexor digitorum profundus to the index finger is not tethered, this test is less reliable for the index finger. All portions of the flexor digitorum superficialis are innervated by the *median nerve.*

Radial and Ulnar Deviators of the Wrist

Radial and ulnar deviation of the wrist are powered primarily by muscles already mentioned. The primary motors for **ulnar deviation** are the *extensor carpi ulnaris* and the *flexor carpi ulnaris,* whereas the primary motors for **radial deviation** are the *flexor carpi radialis,* the *extensors carpi radialis longus and brevis,* and the *abductor pollicis longus.* Resistance testing of these motions, therefore, adds little information to the rest of the examination. However, strength of ulnar and radial deviation can be tested, if desired, with the patient's elbow flexed and the forearm pronated. The patient is asked to make a fist. To test the strength of **ulnar deviation,** the patient is instructed to ulnar-deviate the wrist and resist the examiner's attempts to force it back into radial deviation (Fig. 4–58). Conversely, to test the strength of **radial deviation,** the patient is asked to radial-deviate the wrist and resist the examiner's attempt to force it back into ulnar deviation (Fig. 4–59).

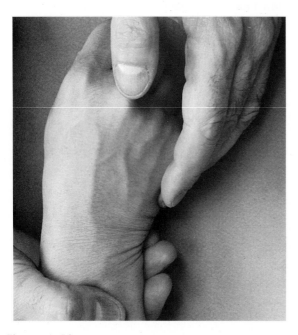

Figure 4–58. Assessing ulnar deviation strength.

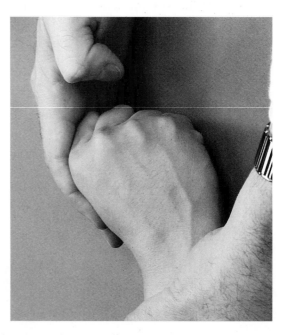

Figure 4–59. Assessing radial deviation strength.

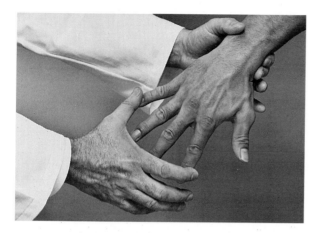

Figure 4–60. Assessing finger abduction strength.

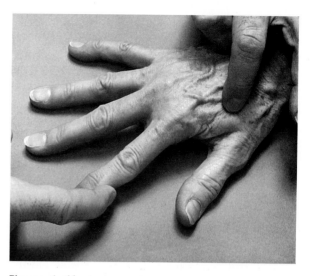

Figure 4–61. Assessing first dorsal interosseous strength in isolation.

Abductors and Adductors of the Fingers

Abduction of the fingers is powered by the *dorsal interossei,* whereas **adduction** is powered by the *volar (palmar) interossei.* All of these muscles are innervated by the *ulnar nerve.* To test the strength of **abduction,** the patient is positioned with the elbows flexed and the forearms pronated. Usually both hands are tested simultaneously for ease of comparison. The patient is instructed to abduct the fingers as far as possible and to maintain that position while the examiner attempts to force the fingers back together with his or her own fingers (Fig. 4–60). The examiner should be able to overcome the strength of the abductors with a feeling of moderate resistance. The **first dorsal interosseous** is by far the largest and most visible of the interossei. If the examiner is uncertain as to whether weakness of the interossei is present, it may be helpful to test the first dorsal interosseous in isolation. This is done with the patient's hand in the same basic position. The patient is instructed to abduct the index finger and to maintain it in that position while the examiner attempts to push it back into adduction (Fig. 4–61). The examiner may palpate the first dorsal interosseous with the index finger of his or her free hand.

The volar interossei are responsible for adduction of the fingers, a relatively weak action. Finger **adduction** strength may be tested by asking the patient to squeeze a file card or piece of paper between the adducted fingers. The patient is then instructed to squeeze the fingers together as tightly as possible in an attempt to prevent the examiner from withdrawing the card (Fig. 4–62). The examiner should sense moderate resistance as the card is withdrawn.

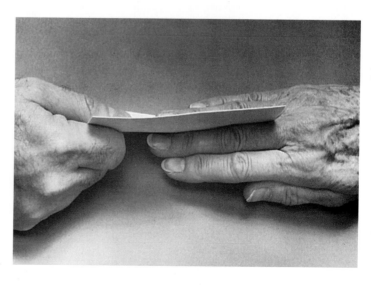

Figure 4–62. Assessing finger adduction strength.

Movements of the Thumb

Thumb extension is powered by the *extensor pollicis longus* and *extensor pollicis brevis,* both of which are innervated by the *posterior interosseous* branch of the radial nerve. Because the extensor pollicis brevis inserts at the base of the proximal phalanx of the thumb, the extensor pollicis longus is the unique extensor of the interphalangeal joint. The strength of the two muscles can be evaluated together by asking the patient to extend the thumb as if hitchhiking. The examiner then presses on the dorsum of the proximal phalanx of the thumb, attempting to force the MCP joint into flexion (Fig. 4–63*A*). The examiner should sense moderate resistance before overcoming the strength of the thumb extensors.

To test the strength of the **extensor pollicis longus** alone, the examiner should isolate the interphalangeal joint. Again, the patient is asked to extend the thumb as if hitchhiking. This time, the examiner stabilizes the proximal phalanx of the patient's thumb between the thumb and the index finger of one hand and attempts to force the interphalangeal joint into flexion by pressing on the patient's thumbnail with the index finger of the other hand (Fig. 4–63*B*). The examiner should sense strong resistance before overcoming the strength of the patient's extensor pollicis longus. *Extensor pollicis longus tendon rupture,* a common event in rheumatoid arthritis and sometimes following fractures of the distal radius, is associated with a complete loss of strength of extension at the interphalangeal joint of the thumb.

Thumb flexion is powered by the *flexor pollicis longus* and the *flexor pollicis brevis.* The flexor pollicis longus is innervated by the *anterior interosseous branch* of the median nerve, whereas the flexor pollicis brevis is innervated partly by the *median nerve* itself after the nerve passes through the carpal tunnel and partly by the *ulnar nerve.* Because the brevis inserts at the base of the proximal phalanx of the thumb and the longus extends to the distal phalanx, the flexor pollicis longus is uniquely responsible for flexion of the interphalangeal joint of the thumb. The strength of thumb flexion can be tested by having the patient flex the thumb across the palm. The patient is then instructed to maintain the thumb in flexion while the examiner attempts to force it back into extension (Fig. 4–64). The examiner should feel moderately strong resistance before being able to overcome the strength of the thumb flexors. *Rupture of the flexor pollicis longus* results in complete loss of flexion strength at the interphalangeal joint of the thumb.

Radial abduction of the thumb is powered by the *abductor pollicis longus* and innervated by

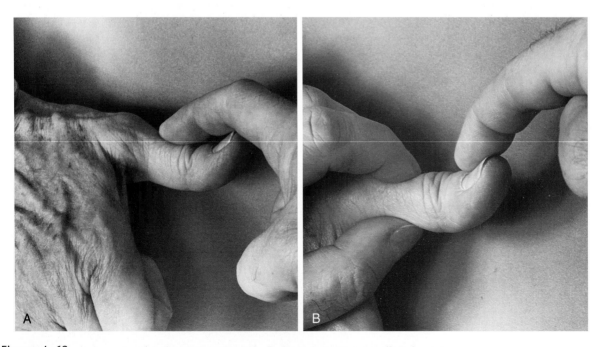

Figure 4–63. *A,* Assessing thumb extensor strength. *B,* Assessing extensor pollicis longus strength in isolation.

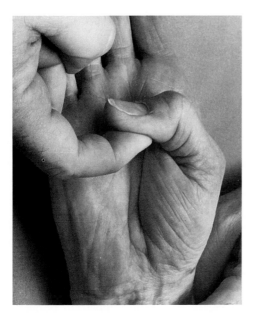

Figure 4–64. Assessing thumb flexion strength.

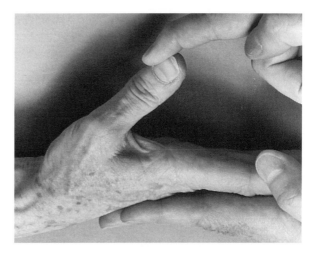

Figure 4–65. Assessing thumb palmar abduction strength.

the *radial nerve,* whereas **palmar abduction** is powered by the *abductor pollicis brevis,* which is innervated by the *median nerve* after the nerve passes through the carpal tunnel. To test thumb **palmar abduction,** the examiner stabilizes the patient's hand in a supinated position and instructs the patient to abduct the extended thumb perpendicular to the palm. The patient is instructed to maintain this abducted position while the examiner tries to force the thumb back toward the palm (Fig. 4–65). Normally, the examiner feels moderate resistance before being able to force the thumb back into the palm. **Radial abduction** may be tested by having the patient

abduct the thumb in the plane of the hand while the hand is lying flat on a table.

Thumb adduction is primarily a function of the *adductor pollicis,* the only one of the four thenar muscles to be innervated solely by the ulnar nerve. There are two ways of testing the adductor pollicis. The first is the reverse of the test for thumb abduction strength. In this case, the examiner's finger is placed against the patient's hand on the palmar aspect of the second metacarpal. The patient is then asked to adduct the thumb against the examiner's finger. The patient is instructed to maintain the thumb in the adducted position while the examiner attempts to pull the thumb back into abduction (Fig. 4–66). In the normal patient, the examiner should feel moderate resistance before being able to overcome the patient's own adductor pollicis.

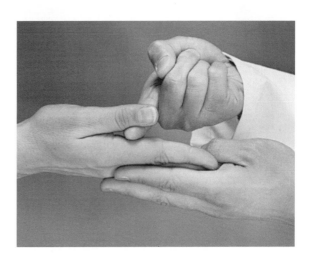

Figure 4–66. Assessing thumb palmar adduction strength.

The adductor pollicis may also be tested using **Froment's test,** which evaluates the strength of *key pinch,* an action powered primarily by the adductor pollicis. To perform Froment's test, the patient is asked to make tight fists with both hands and to place the hands against each other. The extended thumbs are then used to pinch an index card against the radial side of the index fingers. The patient is instructed to pinch the card as tightly as possible and to attempt to prevent the examiner from withdrawing the card (Fig. 4–67A). The patient should normally be able to resist withdrawal of the card while maintaining the interphalangeal joints of the thumbs in extension. If the adductor pollicis of one hand is weak, the patient usually attempts to substitute for the lost strength by firing the flexor pollicis longus. This action causes the interphalangeal joint of the thumb to visibly flex, an action known as **Froment's sign** (Fig. 4–67B). Froment's sign usually signifies an isolated *ulnar nerve palsy,* as the adductor pollicis is innervated by the ulnar nerve, but the flexor pollicis longus is innervated by the median nerve.

True **opposition** of the thumb requires proper function of both the *abductor pollicis brevis* and the *opponens pollicis* muscles. The abductors of the thumb participate in this complex motion by bringing the thumb away from the palm, but it is the opponens pollicis that rotates it so that it faces the other fingers. Because opposition is usually tested by bringing the tips of the thumb and the little finger together, the *opponens digiti minimi* also participates in this action. It is the opponens pollicis, however, that is of primary functional significance and interest. To test the strength of opposition, the examiner asks the patient to touch the tips of the thumb and the little finger together. Because the thumb flexors can bring the tip of the thumb toward the little finger in the absence of opponens function, the examiner should inspect the patient's hand carefully to verify that true opposition is occurring. The patient is then instructed to press the tips of the two fingers together as tightly as possible. The examiner's two index fingers are then hooked around the base of the thumb and the little finger, respectively, and the examiner at-

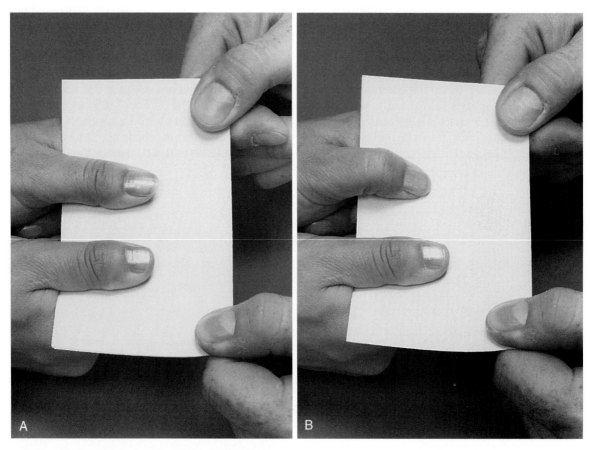

Figure 4–67. Froment's test. *A,* Normal. *B,* Abnormal.

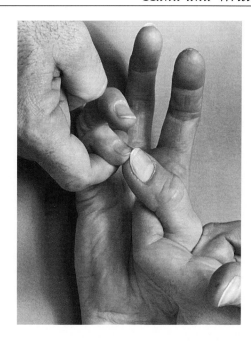

Figure 4–68. Assessing opposition strength.

tempts to pull these two digits apart (Fig. 4–68). In the normal patient, the examiner should encounter considerable resistance but usually is able to break the strength of opposition. Inability to properly oppose the thumb owing to muscular weakness is most commonly the result of a *carpal tunnel syndrome* because the opponens pollicis is innervated by the median nerve. Severe *basilar joint arthritis* can also interfere with proper opposition, however, owing to pain.

SENSATION TESTING

If the **median nerve** is compressed in the carpal tunnel, there may be altered sensation in the median nerve distribution in the hand, which includes the palmar surfaces and the tips of the thumb, the index finger, the long finger, and the radial aspect of the ring finger (Fig. 4–69). This loss is usually evaluated by testing two-point dis-

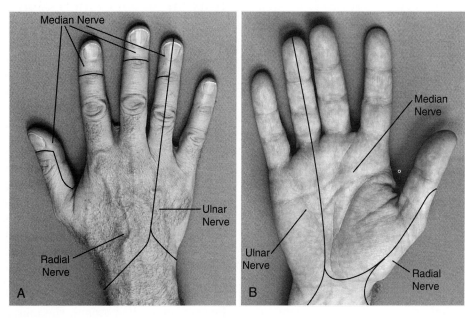

Figure 4–69. Average sensory distribution in the hand. *A*, Dorsum. *B*, Palm.

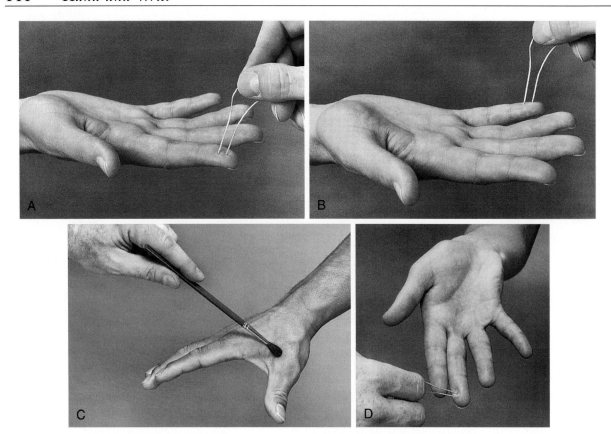

Figure 4–70. Sensation testing. *A*, Median nerve. *B*, Ulnar nerve. *C*, Radial nerve. *D*, Radial digital nerve of the long finger.

crimination at the volar tip of the thumb or index finger (Fig. 4–70*A*). Because the palmar cutaneous branch of the median nerve arises proximal to the carpal tunnel, the palmar base of the thumb is spared.

Ulnar nerve compression in Guyon's canal may lead to altered sensation in the ulnar nerve distribution, including the little finger and the ulnar aspect of the ring finger. This is best evaluated by testing two-point discrimination at the volar tip of the little finger (see Fig. 4–70*B*).

Although the superficial sensory branch of the **radial nerve** supplies the radial dorsum of the hand, it is most likely to be injured proximal to the wrist. This loss can be investigated by testing for light touch or sharp-dull sensation on the dorsum of the first web space (see Fig. 4–70*C*).

Laceration of the **digital nerves** is common. Transection of a digital nerve causes numbness on the same side of the finger as the injured nerve. This numbness is best detected by testing two-point discrimination on the appropriate side of the volar fingertip (see Fig. 4–70*D*).

SPECIAL TESTS

Tests for Nerve Compression

Median Nerve

The most common nerve compression syndrome in the hand and wrist, and probably the most common nerve compression syndrome in the human body, is *carpal tunnel syndrome,* the compression of the **median nerve** within the carpal tunnel at the wrist. The base and sides of the carpal tunnel are a U-shaped bed of carpal bones; the roof is the transverse carpal ligament, a thickening of the antebrachial fascia that connects the hook of the hamate with the tubercles of the scaphoid and trapezium. Through this tunnel runs the median nerve along with nine long flexor tendons of the fingers and thumb. Compression of the median nerve at this location is called *carpal tunnel syndrome* because many different pathologies may be responsible for the compression. Posttraumatic hematoma, rheumatoid synovitis, peripheral edema, and space-occupying tumors are

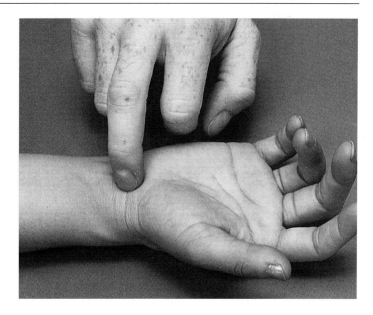

Figure 4–71. Tinel's test of the median nerve.

just a few examples. The adjunctive tests for carpal tunnel syndrome are provocative tests that attempt to evoke or exacerbate the patient's symptoms by increasing the pressure in the carpal tunnel.

TINEL'S TEST. The most basic of these tests is **Tinel's test.** To perform Tinel's test, the examiner places the patient's supinated wrist on a table or supports it with one hand. The examiner then taps briskly with the tip of his or her own long finger over the median nerve between the flexor carpi radialis and the palmaris longus tendons (Fig. 4–71). **Tinel's sign** is considered to be present if this maneuver elicits uncomfortable sensations of pain or electric shocks shooting into the hand. Tinel's sign is present in many cases of carpal tunnel syndrome.

CARPAL TUNNEL COMPRESSION TEST. In the **carpal tunnel compression test,** the examiner supports the patient's supinated wrist with one hand and presses firmly with the opposite thumb or finger over the space between the flexor carpi radialis and the palmaris longus tendons at the distal flexion crease of the wrist. This is the point where the median nerve enters the carpal tunnel (Fig. 4–72). Compression is maintained for 1 minute. Normal individuals may find this mildly uncomfortable. If, however, the compression test elicits symptoms of tingling or numbness in the median nerve sensory distribution in the hand, a carpal tunnel syndrome is usually present. This is the most sensitive test for carpal tunnel syndrome.

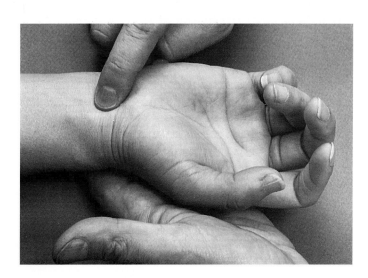

Figure 4–72. Carpal tunnel compression test.

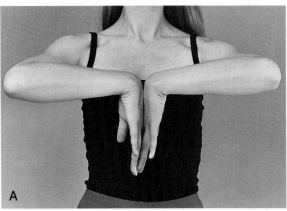
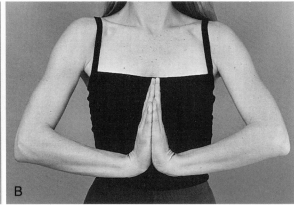

Figure 4–73. *A,* Phalen's test. *B,* Reverse Phalen's test.

PHALEN'S TEST AND REVERSE PHALEN'S TEST. Phalen's test and reverse Phalen's test are additional methods of indirectly compressing the median nerve at the wrist. In **Phalen's test,** the patient is instructed to compress the backs of both hands against each other so that the wrists are flexed a full 90° (Fig. 4–73*A*). In **reverse Phalen's test,** the patient presses the palms of both hands against each other so that both wrists are extended a full 90° (Fig. 4–73*B*). In both tests, the position is maintained for 1 minute. Carpal tunnel syndrome is suspected if either maneuver reproduces the patient's symptoms and causes aching or tingling in the distribution of the median nerve. Many clinicians now consider the carpal tunnel compression test to be more sensitive than either form of Phalen's test and rely on it exclusively.

Ulnar Nerve

ULNAR NERVE COMPRESSION TEST. Running a distant second to carpal tunnel syndrome is **ulnar nerve** compression at the wrist in *Guyon's canal.* Guyon's canal is formed on the ulnar side of the wrist by the pisohamate ligament that connects the pisiform with the hook of the hamate. Through this canal run the ulnar artery and nerve. The most sensitive test for ulnar nerve entrapment at Guyon's canal is the ulnar nerve compression test of the wrist. Analogous to the carpal tunnel compression test, the examiner performs it by compressing the ulnar nerve just radial to the pisiform bone for 1 minute (Fig. 4–74). If this produces tingling or numbness in the distribution of the ulnar nerve, it is evidence

for ulnar nerve compression at Guyon's canal. **Tinel's test** can also be used to screen for ulnar nerve compression at this site. In this case, the examiner supports the supinated hand and taps with the tip of the opposite long finger over the ulnar nerve (Fig. 4–75).

Stability Testing

INTERPHALANGEAL JOINTS. The collateral ligaments of the interphalangeal joints of the thumb and fingers are tested in a manner analo-

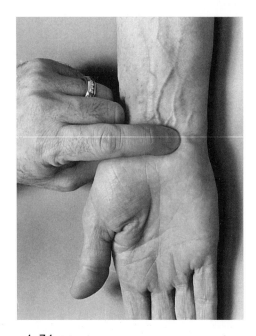

Figure 4–74. Ulnar nerve compression test at the wrist.

gous to that used for testing the collateral ligaments of the knee. The **DIP and PIP joints of the fingers** and the **interphalangeal joint of the thumb** are all tested in the same fashion. Of these joints, the PIP joints of the fingers are the most likely to suffer damage to the collateral ligaments.

To test the ulnar collateral ligament of the *PIP joint of the index finger,* for example, the proximal phalanx of the finger to be tested is stabilized between the thumb and the index finger of the examiner's own hand. The thumb and index finger of the examiner's other hand are then used to grasp the middle phalanx of the same finger. While maintaining the position of the interphalangeal joint at 30° of flexion, the examiner attempts to deviate the distal portion of the finger in the direction of the patient's thumb. This maneuver puts the ulnar collateral ligament under tension (Fig. 4–76A).

In a normal finger, virtually no movement is felt between the middle and the proximal phalanges at the PIP joint when this stress is applied. If a mild sprain of the ulnar collateral ligament is present, this stress produces pain on the ulnar side of the joint but the stability of the joint

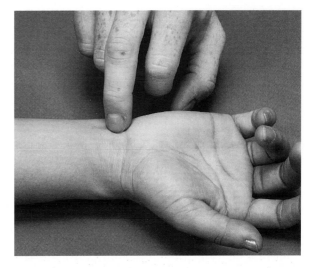

Figure 4–75. Tinel's test of the ulnar nerve at the wrist.

remains normal. In more severe sprains the ulnar side of the joint separates, allowing the joint to angulate 20° or 30°. The **interphalangeal joint of the thumb** is tested in an analogous manner (Fig. 4–76B).

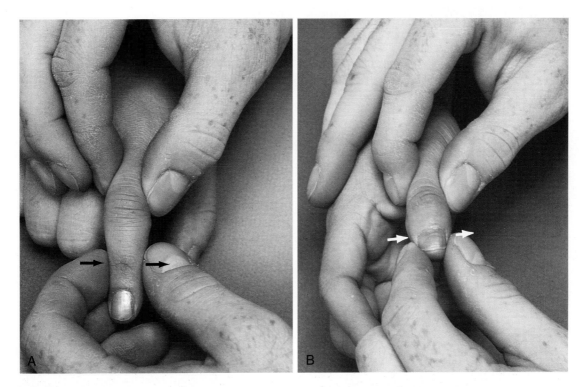

Figure 4–76. *A,* Stability test of the ulnar collateral ligament of the proximal interphalangeal joint of the index finger (*arrows* indicate the direction of force applied to the middle phalanx). *B,* Stability testing of the ulnar collateral ligament of the interphalangeal joint of the thumb (*arrows* indicate the direction of force applied to the distal phalanx).

METACARPOPHALANGEAL JOINTS. The collateral ligaments of the **MCP joints** are a bit more complicated to test. Because the collateral ligaments are loose in extension to permit the normal motion of abduction, the ligaments must be tested with the joint fully flexed so that the collateral ligaments are under tension.

To test the *ulnar collateral ligament of the index finger,* for example, the examiner grasps the proximal phalanx of the patient's index finger in one hand and the proximal phalanx of the adjacent long finger in the other. The examiner flexes both MCP joints to 90° to tighten the collateral ligaments and then attempts to separate the two fingers (Fig. 4–77). The examiner feels for any abnormal laxity at the MCP joint and notes the angle that the deviated index finger makes with the adjacent long finger.

In the normal patient, a small amount of separation between the index and the long fingers occurs owing to rotation of the metacarpals or minor degrees of residual laxity in the collateral ligaments, but the angle between the two adjacent fingers should not exceed 15° or 20°. In the presence of a mild sprain of the ulnar collateral ligament, this stress reproduces the patient's pain on the ulnar side of the metacarpal head, but stability feels normal. In more severe injuries of the ulnar collateral ligament of the MCP joint, the resistance of the collateral ligament feels spongy and the bones appear to separate more than in the normal hand. If the feeling of an

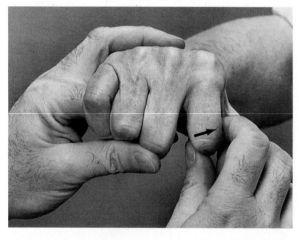

Figure 4–77. Stability testing of the ulnar collateral ligament of the metacarpophalangeal joint of the index finger (*arrow* indicates the direction of the force applied to the index finger).

endpoint is completely lacking, or if the angle between the index and the long fingers exceeds 35°, a complete rupture of the ulnar collateral ligament of the MCP joint of the index finger is present. Most injuries to the collateral ligaments of the MCP joints are traumatic, but in *rheumatoid arthritis* the radial collateral ligaments stretch out gradually as the subluxing extensor tendons pull the fingers into ulnar deviation.

The collateral ligaments of the **MCP joint of the thumb** are tested in a manner almost identical to that just described for the MCP joints of the fingers. In the thumb, the vast majority of these injuries occur to the ulnar collateral ligament; injuries to the radial collateral ligament are uncommon. In many individuals, the MCP joint of the thumb cannot flex to 90°. Flexing the joint to the maximal amount possible, however, tenses the collateral ligaments and allows for proper testing.

To test the **ulnar collateral ligament of the thumb,** the examiner fully flexes the patient's thumb at the MCP joint by grasping the proximal phalanx (Fig. 4–78*A*). The examiner then pushes the thumb away from the index finger, thus tensing the ulnar collateral ligament (Fig. 4–78*B*). In some individuals, some laxity of the ulnar collateral ligament is felt before the ligament tightens fully and firmly resists further motion.

In the normal thumb, this laxity is usually limited to 15° or less. If a mild sprain of the ulnar collateral ligament is present, this maneuver reproduces the patient's pain on the ulnar side of the joint, but no abnormal laxity is felt. In more severe degrees of ligament injury, the ulnar side of the joint is felt to separate as the thumb is pushed away from the index finger. Asymmetric deviation of the joint of more than 30° reflects a severe injury to the ulnar collateral ligament. In the most severe injuries, virtually no resistance is perceived and the examiner may feel that the thumb can be pushed to the side almost without restriction.

Radial collateral ligament injuries of the MCP joint of the thumb are unusual. When they do occur, abnormal laxity can be evaluated by a similar test conducted by applying force in the opposite direction.

BASILAR JOINT. Instability of the basilar joint of the thumb may occur, and it is often associated with arthritis. The test for instability of the basilar joint is called the **shuck test.** To perform

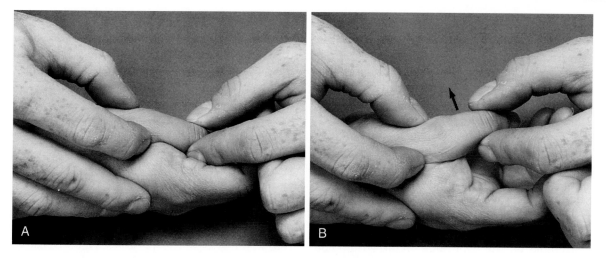

Figure 4–78. *A* and *B*, Stability testing of the ulnar collateral ligament of the thumb (*arrow* indicates the direction of the force applied to the proximal phalanx of the thumb).

the shuck test, the patient's forearm is placed in a position of neutral rotation so that the dorsum of the thumb faces upward.

To test the right thumb, for example, the examiner's right hand grasps the first metacarpal of the patient's thumb between the examiner's own thumb and the index and long fingers. The examiner's thumb is placed proximally at the base of the first metacarpal so that it can feel the relative positions of the base of the first metacarpal and the trapezium. Because the basilar joint may already be subluxed, the examiner then pushes downward on the patient's first metacarpal and notes how much translation occurs in relationship to the trapezium (Fig. 4–79). In the normal

patient, only 1 mm or 2 mm of translation is possible; if the joint is subluxed, greater translation is perceived.

Now that the joint is in a maximally reduced position, the examiner reverses the process, attempting to lever the base of the metacarpal upward and away from the trapezium. The examiner assesses how much total translation is present and compares it with the opposite thumb. If there is a noticeable difference in the amount of translation between the two sides or if the translation is uncomfortable to the patient, then the joint is subluxable. If crepitus is felt during the translation, then arthritis is probably also present in the joint.

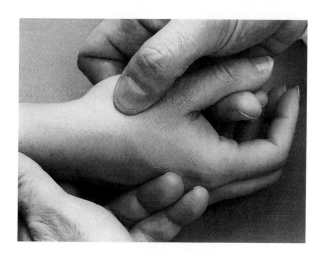

Figure 4–79. Shuck test for basilar joint instability.

CARPAL INSTABILITY. The concept of carpal instability is a subject of relatively recent interest and investigation. This is an area in which knowledge continues to expand. Several tests for carpal instability have been described and are in current use.

The **scaphoid shift test (Watson's test)** for *scapholunate instability* is probably the most widely known. It is designed to detect abnormal motion between the scaphoid and the lunate due to damage to the scapholunate ligament. To test the patient's right wrist, for example, the examiner's right hand grasps the patient's right hand, placing the examiner's thumb on the tubercle of the scaphoid on the volar side of the wrist. The patient's wrist is placed in a position of dorsiflexion and ulnar deviation (Fig. 4–80A). Pressing upward on the scaphoid tubercle, the examiner gently brings the wrist into a position of volar flexion and radial deviation (Fig. 4–80B). In the normal patient, this maneuver should produce smooth movement and minimal discomfort. In the presence of scapholunate instability, the examiner notes a popping sensation as the dorsal proximal pole of the scaphoid subluxes over the dorsal rim of the distal radius. The examiner's thumb then releases its pressure from the scaph-

oid tubercle, allowing the scaphoid to reduce (Fig. 4–80C). If this sequence reproduces the patient's pain and the pain is relieved when the pressure on the scaphoid is released, further evidence of scapholunate instability is present.

The **lunotriquetral ballottement test** was developed to detect instability of the *lunotriquetral joint* caused by injury. This test is performed with the patient's elbow flexed and forearm pronated. The goal of the test is to control the lunate and triquetrum separately so that they can be moved in relation to each other. To test the patient's right hand, for example, the examiner's left hand grasps the patient's right wrist with the examiner's left thumb over the triquetrum and the examiner's left index finger on the volar surface of the pisiform. The examiner's right hand then grasps the wrist from the other side, the examiner's right thumb being placed over the dorsum of the patient's lunate and the examiner's right index finger over the volar surface of the carpal tunnel. The examiner then attempts to displace the lunate and triquetrum in relation to each other (Fig. 4–81). To do this, the examiner's right hand pulls upward while the examiner's left hand pushes downward. This process is then

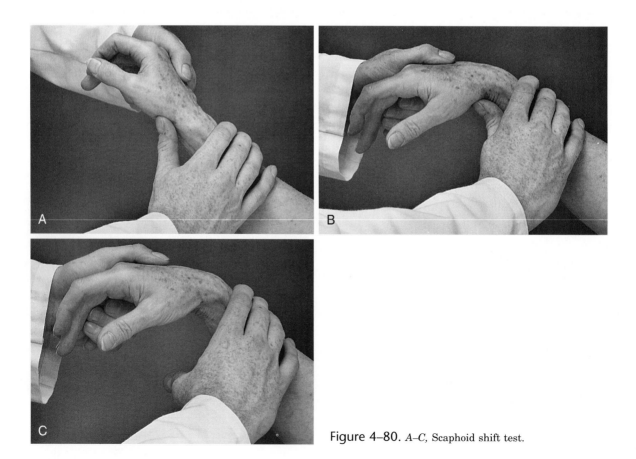

Figure 4–80. *A–C,* Scaphoid shift test.

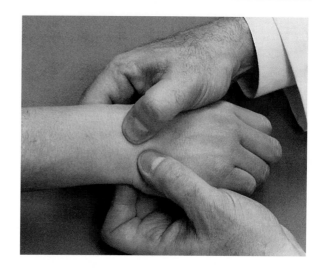

Figure 4–81. Lunotriquetral ballottement test.

reversed, pushing downward with the right hand and upward with the left hand. In the normal patient, very little movement or discomfort is noted. If significantly more translation is noted than in the opposite wrist, lunotriquetral instability should be suspected. If this maneuver reproduces the patient's pain or results in a grinding sensation, this is further evidence that lunotriquetral instability is responsible for the patient's symptoms.

Midcarpal instability is the most difficult of the wrist instabilities to detect and interpret. When midcarpal instability is present, the proximal and distal rows of carpal bones do not move synchronously in relation to each other as the wrist progresses from radial to ulnar deviation. Instead, a jump, a catch, or a clunk is felt in the middle of the joint motion. For the **midcarpal instability test,** the patient is positioned with

the elbow flexed and forearm pronated. To test the patient's right wrist, for example, the examiner's left hand grasps the patient's right hand and the examiner's right hand grasps the patient's right forearm. The examiner places the patient's wrist in a position of ulnar deviation and loads the patient's wrist by pushing the hand proximally toward the forearm (Fig. 4–82A). While maintaining this loading, the patient's wrist is slowly moved into radial deviation (Fig. 4–82B). In the normal wrist, this movement should proceed smoothly, accompanied by no significant jumping, catching, or clunking sensations. If midcarpal instability is present, the examiner usually sees or feels the midcarpal joint jump, catch, or clunk as the wrist moves into radial deviation. Pushing upward on the volar surface of the pisiform should correct the subluxation and cause the clunk to disappear.

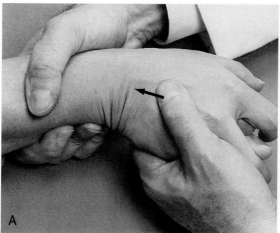
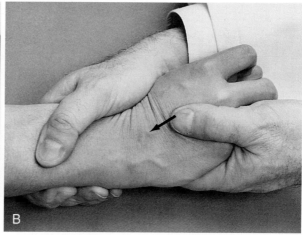

Figure 4–82. *A* and *B,* Midcarpal instability test (*arrows* indicate the direction of the applied compression force).

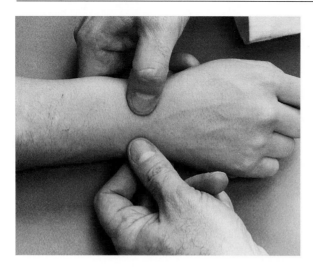

Figure 4–83. Piano key test of the distal radioulnar joint.

DISTAL RADIOULNAR JOINT. Instability can also exist in the distal radioulnar joint. Most commonly, the head of the ulna subluxes dorsally in relation to the radius when the forearm is in the pronated position. The test for instability in the distal radioulnar joint is sometimes called the **piano key test.** To perform it, the patient is placed in a position of elbow flexion and forearm pronation. To test the right wrist, for example, the examiner grasps the patient's ulnar head between the thumb and the index finger of his or her own left hand and the distal radius between the thumb and the index finger of his or her own right hand. The examiner then translates the distal ulna up and down in relation to the distal radius (Fig. 4–83). The examiner compares the amount of translation with the patient's other wrist and notes whether clicking, popping, or pain is produced. The finding of increased translation, compared with the opposite wrist, accompanied by clicking, popping, or pain suggests the presence of symptomatic instability of the distal radioulnar joint. The examiner can also stress the distal radioulnar joint by compressing the distal ulna against the distal radius with one hand while passively pronating and supinating the patient's forearm with the other hand (Fig. 4–84). If this maneuver produces pain, popping, or grinding at the distal radioulnar joint, then arthritis or instability of the distal radioulnar joint is probably present. This maneuver may be called the **distal radioulnar joint compression test.**

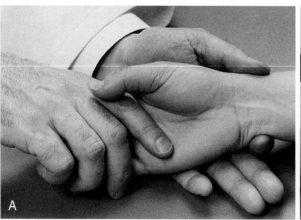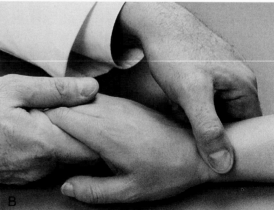

Figure 4–84. *A* and *B,* The distal radioulnar joint compression test.

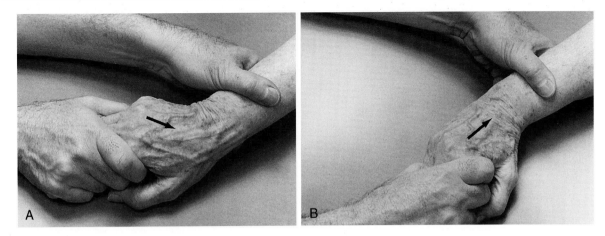

Figure 4–85. *A* and *B,* Triangular fibrocartilage complex (TFCC) compression test (*arrows* indicate the direction of the applied compression force).

Triangular Fibrocartilage Complex Compression Test

If tenderness just distal to the ulnar head has raised the suspicion of injury to the TFCC, the examiner can further investigate this possibility with the **TFCC compression test.** To perform this test, the patient's forearm is placed in a pronated position with the elbow flexed. To test the right wrist, for example, the examiner's right hand grasps the patient's right hand and the examiner's left hand stabilizes the patient's forearm. The wrist is then loaded by compressing the hand proximally against the forearm, and the

wrist is moved repeatedly back and forth from radial deviation to ulnar deviation (Fig. 4–85). In the presence of a symptomatic TFCC tear, this maneuver usually produces painful clicking and popping. Although this test is similar to the midcarpal instability test, the sensation of popping and clicking of the TFCC is very different from the jumping or clunking sensation produced by midcarpal instability.

Grind Test

The **grind test** is a provocative test to elicit symptoms of *basilar joint arthritis.* To examine the patient's right thumb, for example, the examiner grasps the patient's right first metacarpal between the thumb, the index finger, and the long finger of the examiner's right hand. The examiner's right thumb then pushes down on the dorsum of the base of the first metacarpal. This action has the effect of reducing the basilar joint in case it is subluxed. This reduction maneuver is the first part of the shuck test, as described previously. While maintaining the basilar joint in reduction, the examiner loads the basilar joint by pushing the first metacarpal proximally and then rotating the metacarpal in a circular fashion (Fig. 4–86). This portion of the examination is known as the grind test. If the circumduction maneuver reproduces the patient's pain or results in a palpable grinding sensation, this is evidence for degenerative arthritis of the basilar joint.

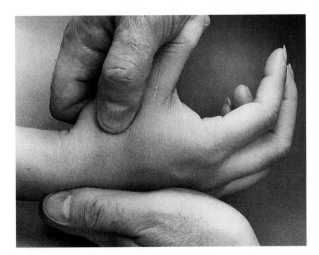

Figure 4–86. Grind test of the basilar joint.

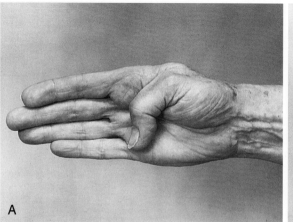
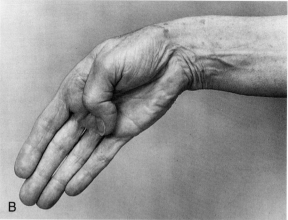

Figure 4–87. *A* and *B*, Finkelstein's test.

Finkelstein's Test

The **Finkelstein test** is a provocative test to evoke the symptoms of *de Quervain's disease,* the eponym for tenosynovitis of the first dorsal compartment tendons: the abductor pollicis longus and extensor pollicis brevis. Finkelstein's test is usually performed with the patient's elbow flexed and the forearm in a position of neutral rotation so that the dorsal surface of the thumb faces upward. The patient is then instructed to flex the thumb across the palm (Fig. 4–87*A*) and then to ulnar-deviate the wrist (Fig. 4–87*B*). In the normal patient, this maneuver should not be uncomfortable. In the presence of de Quervain's disease, this maneuver usually produces a severe exacerbation of the patient's pain. Many authors recommend performing the ulnar deviation passively, but this may be excessively painful for a patient with de Quervain's tenosynovitis.

Transillumination

Transillumination is a technique for verifying that a protruding mass at the wrist or the hand is a ganglion cyst. The transillumination test is not useful for tiny ganglia. Transillumination of a ganglion is best performed in a darkened room. The examiner places the lighted end of a penlight flashlight against the cutaneous surface of the mass. If the mass is indeed a ganglion, the light should be seen to pass through it, changing the glow of the light from a round to a dumbbell-shaped globe. This demonstrates that the mass is indeed a cyst filled with fluid, and thus it is almost certainly a ganglion. If, on the other hand, the mass does not transmit the light, it is probably a solid mass and not a ganglion.

Evaluation of Circulation

CAPILLARY REFILL. The most basic test for evaluating the circulation to the fingers is to assess the **capillary refill.** Circulation to the fingers or the hands in general may be compromised by peripheral vascular disease, Raynaud's disease, or local arterial injury. Capillary refill is assessed with the patient's hand pronated. The examiner first notes the color of the nailbed of the finger to be evaluated. Normally, the nailbed should have a healthy pink tinge, reflecting good capillary perfusion. The examiner then compresses the patient's fingertip between the examiner's own thumb and index finger for a few seconds (Fig. 4–88*A*). This compression serves to empty most of the blood from the capillaries of the patient's fingertip. The examiner then suddenly uncovers the patient's nailbed and observes its color (Fig. 4–88*B*). When the patient's nailbed is first uncovered, it should appear blanched compared with the other fingers and compared with its previous color. The normal pink color should, however, return to the nailbed within 2 seconds or 3 seconds. If reperfusion occurs more slowly than this, circulation to the finger is compromised. Examination of the other digits allows the examiner to determine whether the problem is confined to one particular finger or affects the entire hand.

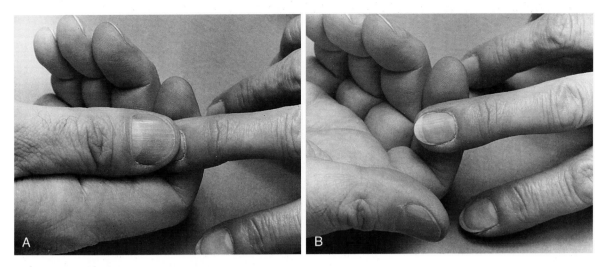

Figure 4–88. *A* and *B,* Assessing capillary refill.

ALLEN'S TEST. Allen's test is designed to determine whether both the **radial** and the **ulnar arteries** contribute significantly to the perfusion of the hand. This information is important to know before performing a procedure that might injure one of the arteries, such as inserting an arterial line into the radial artery or surgically approaching the scaphoid tubercle from its volar aspect.

The Allen test is performed with the patient's elbow flexed and forearm supinated. The examiner locates the radial and ulnar pulses as described in the Palpation section and places a thumb over each. The normal color of the patient's fingers and palm is noted (Fig. 4–89*A*). The patient is then instructed to open and close the hand three times and then make a tight fist (Fig. 4–89*B*). This action has the effect of

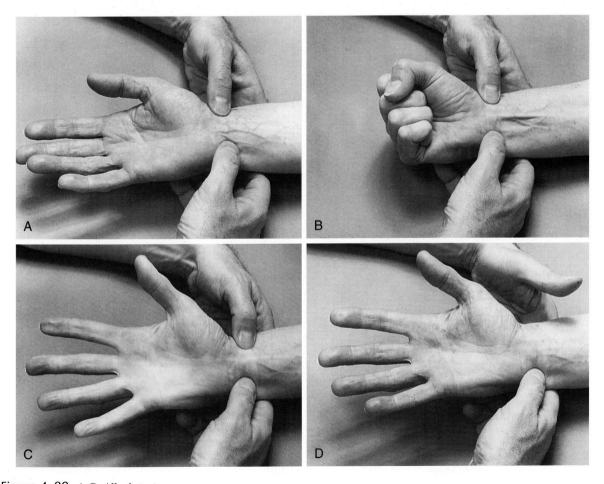

Figure 4–89. *A–D,* Allen's test.

exsanguinating much of the blood from the patient's hand. The radial and ulnar arteries are then simultaneously compressed beneath the examiner's thumbs. The patient is then instructed to open the hand. Immediately after opening, the hand should appear blanched because the examiner is occluding inflow from both arteries (Fig. 4–89C). The examiner then quickly releases compression from one of the arteries and observes the color of the hand (Fig. 4–89D). If the released artery is contributing significantly to perfusion, the normal color of the palm and volar fingers should return within a few seconds.

The test is then repeated, this time releasing the other artery while maintaining compression on the artery that was previously released. Again, the time required for perfusion to return to the hand is noted. In about 80% of normal individuals, the ulnar artery predominates over the radial artery. However, both arteries should be able to perfuse the hand in the majority of individuals. If the return of color to the palm is significantly prolonged after the release of either artery, the examiner should conclude that perfusion from that artery is reduced.

The Allen test can also be used for assessing the relative contributions of the two **digital arteries** to an individual finger. In this case, the examiner observes the normal resting color of the finger in question and has the patient exsanguinate it by flexing the finger tightly. The examiner then obstructs both digital arteries by compressing at both sides at the base of the finger (Fig. 4–90A). Because the digital arteries are closer to the volar than the dorsal surface of the fingers, the examiner's thumbs should be positioned to compress from the volar surface. The patient is then instructed to extend the finger (Fig. 4–90B). The examiner then releases compression from one of the digital arteries and observes the time required for normal color to return to the finger (Fig. 4–90C). As with the Allen test of the hand,

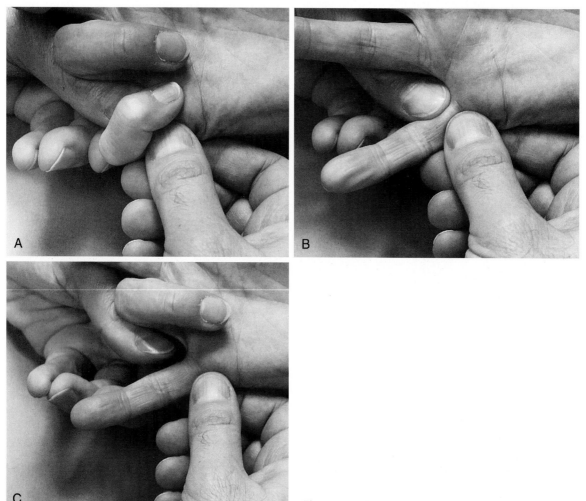

Figure 4–90. *A–C,* Allen's test of the digital arteries.

TABLE 4–1.
PHYSICAL FINDINGS IN COMMON CONDITIONS OF THE HAND AND WRIST

Degenerative Arthritis of the Fingers

Heberden's nodes (most common)
Bouchard's nodes (common)
Mucous cysts (occasional)
Decreased motion at involved interphalangeal joints
Instability of involved joints (occasional)

Basilar Joint Arthritis

Swelling and tenderness of the basilar joint
Subluxation of the basilar joint (shuck test) (more severe cases)
Reduced motion at the basilar joint (palmar abduction, opposition)
Weakened opposition and grip strength
Abnormal grind test
Hyperextension of the first metacarpophalangeal joint (more severe cases)

Carpal Tunnel Syndrome

Median nerve compression test abnormal (most sensitive test)
Tinel's sign over the median nerve (frequent)
Phalen's and reverse Phalen's tests reproduce symptoms (variable)
Abnormal sensation (two-point discrimination) in the median nerve distribution (more severe cases)
Thenar eminence softened and atrophied (more severe cases)
Weakened or absent opposition (more severe cases)

De Quervain's Stenosing Tenosynovitis

Tenderness and swelling over the first dorsal compartment at the radial styloid
Finkelstein's test aggravates pain

Ganglion

Palpable mass (may be firm or soft)
Most common locations: the volar hand at the web flexion crease of the digits or the transverse palmar crease, the dorsal wrist near the extensor carpi radialis longus and brevis tendons, the volar wrist near the radial artery
Mass transilluminates (larger ganglia)

Dupuytren's Disease

Palpable nodules in palmar aponeurosis, most commonly affecting the ring finger or the little finger
Secondary flexion contracture of the metacarpophalangeal and, occasionally, proximal interphalangeal joint

Rheumatoid Arthritis

Boggy swelling of multiple joints (metacarpophalangeal joints and wrist joint most commonly involved)
Boggy swelling of the tenosynovium of the extensor tendons over the dorsum of the wrist and the hand (common)
Boggy swelling of the tenosynovium of the flexor tendons on the volar surface of the wrist (common)
Secondary deformities in more severe cases, such as ulnar deviation of the metacarpophalangeal joints and swan neck and boutonnière deformities
Secondary rupture of extensor or flexor tendons (variable)

Flexor Tendon Sheath Infection

Cardinal signs of Kanavel present
Finger held in flexed position at rest
Swelling along the volar surface of the finger
Tenderness of the volar surface of the finger along the course of the flexor tendon sheath
Pain exacerbated by passive extension of the involved finger

Injury to the Ulnar Collateral Ligament of the Metacarpohalangeal Joint of the Thumb (Skier's or gamekeeper's thumb)

Swelling and tenderness over the ulnar aspect of the first metacarpophalangeal joint
Pain exacerbated by stress of the ulnar collateral ligament
Increased laxity of the ulnar collateral ligament (more severe injuries)
Rotational deformity of the thumb (chronic cases)

Ulnar Nerve Entrapment at the Wrist

Compression of the ulnar nerve at Guyon's canal reproduces symptoms (most sensitive test)
Abnormal Tinel's sign over Guyon's canal (variable)
Weakness of intrinsic muscles (finger abduction or adduction) (more severe cases)
Atrophy of the interossei and the hypothenar eminence (more severe cases)
Abnormal sensation in the little finger and the ulnar aspect of the ring finger (variable)
Abnormal Froment's sign (variable)

Scapholunate Instability

Swelling over the radial wrist
Tenderness of the dorsal wrist over the scapholunate ligament
Scaphoid shift test produces abnormal popping and reproduces the patient's pain

---

the procedure is then repeated for the other digital artery so that the relative contributions of the two vessels can be compared.

The physical findings in common conditions of the hand and wrist are summarized in Table 4–1.

Bibliography

Backdahl MJ: The caput ulnae syndrome in rheumatoid arthritis. Acta Rheumatol Scand. 1963; 5(suppl):1–75.

Burkhart SS, Wood MB, Linscheid RL: Posttraumatic recurrent subluxation of the extensor carpi ulnaris tendon. J Hand Surg [Am]. 1982; 7:1–3.

Burton RI: Basal joint arthrosis of the thumb. Orthop Clin North Am. 1973; 4:347–348.

Coleman HM: Injuries of the articular disk at the wrist. J Bone Joint Surg Br. 1960; 42:522–529.

Cooney WP: Tears of the triangular fibrocartilage of the wrist. In Cooney WP, Linscheid RL, Dobyns JH, eds. The Wrist: Diagnosis and Operative Treatment. St. Louis, CV Mosby, 1998:710–742.

Durkan JA: A new diagnostic test for carpal tunnel syndrome. J Bone Joint Surg Am. 1991; 73:535–538.

Finkelstein H: Stenosing tenosynovitis at the radial styloid process. J Bone Joint Surg. 1930; 30:509.

Flatt AE: Care of the arthritic hand. St. Louis, CV Mosby, 1982.

Kleinman W: The ballottement test. American Society for Surgery of the Hand Correspondence Newsletter. 1985:51.

Lichtman DM, Schneider JR, Swafford AR, Mack GR: Ulnar midcarpal instability—clinical and laboratory analysis. J Hand Surg [Am]. 1981; 6:515–523.

Palmer AK: The distal radioulnar joint. Orthop Clin North Am. 1984; 15:321–335.

The pelvis is a complex bony structure that is formed by the joining of seven individual components. On each side of the pelvis, the ilium, the ischium, and the pubis fuse together to become a pelvic, or innominate, bone. The right and left pelvic bones join each other anteriorly at the pubic symphysis and join the sacrum posteriorly at the sacroiliac joints to form a closed ring. As with the skull and the ribs, the pelvic ring protects vital internal structures. The primary orthopaedic function of the pelvis, however, is to serve as a stable central base for human locomotion. The pelvis provides a foundation for the spine and upper body and the point of origin or insertion for many muscles of the thorax, the hip, and the thigh.

The hip consists of the femoral head, the most proximal aspect of the femur, and the acetabulum, a socket located in the center of the lateral surface of the pelvis. Portions of the ilium, the ischium, and the pubis coalesce during skeletal development to form the acetabulum. The great depth of the acetabulum combines with the strong iliofemoral ligaments to make the hip a very stable joint. Despite this great stability, the ball-and-socket design of the hip joint allows considerable motion in three planes. The hips provide stable support for the pelvis and upper body while still allowing the lower extremities to assume a tremendous variety of positions in space. Distal to the hip, the femoral shaft undergirds the muscles of the thigh, serving as the site of origin and insertion for many of the muscles required for normal ambulation.

Inspection

SURFACE ANATOMY

Anterior Aspect

The bony landmarks of the pelvis are easily identified in the average patient (Fig. 5–1). In the presence of obesity, the pendulous abdominal fat, or panniculus, tends to obscure these landmarks. When such patients are examined in the supine position, the panniculus tends to shift superiorly and to expose more of the normal anatomy.

PELVIS. The most prominent feature of the pelvis is the arching superior margin of the ilium, known as the **iliac crest.** The iliac crest is visible in many patients and palpable in most. In obese patients, it lies immediately beneath the abdominal fold at the waist. As its name implies, the **anterior superior iliac spine** (ASIS) is the anterior terminus of the iliac crest. The ASIS serves as the site of origin for the **inguinal ligament,** a fibrous band that traverses the anterior pelvis and inserts just lateral to the pubic symphysis on a small prominence of the pubis known as the **pubic tubercle.** The inguinal ligament serves as the insertion for some of the abdominal muscles, and its fascia envelops the round ligament in women and the spermatic cord in men. The ASIS also serves as the origin for the **sartorius** muscle, which is visible in lean or muscular individuals. The sartorius courses obliquely across the anterior thigh to insert on the proximal medial tibia as the outer layer of the pes anserinus.

The ASIS may be used to reference the location of the **lateral femoral cutaneous nerve,** which is not normally visible. The lateral femoral cutaneous nerve exits the pelvis and enters the anterolateral thigh about 2 cm medial to the ASIS. This is the site at which the nerve may be compressed by tight clothing, leading to the uncomfortable condition known as *meralgia paresthetica.*

Further medially, the femoral nerve, artery, and vein pass deep to the inguinal ligament as they enter the anterior thigh. These structures are not directly visible, although the pulsations of the artery may be seen in a lean patient. In others, the **femoral artery** should be palpable just medial to the midpoint of the inguinal ligament. The **femoral nerve** is just lateral to the artery, and the **femoral vein** is just medial to it. After passing beneath the inguinal ligament, the neurovascular structures pass through the *femoral triangle.* The boundaries of the femoral triangle, which may be visible, include the inguinal ligament superiorly, the sartorius muscle laterally, and the adductor longus muscle medially.

The **tensor fascia lata** is a superficial muscle that arises from the anterior portion of the iliac crest and inserts into the fascia lata, or enveloping fascia, of the lateral thigh. Its muscle belly

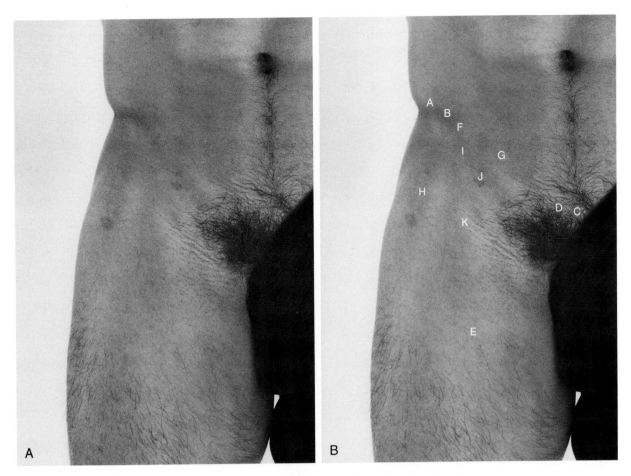

Figure 5–1. *A* and *B*, Anterior aspect of the hip and pelvis. A, iliac crest; B, anterior superior iliac spine; C, pubic symphysis; D, pubic tubercle; E, sartorius; F, lateral femoral cutaneous nerve; G, femoral artery; H, tensor fascia lata; I, anterior inferior iliac spine; J, hip joint; K, lesser trochanter.

is visible anteriorly in lean individuals, forming the lateral contour of the proximal thigh.

The **anterior inferior iliac spine** (AIIS) lies just medial and inferior to the ASIS. This small bony prominence is not normally visible because it is obscured by the sartorius. It serves as the origin for a portion of the rectus femoris muscle, the only component of the quadriceps femoris muscle group to arise superior to the hip joint.

The medial portion of each pelvic bone is formed by the **pubis.** The contours of the pubic bone are not normally visible. The upper portion of the pubis is known as the *superior pubic ramus.* The two pubic bones join together at the midline in a fibrocartilaginous joint called the **pubic symphysis.** The *pectineus* muscle inserts along the superior pubic ramus, and the *pyramidalis* and *rectus abdominis* muscles insert near the pubic symphysis. Although not visible, the pubic symphysis can usually be palpated in the midline at the superior margin of the normal area of growth of pubic hair. The disruption of the two halves of the pelvis may occur as a result of high velocity trauma. Pelvic disruption is often associated with fractures of the pubic ramus or dissociation of the pubic symphysis.

HIP JOINT. Although the hip joint itself lies deep to the muscles of the pelvis and thigh, the visible anterior landmarks of the pelvis can be used to identify the location of the hip joint. To do so, the examiner first locates the pulse of the femoral artery. This should be palpable approximately midway between the ASIS and the pubic tubercle. The hip joint itself is located 2 cm lateral and 2 cm distal to the point at which the femoral pulse is palpable beneath the inguinal ligament. Pain arising from pathology of the hip joint, such as osteoarthritis, usually is localized to this site and often is described by the patient as "groin pain."

THIGH. The **quadriceps** muscle group constitutes the primary bulk of the anterior thigh (Fig. 5–2). The quadriceps consists of four distinct muscles that coalesce as they insert into the superior pole of the patella and, ultimately, through the patellar tendon, into the tibial tubercle. The **rectus femoris** muscle arises partly from the AIIS and partly from the anterior hip capsule and constitutes the central bulge of the thigh. The other three components of the quadriceps all arise below the hip joint. The **vastus interme-**

161

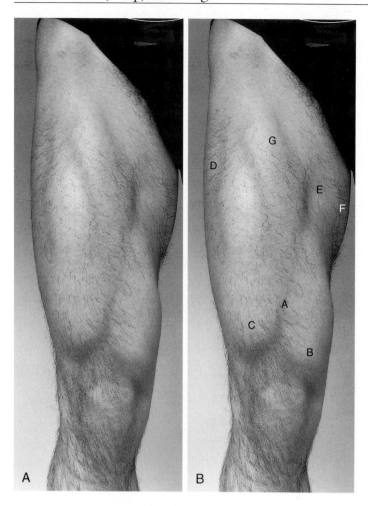

Figure 5–2. *A* and *B,* Anterior aspect of the thigh. A, rectus femoris; B, vastus medialis; C, vastus lateralis; D, iliotibial tract; E, adductor longus; F, gracilis; G, sartorius.

dius is located deep to the rectus femoris and is not separately visible. Flanking the medial border of the rectus femoris lies the **vastus medialis,** and the **vastus lateralis** fills out the lateral contour of the anterior thigh. In a lean or muscular individual, these muscle bellies may be clearly distinguishable. The lateral border of the thigh has a straight contour that is created by the **iliotibial tract,** which borders the vastus lateralis muscle. In the distal third of the thigh, the iliotibial tract narrows down and angles toward its insertion on the tubercle of Gerdy.

The adductor longus and gracilis muscles comprise the medial contour of the thigh. The **adductor longus** originates from the pubis and inserts on the linea aspera of the femur. The **gracilis** also arises from the pubis and runs the length of the medial thigh until it inserts as a narrow tendon on the tibia as part of the pes anserinus.

Lateral Aspect

PELVIS AND HIP. Viewed from the lateral position, the most prominent landmark of the pelvis is the arching contour of the **iliac crest** (Fig.

5–3). The position of the pelvis is traditionally judged by the orientation of *Nelaton's line,* an imaginary line drawn from the posterior superior iliac spine (PSIS) to the ASIS. In the standing patient, the ASIS is normally somewhat lower than the PSIS, giving Nelaton's line a downward slant.

From the lateral perspective, the examiner is looking directly at the prominence created by the principal abductor of the hip, the gluteus medius. The **gluteus medius** arises from the superior portion of most of the iliac wing and inserts on the greater trochanter. Anterior to the gluteus medius, the **tensor fascia lata** arises from the most anterior portion of the iliac crest and constitutes the anterior border of the lateral aspect of the hip. Posterior to the gluteus medius, the bulky **gluteus maximus** muscle arises from the posterior ilium and adjacent sacrum. The belly of the gluteus maximus constitutes the familiar rounded contour of the buttock.

THIGH. Distal to the pelvic area, the **vastus lateralis** and the **biceps femoris** muscles constitute the anterior and the posterior contours of the thigh, respectively (Fig. 5–4). The most

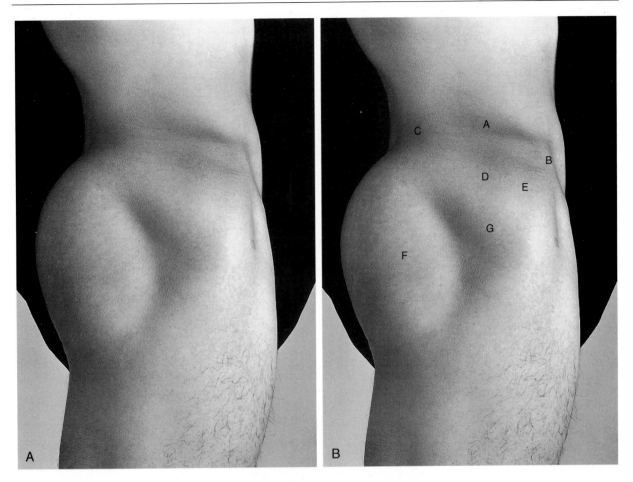

Figure 5–3. *A* and *B,* Lateral aspect of the hip and pelvis. A, iliac crest; B, anterior superior iliac spine; C, posterior superior iliac spine; D, gluteus medius; E, tensor fascia lata; F, gluteus maximus; G, greater trochanter.

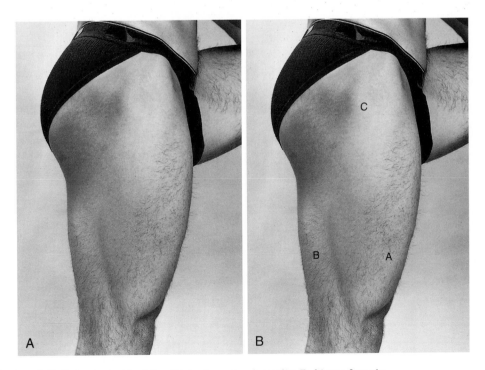

Figure 5–4. *A* and *B,* Lateral aspect of the thigh. A, vastus lateralis; B, biceps femoris; C, greater trochanter.

prominent bony landmark is the **greater trochanter** of the proximal femur. The greater trochanter projects laterally to provide increased leverage for the gluteus medius and the gluteus minimus muscles that insert there. These critical muscles not only abduct the femur but also, more importantly, prevent drooping of the pelvis when the opposite limb is lifted from the ground during normal ambulation. The contour of the greater trochanter is somewhat obscured by the overlying fascia lata, although the prominence it creates is still usually quite noticeable. It should lie just distal to the midpoint of Nelaton's line. Between the fascia lata and the greater trochanter lies the **trochanteric bursa,** which facilitates the back-and-forth motion of the fascia lata across the greater trochanter during normal gait. Pain that localizes to the vicinity of the greater trochanter usually arises from trochanteric bursitis or gluteus medius tendinitis, rather than pathology of the hip joint itself.

Posterior Aspect

PELVIS AND HIP. The posterior aspect of the pelvis is again dominated by the curve of the **iliac crest** (Fig. 5–5). The posterior border of the crest is seen to curve posteriorly and medially to its point of termination, the PSIS. Relatively little soft tissue overlies the PSIS; consequently, its presence is often indicated by a dimple in the overlying skin. The PSIS overhangs the **sacroiliac joint,** which is located just distal to it. The sacroiliac joint is not normally visible, although it can be palpated as a longitudinal prominence proceeding distally from the PSIS. The other landmarks of the posterior hip and pelvis are mostly obscured by the great bulk of the **gluteus maximus,** the principal extensor of the hip, which originates from the posterior portion of the iliac crest and inserts into both the fascia lata and the linea aspera of the posterior femur. The area of the **sacrum** is visible as a triangular

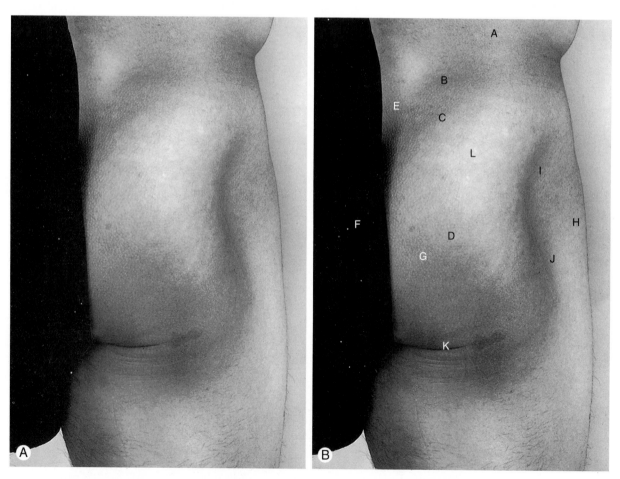

Figure 5–5. *A* and *B,* Posterior aspect of the hip and pelvis. A, iliac crest; B, posterior superior iliac spine; C, sacroiliac joint; D, gluteus maximus; E, sacrum; F, coccyx; G, ischial tuberosity; H, greater trochanter; I, piriformis; J, quadratus femoris; K, gluteal fold; L, sciatic notch.

depression between the two great prominences created by the gluteus maximus muscles. The sacrum tapers distally to the **coccyx,** which is palpable beneath the top of the midline crease of the buttocks.

The ischium is the most inferior of the three bones that constitute the innominate, or pelvic, bone. Its inferior contour, the **ischial tuberosity,** constitutes the inferiormost portion of the pelvis. The ischial tuberosity is not normally visible, but it is palpable in the inferior medial buttock deep to the gluteus maximus. It serves as the origin for the hamstrings, the principal flexors of the knee, and a portion of the adductor magnus.

Although the gluteus maximus obscures the deeper muscles of the posterior hip, their position can be estimated through knowledge of their relationship to the **greater trochanter,** whose prominence can usually be identified from the posterior perspective. A group of four short external rotators arises from the pelvis and inserts in a relatively small area on the superior portion of the greater trochanter. From superior to inferior they are the **piriformis,** the **superior ge-**mellus, the **obturator internus,** and the **inferior gemellus.** Tendinitis in these structures can be a source of posterior hip pain, and the piriformis is thought to sometimes compress the *sciatic nerve,* which emerges from beneath it. Two other transversely oriented muscles, the **obturator externus** and the **quadratus femoris,** insert further distally on the posterior margin of the greater trochanter. They are less likely than the external rotators to be implicated as a source of hip pain.

The transverse crease that forms at the junction of the buttock and the posterior thigh is known as the **gluteal fold.** These folds, which are formed as the gluteus maximus inserts into the posterior aspect of the proximal femur, are normally symmetric. Abnormalities of the hip, such as arthritis with hip joint subluxation or congenital hip dysplasia, cause the gluteal folds to appear asymmetric.

THIGH. The lateral margin of the posterior thigh is defined by the iliotibial tract (Fig. 5–6). The visible muscle bulk consists primarily of the three hamstring muscles: the biceps femoris, the

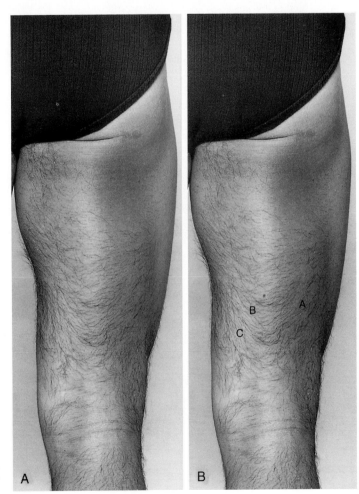

Figure 5–6. *A* and *B,* Posterior aspect of the thigh. A, biceps femoris; B, semitendinosus; C, semimembranosus.

semimembranosus, and the semitendinosus. The **biceps femoris,** the sole lateral hamstring, originates from both the ischial tuberosity and the proximal femur and courses distally to a complex insertion on the fibular head. The other two hamstrings originate exclusively from the ischial tuberosity. The **semimembranosus** courses distally to its own complex insertion on the posteromedial tibia just distal to the joint line. The **semitendinosus** is superficial and lateral to the bulk of the semimembranosus. It tapers distally to a long narrow tendon that curves around the medial tibia to insert anteriorly as the third component of the pes anserinus. The semitendinosus and biceps tendons are usually visible, especially if the knee is flexed against resistance (Fig. 5–7). Because the hamstrings traverse both the hip and the knee joints, they function as both principal flexors of the knee and auxiliary extensors of the hip. Passive flexion of the hip, therefore, tightens the hamstrings and thus may limit knee extension, whereas passive extension of the knee may cause involuntary hip extension by the same mechanism.

Medial Aspect

THIGH. The medial thigh is bordered by the **vastus medialis** and **sartorius** anteriorly and by the **hamstrings** posteriorly (Fig. 5–8). Between these margins are located the adductor magnus, the adductor longus and the gracilis muscles. The **adductor magnus** originates from the ischial tuberosity and inferior pubic ramus and inserts on the femur in two places: the linea aspera of the posterior femoral shaft and above the medial epicondyle in the area often referred to as the **adductor tubercle.** The adductor magnus is the bulkiest of the adductor muscles. The **adductor longus** arises from the anterior pubis near the pubic symphysis and inserts on the linea aspera. The adductor longus is the most distinctly visible of the adductors. Its proximal portion stands out in the medial groin when the leg is maximally abducted or placed in the figure-four position (Fig. 5–9). The **gracilis** originates on the medial pubis and inserts on the tibia, where, along with the overlying sartorius and adjacent semitendinosus tendons, it forms the pes anserinus.

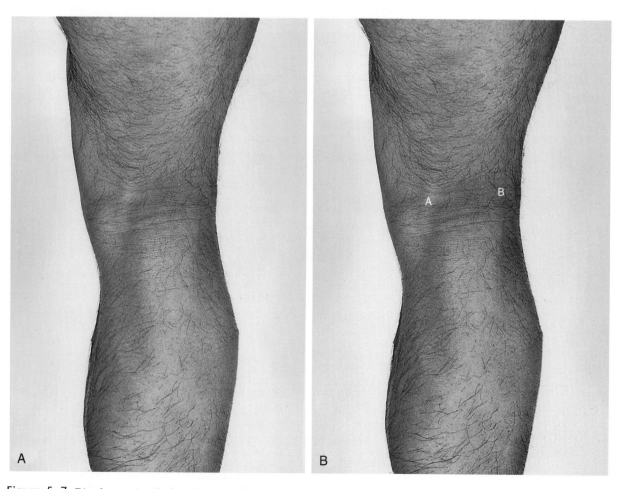

Figure 5–7. Distal posterior thigh with resisted knee flexion. A, Semitendinosus. B, Biceps femoris.

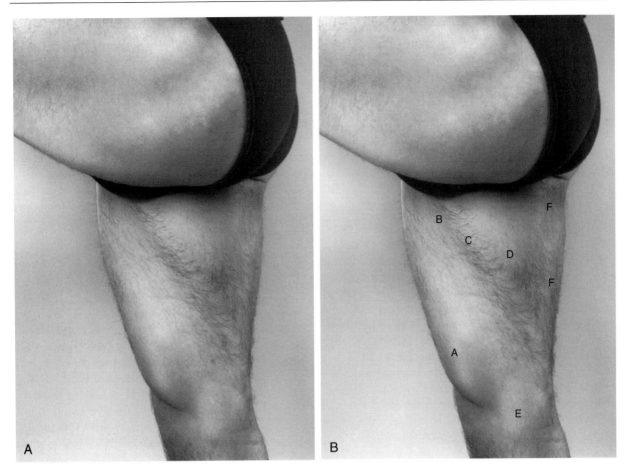

Figure 5–8. *A* and *B,* Medial aspect of the thigh. A, vastus medialis; B, adductor longus; C, gracilis; D, adductor magnus; E, adductor tubercle; F, hamstrings.

ALIGNMENT

Two aspects of alignment are usually associated with a hip examination: evaluation for **leg length discrepancy** (lower limb length discrepancy) and evaluation for **rotational malalignment** of the lower limbs. Both of these qualities

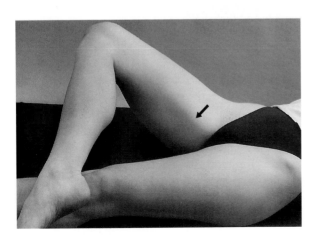

Figure 5–9. Figure-four position brings out the contour of the adductor longus *(arrow)*.

may be affected by factors outside of the hip, the pelvis, and the thigh. For purposes of coherence and continuity, these other factors are discussed here.

Leg Length Discrepancy

Differences in the lengths of a patient's lower limbs are usually described as leg length discrepancies, although lower limb length discrepancies would really be more accurate because the overall lengths of the lower extremities are what are being compared.

PELVIC OBLIQUITY. Abnormalities of limb length usually result in obliquity of the pelvis; therefore, a check for **pelvic obliquity** is an excellent starting point to begin the alignment examination. In a normal patient, the two sides of the pelvis should be level with each other when the patient is standing. To check for pelvic obliquity, the patient is asked to stand facing away from the examiner. The patient should be barefoot, with the knees fully extended and the feet together. The examiner then places a finger or two of each hand on each of the patient's iliac crests and imagines a line drawn between the two crests (Fig. 5–10). Pelvic obliquity is present when this imaginary line is not parallel to the floor. The many possible causes of obliquity can be divided into two large groups: factors resulting in a true leg length discrepancy and factors resulting in a functional, or apparent, leg length discrepancy.

TRUE VERSUS FUNCTIONAL LEG LENGTH DISCREPANCY. In a **true leg length discrepancy,** the actual length of the patient's two lower limbs, when measured from the femoral heads to the plantar surfaces of the feet, is different. In a **functional leg length discrepancy,** or **apparent leg length discrepancy,** the patient's two lower limbs, as measured from the femoral heads to the plantar surfaces of the feet, are identical in length; however, other factors, such as joint or muscle contractures, cause one of the lower limbs to function as if it were shorter or longer than the other.

The *true leg length discrepancy* is caused by abnormalities that result in one of the bones of the lower limb actually being shorter or longer than its counterpart on the other side, such as varus or valgus deformities of the femoral neck, congenital anomalies of the femur or tibia, or

growth disturbances of the femur or tibia. Possible causes of a *functional leg length discrepancy* include contractures at the lumbosacral junction due to scoliosis or other causes, posttraumatic deformities of the pelvis, and abduction or adduction contractures of the hip or flexion contracture of the knee.

In evaluating a case of pelvic obliquity, the examiner should have three goals: (1) to determine whether a true leg length discrepancy or an apparent limb length discrepancy is present, (2) to determine the source of the discrepancy, and (3) to determine the magnitude of the discrepancy.

DIRECT MEASUREMENT. To distinguish between a true and a functional leg length discrepancy, the patient is asked to lie supine on the examination table with the body as straight as possible. To check for a **true leg length discrepancy,** the examiner then identifies the patient's right ASIS and places the free end of a tape measure on it. The patient is asked to hold the end in place so that the examiner can unwind the tape measure in a straight line toward the distal tip of the right medial malleolus (Fig. 5–11). The examiner records the distance and performs the same measurement on the left lower extremity. If the lengths differ significantly, a true leg length discrepancy is present. Differences of 5 mm or less are difficult to accurately assess with this method of measurement.

If the ASIS to medial malleolus distances are virtually identical, then the true leg lengths are equal and a functional leg length discrepancy may be present. To check for a **functional leg length discrepancy,** the examiner measures the distance from the patient's umbilicus to the tip of each medial malleolus (Fig. 5–12). If the ASIS to medial malleolus lengths are equal but the umbilicus to medial malleolus lengths are different, a functional leg length discrepancy is present.

BLOCK METHOD. Two other methods are available for quantitating a true leg length discrepancy. In the **block method,** blocks or books of various thicknesses may be placed under the shorter limb of the standing patient until the pelvic obliquity is eliminated and the imaginary line between the iliac crests is parallel to the floor. Measuring the thickness of material necessary to level the pelvis yields a fairly accurate estimate of the leg length discrepancy.

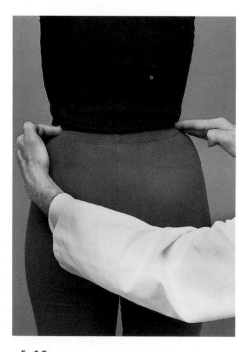

Figure 5–10. Assessing pelvic obliquity.

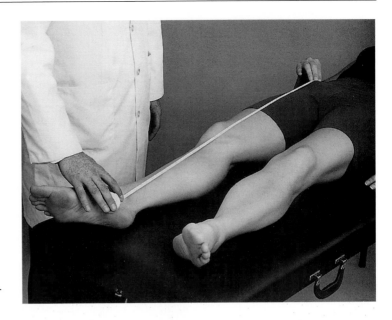

Figure 5–11. Measuring a true leg length discrepancy.

VISUAL METHOD. The last method for quantitating leg length discrepancy, the **visual method,** is particularly useful when the discrepancy is fairly small. It is also useful as a screening method when no measurement devices are available. The patient lies supine on the examination table and the examiner stands at the foot of the examination table. The examiner aligns the patient as straight as possible and, grasping the patient's feet, shifts the lower extremities until a line drawn straight between them also passes straight down the center of the patient's body (Fig. 5–13*A*). The examiner then compares the position of the two medial malleoli (Fig. 5–13*B* and *C*). If one is proximal or distal to the other, a leg length discrepancy exists. The difference in the position of the two malleoli is the magnitude of the leg length discrepancy.

ABDUCTION CONTRACTURE. Figures 5–14*A* through 5–15*B* illustrate how an abduction or adduction contracture of the hip can produce a functional limb length discrepancy. In Figure 5–14*A*, the model is simulating an **abduction contracture** of the hip, a condition in which tightness of the hip abductor muscles prevents the

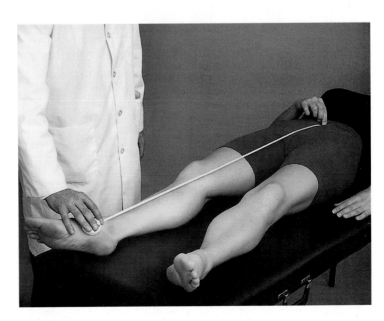

Figure 5–12. Measuring a functional leg length discrepancy.

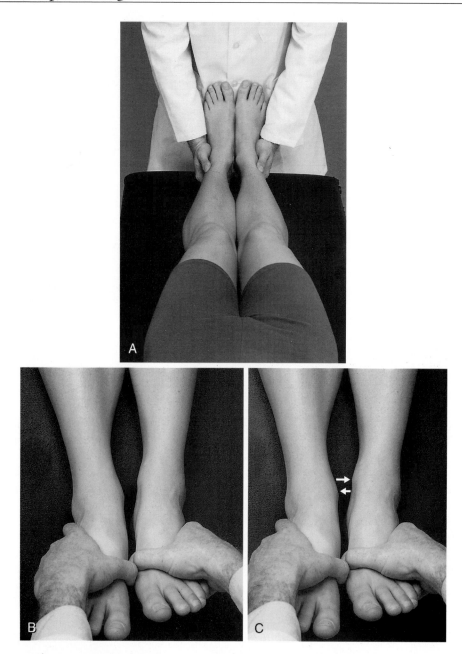

Figure 5–13. Visual method for assessing leg length discrepancy. *A,* Technique. *B* and *C,*
Closeup, comparing medial malleoli (*arrows* in *C*).

patient's hip from being adducted to the neutral
(0°) position. In order to align the involved limb
perpendicular to the floor, the patient has to drop
the pelvis on the involved side. This causes the
involved limb to be functionally long. Placing a
lift on the uninvolved side compensates for the
patient's functional lengthening of the involved
side, although the pelvis is oblique (Fig. 5–15*B*).
In the absence of a lift, patients may also
shorten the involved limb by flexing the ipsilateral knee.

ADDUCTION CONTRACTURE. In Figure 5–
15*A*, the model is simulating an **adduction contracture** of the left hip. In this case, contracture
of the adductor muscles prevents the involved
hip from being abducted to at least a neutral
position. In this case, the lower extremities may
be brought into proper alignment by placing a
lift on the involved side (see Fig. 5–15*B*). Again,
this compensates for the contracture although it
causes an oblique pelvis. In the absence of a lift,
the patient may intuitively compensate for the

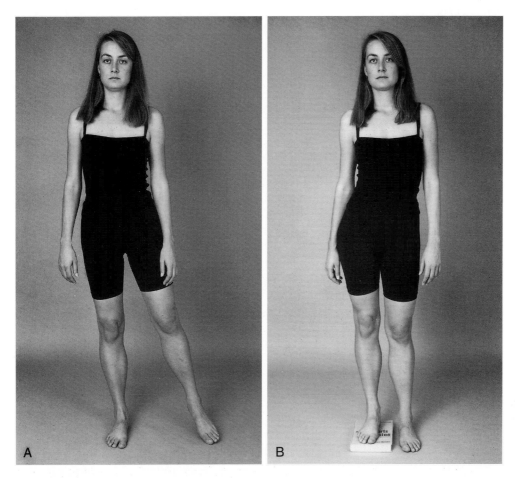

Figure 5–14. *A*, Simulated abduction contracture of the left hip. *B*, Compensation with lift under the right foot.

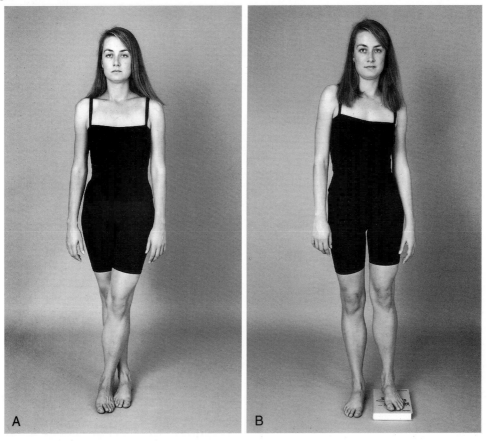

Figure 5–15. *A*, Simulated adduction contracture of the left hip. *B*, Compensation with lift under the left foot.

171

functional leg length discrepancy by flexing the contralateral knee or walking on the toes of the short limb.

FEMORAL VERSUS TIBIAL DISCREPANCY. If a true leg length discrepancy is present, further examination may determine whether the discrepancy is in the femur or the tibia. To detect a **femoral length discrepancy,** the patient lies supine on the examination table with the hips and the knees flexed to 90°. If one femur is longer than the other, the patient's knees rest at different heights from the examination table (Fig. 5–16). To detect a **tibial length discrepancy,** the patient is positioned prone with the knees again flexed to 90°. If the tibias differ in length, the soles of the patient's feet rest at different heights above the examination table (Fig. 5–17). Although uncommon, shortening in the hindfoot (talus or calcaneus) can also produce this appearance. In that case, comparing the resting position of the malleoli reveals that the tibial lengths are equal.

Flexion Contracture

Examining the standing patient from the side permits the detection of any abnormalities of pelvic rotation in the sagittal plane. Figure 5–18 illustrates how a **hip flexion contracture** can produce such an abnormality. Figure 5–18*A* shows normal sagittal alignment. In Figure 5–18*B,* the model is simulating a flexion contracture of the hips. To compensate for such an inability to fully extend the hips, a patient hyperextends the lumbar spine, as demonstrated in Figure 5–18*C.* This results in **hyperlordosis,** in which the abdomen and buttocks are more prominent than normal. When hip flexion contractures become more severe, the patient is unable to stand fully erect.

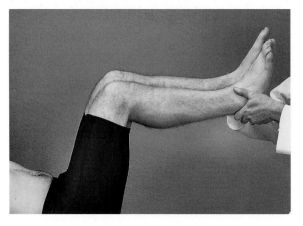

Figure 5–16. Comparing femoral lengths.

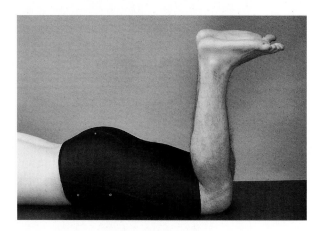

Figure 5–17. Comparing tibial lengths.

Rotational Malalignment

RESTING POSITION. In the setting of acute trauma, the patient is often first encountered in the supine position. In this situation, the **resting position** of the limb often alerts the clinician to the probable diagnosis. When a *posterior dislocation* of the hip is present, for example, the hip assumes a flexed and internally rotated position. An external rotation deformity, on the other hand, may reflect an *anterior dislocation* or a *fracture* of the hip or femur. A variable amount of apparent shortening of the limb is present as well, depending on the exact nature of the injury.

IN-TOEING/OUT-TOEING. In the ambulatory patient, the examiner may screen for rotational malalignment of the lower limbs by inspecting the standing patient from the front. When the patient is standing in a relaxed position, the feet should normally point outward approximately 10° to 20° from the straight-ahead position (Fig. 5–19). Deviation from this position while standing may be due to a rotational abnormality of the femur, the tibia, or the foot. Whatever the cause, rotational malalignment is usually named by the resulting position of the foot. Thus, an abnormality that produces internal rotation of the lower limb is called **in-toeing,** and an abnormality that produces external rotation of the lower limb is called **out-toeing.** Asking the patient to walk directly toward the examiner is another way to observe the patient's natural foot placement.

FEMORAL VERSION. When in-toeing or out-toeing is observed, additional tests may help the examiner determine whether the abnormality lies in the femur, tibia, or the foot. Rotational malalignment of the femur is usually due to variations in the version of the femoral neck. The **version** of the femoral neck refers to the angle that the femoral neck makes in relation to the

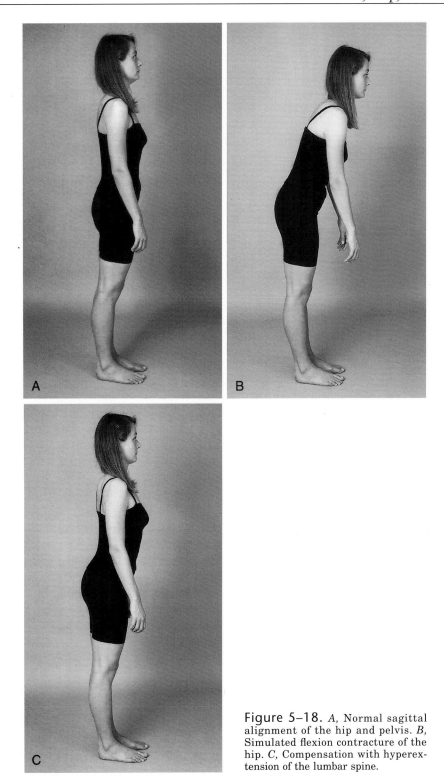

Figure 5-18. *A,* Normal sagittal alignment of the hip and pelvis. *B,* Simulated flexion contracture of the hip. *C,* Compensation with hyperextension of the lumbar spine.

coronal plane of the rest of the femur. This coronal plane is usually taken to be the plane defined by the posterior aspect of the two femoral condyles, and it may be estimated from the flexion axis of the knee. A normal femoral neck is anteverted about 8° to 15°; that is, it angles forward

8° to 15° from the plane defined by the posterior aspect of the femoral condyles.

When the femoral neck angles forward more than this, the patient is said to have **increased femoral anteversion.** A patient with increased femoral anteversion tends to stand with the limb

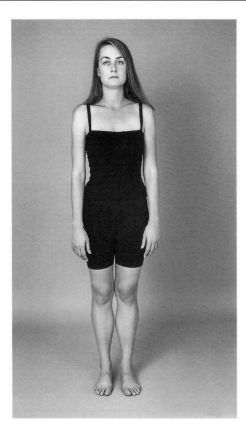

Figure 5–19. Normal standing position.

in an internally rotated position, producing in-toeing. If, however, an increased femoral anteversion is compensated by increased external rotation of the tibia, the patient does not exhibit in-toeing but rotational malalignment of the knee instead. This is described in Chapter 6, Knee.

If the femoral neck is angled less than 8° to 15° anterior to the coronal plane of the femur, the patient is said to have **decreased femoral anteversion** or **femoral retroversion.** The patient with decreased femoral anteversion tends to stand with the limb in an externally rotated position, producing out-toeing. Decreased femoral anteversion is less common than increased femoral anteversion; it may be found among ballet dancers, who are required to perform with their feet in the turned-out position.

The amount of femoral anteversion present is most precisely assessed by complex radiographic methods. However, **Craig's test** may be used to estimate the amount of femoral anteversion present. To perform Craig's test, the patient is positioned prone on the examining table, with the ipsilateral knee flexed 90°. The examiner palpates the lateral prominence of the greater trochanter with one hand while controlling the rotation of the limb with the other. An imaginary

vertical line serves as the reference for this test. The limb is then rotated until the lateral prominence of the greater trochanter is felt to be maximal (Fig. 5–20). The angle made between the axis of the tibia and the vertical is considered an approximation of the femoral anteversion. It normally varies between 8° and 15°. This is also known as the **Ryder method** for measuring femoral anteversion.

TIBIAL TORSION. Rotational abnormalities of the tibia may also produce in-toeing or out-toeing. In the normal individual, about 20° of external **tibial torsion** is present. This means that the axis of the ankle joint is externally rotated about 20° compared with the axis of the knee joint. Uncompensated external tibial torsion beyond this amount favors out-toeing, whereas less external tibial torsion, or actual internal tibial torsion, favors in-toeing. Tibial torsion can also be estimated with the patient lying prone on the examination table, the knees flexed 90°, and the tibias held vertical. The patient's ankles are held in a neutral position at right angles to the tibias. In this position, the flexion axis of the knees should be perpendicular to the length of the table (Fig. 5–21A). The examiner looks down on the patient's feet from above, estimating the angle that the medial border of the foot makes with the longitudinal axis of the thighs (Fig. 5–21B). Normally, the medial border of the foot should be externally rotated about 20° from the longitudinal axis of the table. Variations from this amount are described as increased or decreased external tibial torsion. As in the femur, rotational malalignment of the tibia may be a developmental anomaly or the sequela of a malunited fracture.

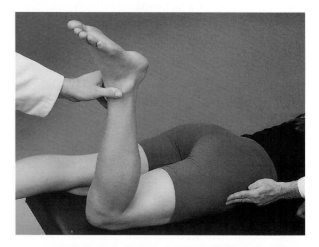

Figure 5–20. Craig's test for measuring femoral anteversion. To avoid obscuring the patient, an assistant is palpating the greater trochanter in this photograph.

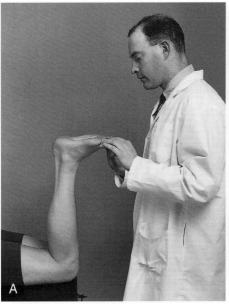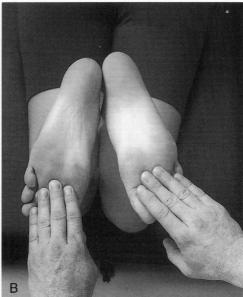

Figure 5–21. *A* and *B,* Assessing tibial torsion.

FOOT ABNORMALITIES. The final potential cause of in-toeing or out-toeing is an abnormality of the foot. When this is the case, a clear-cut foot deformity is usually present. The most common example of this is the in-toeing associated with the **forefoot adductus** deformity of an incompletely corrected *clubfoot.*

GAIT

Anterior and Posterior Perspectives

ABDUCTOR MUSCLE FUNCTION. Observation of the pelvis during gait reveals abnormalities that may not be appreciated during a static standing examination. Owing to the symmetric design of human anatomy, the body's center of gravity passes midway between the hips through the pubic symphysis. When one foot is lifted from the ground, the center of gravity generates a downward force that tends to drop the pelvis toward the side where the foot has been lifted (Fig. 5–22). This effect is similar to what would happen if a leg were removed from a stool, causing the stool to fall toward the side of the removed leg.

In humans, the gluteus medius and minimus muscles counteract the tendency of the pelvis to fall toward the opposite side by pulling it toward the greater trochanter of the weightbearing limb. These abductor muscles must be very strong because they are working at a mechanical disad-

vantage. When one lower limb is lifted off the ground to take a step, the entire upper body must be balanced on the femoral head of the weightbearing limb. The weight of the upper body can be assumed to act through its center of gravity, which passes through the pubic symphysis. The distance from the abductor muscles to the femoral head is only about half the distance from the center of gravity to the femoral head; consequently, the abductor muscles must pull with a force approximately twice the patient's upper body weight to counterbalance it. This system seems to work quite well in normal individuals, although it generates tremendous forces across the weightbearing hip joint. With the weight of the patient's upper body bearing down on one side of the femoral head and the abductor muscles pulling at a force twice the patient's upper body weight on the other side, a compressive force of three times the weight of the patient's upper body is transmitted across the weightbearing femoral head with every step.

TRENDELENBURG'S GAIT. This precariously balanced system can break down in several ways. If the gluteus medius and minimus are not quite strong enough to counterbalance the patient's upper body weight, the pelvis tends to droop toward the floor when the patient is bearing weight on the weak limb. This results in an exaggerated up-and-down motion of the pelvis during ambulation known as **Trendelenburg's gait** (Fig. 5–23). In a Trendelenburg gait, the patient's pelvis sags

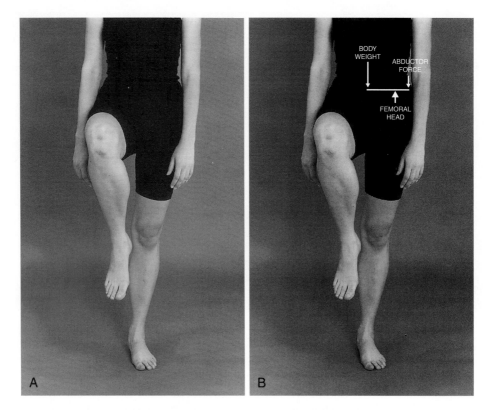

Figure 5–22. *A* and *B*, Diagram of forces across the hip during single-leg stance.

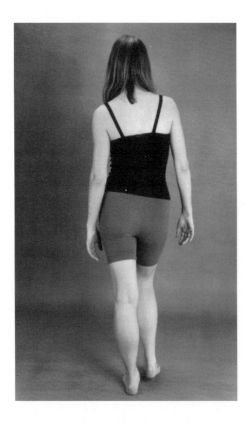

Figure 5–23. Trendelenburg's gait.

every time the patient lifts the uninvolved limb to take a step.

ABDUCTOR LIMP. If the abductor muscles are even weaker, further modifications of gait need to be made to prevent the patient from falling over when bearing weight on the involved limb. By leaning over toward the side of the weight-bearing limb, the patient brings his or her center of gravity closer to the femoral head. This decreases the leverage of the patient's upper body weight and thus decreases the counterbalancing force that needs to be exerted by the abductor muscles. The corresponding gait abnormality, with its dramatic shift of body position, is often known as an **abductor limp** or **abductor lurch** (Fig. 5–24). When compensation of this sort is necessary in both hips, the side-to-side shifting of the patient's upper body during ambulation is quite dramatic.

An abductor limp may also be present in a patient with a painful hip joint but otherwise normal abductor strength. This is because shifting the center of gravity of the upper body to a position closer to the femoral head reduces the counterbalancing force required in the abductor

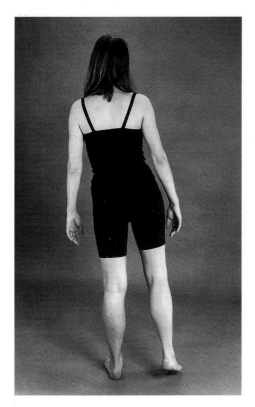

Figure 5–24. Abductor limp (lurch).

muscles, thus dramatically reducing the compressive force across the painful hip joint. Close examination of these patients reveals no evidence of a pelvic droop or of abductor weakness. This gait abnormality is common in osteoarthritis of the hip.

PELVIC ROTATION. Some **pelvic rotation** in the **coronal plane** occurs during normal gait and is exaggerated in some pathologic conditions of the hip joint, such as muscle weakness or hip arthritis, resulting in a waddling appearance when the patient walks. Pelvic rotation in the **transverse plane** is also normal during gait, and it occurs as each lower extremity swings forward to accept the body weight of the next step.

Lateral Perspective

FLEXION CONTRACTURE. Observing the patient from the lateral perspective during gait reveals abnormalities in hip flexion and extension. As previously mentioned, a **flexion contracture** of the hip may produce an increase in the normal lumbar lordosis or a forward-stooping posture. A

short stride length may become apparent owing to the patient's inability to fully flex and extend the contracted or arthritic hip. Excessive lumbar flexion and extension may be noticed as the patient attempts to maintain a normal stride length by increasing the motion of the lumbar spine.

GLUTEUS MAXIMUS LURCH. A **gluteus maximus lurch** occurs in patients who have a weak gluteus maximus. The gluteus maximus normally locks the hip in extension as the contralateral limb is advanced for the next step. A patient with a weak gluteus maximus may thrust the pelvis forward and trunk backward, shifting the center of gravity posterior to the hip and thereby reducing the force that the gluteus maximus needs to generate to lock the hip in extension (Fig. 5–25).

RANGE OF MOTION

Pelvis

Two types of motion are associated with the pelvis. The first type includes the motions that occur between the pelvic bones themselves at the pubic

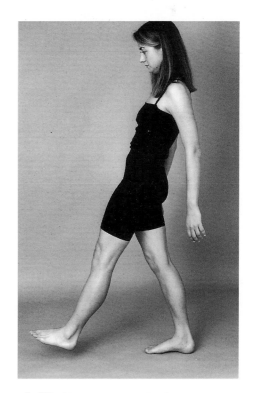

Figure 5–25. Gluteus maximus lurch.

symphysis and sacroiliac joints. These are small motions that are difficult to detect by external examination. The second type of motion involves changes in the position of the entire pelvis in space and in relation to the rest of the body. The movement that permits this change in pelvic position occurs at the joints of the adjacent lumbar spine and hips.

Flexion and extension of the pelvis occur in the sagittal plane and involve rotation of the entire pelvis around an imaginary transverse axis. This is the predominant pelvic motion detectable during gait and with flexion during the physical examination. During **pelvic flexion,** the superior pelvis rotates posteriorly, whereas during **pelvic extension,** the superior pelvis rotates anteriorly. **Pelvic flexion** is produced by flexion of the lumbar spine combined with reciprocal extension of the hips (Fig. 5–26*A*), whereas **pelvic extension** is produced by extension of the lumbar spine combined with reciprocal flexion of the hips (Fig. 5–26*B*). Abnormal limitation of pelvic flexion and extension may result in a shortened stride length when walking, particularly when accompanied by arthritis or contractures about the hip joint.

Hip

As a ball-and-socket joint, the hip is second only to the shoulder in the range and complexity of its potential motion. The hip's potential movement is conventionally divided into three movement pairs: flexion-extension, abduction-adduction, and internal rotation–external rotation.

In evaluating hip range of motion (ROM), it is important to distinguish movement that occurs in the hip joint itself from complementary or compensatory motion that occurs in the adjacent lumbar spine and between the lumbar spine and the pelvis. This is accomplished either by stabilizing the pelvis or by taking care to detect accompanying pelvic motion as soon as it occurs. Active and passive ROM at the hips are usually evaluated together. Because the possible motions are complex and potentially confusing, the exam-

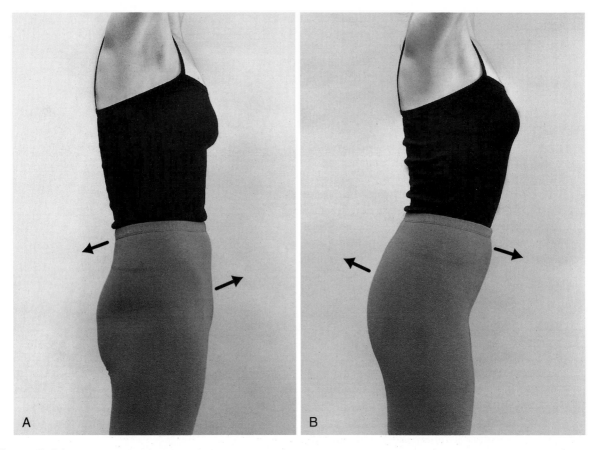

Figure 5–26. *A,* Pelvic flexion. *B,* Pelvic extension. (*Arrows* show direction of motion.)

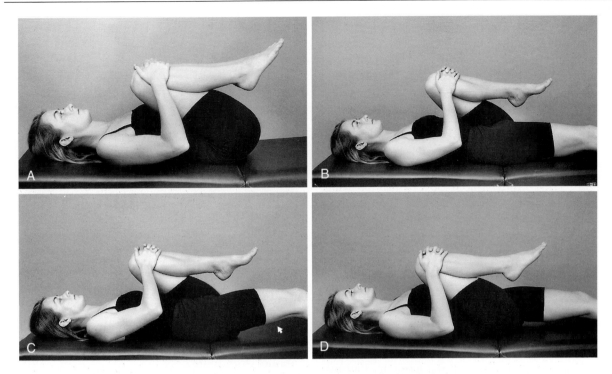

Figure 5–27. Thomas test. *A,* Preparation. *B,* Assessing extension of the right hip. *C,* Demonstrating flexion contracture of the right hip *(arrow). D,* Assessing flexion of the right hip.

iner usually guides the patient's active execution of the ROM maneuvers and passively assists when necessary.

FLEXION AND EXTENSION. Anterior motion in the sagittal plane is defined as hip **flexion,** whereas posterior motion is defined as **extension.** These are the hip motions that are most vital to normal ambulation and sitting. Luckily, they are usually the last to be restricted by the stiffness that often accompanies osteoarthritis of the hip. Significant loss of flexion and extension at the hip places increased stress on the lumbar spine and produces severe gait abnormalities.

Hip flexion and extension are usually assessed with a method called the **Thomas test.** The Thomas test seeks to control flexion and extension of the pelvis and thereby assess the true ROM arising from the hip joint. This is particularly important owing to the considerable ability of the lumbar spine to mimic hip flexion and extension.

The Thomas test for flexion and extension of the hip is performed with the patient lying supine on the examination table. The patient is encouraged to flex both hips until the knees touch the chest; the examiner assists as necessary (Fig. 5–27A). The patient or the examiner maintains the patient's knees positioned tightly against the patient's chest. This maneuver locks the pelvis in maximal flexion, eliminating the ability of the lumbar spine to extend. The hip to be tested for **extension** is then released and allowed to extend to the table while the opposite hip remains tightly held against the patient's chest (Fig. 5–27B).

In a normal patient, the extending thigh should be able to touch the examination table. This is considered neutral or 0° of extension. If the hip being tested is unable to extend enough to allow the thigh to reach the table, a flexion contracture (loss of extension) is said to be present (see Fig. 5–27C). The flexion contracture can be quantitated by estimating or measuring with a goniometer the angle formed by the central axis of the thigh and the top of the examining table.

To measure **flexion,** both knees are again positioned against the patient's chest. The contralateral thigh is now allowed to fall to the examination table while the thigh of the hip being tested is kept in maximal flexion. The angle between the table and the midline of the thigh being examined represents the maximal amount of flexion and can be measured or estimated (see Fig. 5–27D). In normal patients, at least 110° of hip flexion should be present.

During the Thomas test, one hip is positioned in maximal flexion while the other is positioned in maximal extension. Because it is customary to measure the ROM in both hips, the maximal flexion of one hip can be measured at the same time that the extension of the opposite hip is being gauged, thus minimizing the number of maneuvers necessary to test the flexion and extension of both hips.

Extension past 0° may be assessed with the patient lying prone (Fig. 5–28). In this position, it is important to guard against the patient's natural tendency to augment true hip extension by hyperextending the lumbar spine.

ABDUCTION AND ADDUCTION. Abduction

and **adduction** may be assessed in two positions: (1) with the hips extended and (2) with the hips flexed. For both these assessments, the patient is positioned supine on the examination table. Because the pelvis is capable of motion in a fashion that would supplement abduction and adduction, the examiner must observe for such complementary motion of the pelvis when assessing these movements.

To test **abduction in extension,** the examiner stands at the side of the examination table facing the supine patient. One of the examiner's hands grasps the patient's ankle while the examiner's other hand is placed lightly on the ASIS. This allows the examiner to detect any complementary motion of the pelvis during abduction. The examiner then passively abducts the patient's lower extremity away from the midline until the pelvis is just felt to start moving (Fig. 5–29). The angle between the axis of the thigh and the midline of the patient at this point is considered to be the maximal amount of abduction present.

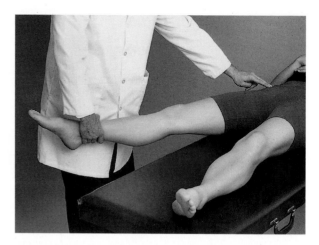

Figure 5–29. Hip abduction in extension.

Most patients' hips should be able to abduct to about 45° in the extended position, and some can abduct even more.

To test **adduction in extension,** the examiner reverses direction and adducts the patient's lower extremity as far as possible. On reaching the midline, it is necessary to flex the hip slightly to allow the extremity being examined to pass in front of the contralateral limb. Again, the limb is adducted until complementary motion of the pelvis is perceived to begin by the hand placed on the ASIS (Fig. 5–30). The angle between the midline of the extremity being tested and the midline of the patient is considered to be the amount of adduction present. Normal adduction in the extended position is about 30°.

Abduction and adduction may also be tested with the hip in the flexed position. This is usually done by instructing the patient to draw the extremity being tested up toward his or her chest until the foot is adjacent to the contralateral knee. To test **abduction in flexion,** the hip is then allowed to fall outward into a position of abduction; the examiner assists as necessary. One of the examiner's hands is placed on the ASIS to detect pelvic rotation supplementing the abduction of the hip (Fig. 5–31). The amount of abduction present is assessed by estimating the angle between the patient's thigh and an imaginary vertical plane drawn down the midline of the patient's body. To measure **adduction in flexion,** the examiner grasps the patient's knee and adducts the thigh back across the midline while gently pressing posteriorly on the ipsilateral ASIS to prevent the pelvis from rotating (Fig. 5–32). The range of abduction and adduction in the flexed position is similar to the range when measured in extension.

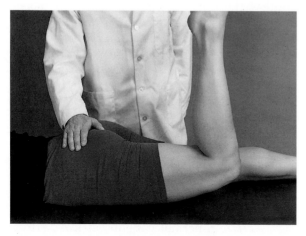

Figure 5–28. Prone hip extension.

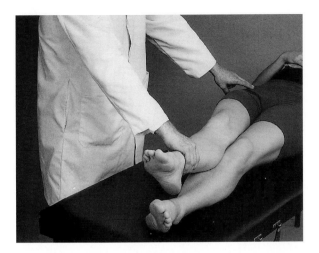

Figure 5–30. Hip adduction in extension.

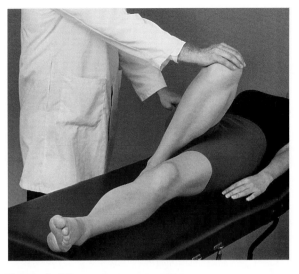

Figure 5–32. Hip adduction in flexion.

ROTATION. Hip rotation also may be measured in both the flexed and the extended positions. The rotational motions observed in these two positions may differ owing to soft tissue contractures about the hip. The rotational ROM in extension affects foot placement (in-toeing or out-toeing) during ambulation, and thus it is physiologically more important. The loss of external rotation in the flexed position may manifest itself by difficulty trimming the toenails or putting on shoes. Patients with early *degenerative arthritis of the hip joint* frequently lose rotation in the affected hip before losing flexion or abduction. In addition, they often report groin pain at the limits of passive hip rotation. A careful assessment of hip rotation allows the examiner to detect degenerative changes in the hip at an early stage.

Hip **rotation in extension** may be assessed in either the supine or the prone position. To assess rotation in the **supine position,** the patient is asked to lie comfortably on the examination table with the hips and knees extended. Before beginning the examination, note the **resting position** of the lower extremities. Normally, the weight of the thigh should cause the hips to externally rotate about 30°, and an imaginary line drawn along the medial border of the foot can be used as a pointer to indicate the position of rotation present. An acute or chronic *slipped capital femoral epiphysis* causes the involved hip to rest in a position of increased external rotation. A malunited hip fracture can cause a similar external rotation deformity in an older patient.

To assess the maximal passive **external rotation** possible, the examiner grasps the patient's feet, then uses them to fully externally rotate the lower extremities at the hip (Fig. 5–33). The orientation of the medial border of the foot may be used to estimate the amount of external rotation present. This normally averages about 45°. The examiner then internally rotates the entire limb and estimates the amount of **internal rotation** present (Fig. 5–34). This is usually less than the amount of available external rotation and averages about 35°. An increase in internal rotation at the expense of external rotation may indicate *increased femoral anteversion* (internal femoral torsion), which is twice as common in females. Conversely, external rotation that is increased at the expense of internal rotation may

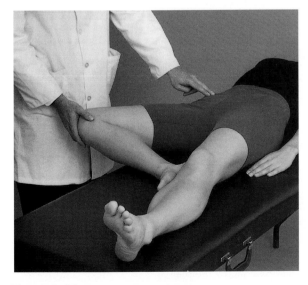

Figure 5–31. Hip abduction in flexion.

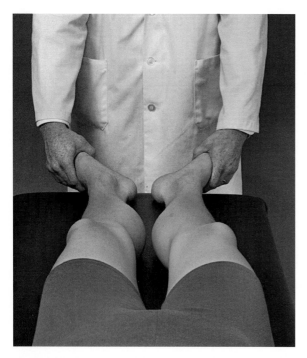

Figure 5–33. Hip external rotation in extension, supine position.

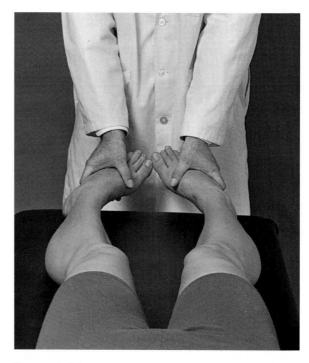

Figure 5–34. Hip internal rotation in extension, supine position.

indicate *femoral retroversion* (external femoral torsion), a common sequela of *slipped capital femoral epiphysis*. *Developmental dysplasia* of the hip may also result in increased external rotation.

Hip **rotation in extension** may also be assessed with the patient in the **prone position**. In this case, the patient's knees are flexed and the axis of the tibia is used as the indicator of the

amount of rotation present (Fig. 5–35*A*). If this method of measurement is selected, the examiner must remember that during **internal rotation** of the hip, the foot moves away from the midline, whereas during **external rotation** of the hip, the foot moves across the midline.

Hip **rotation in flexion** may be measured with the patient supine or seated. For the supine examination, the examiner grasps the patient's

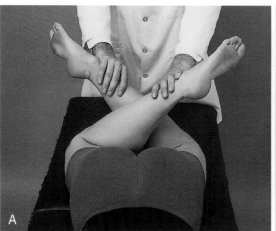
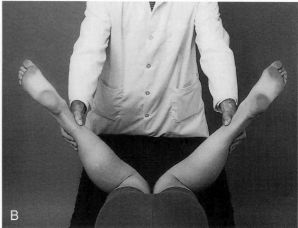

Figure 5–35. Hip rotation in extension, prone position. *A,* External rotation. *B,* Internal rotation.

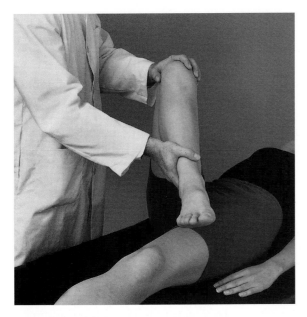

Figure 5–36. Hip external rotation in flexion.

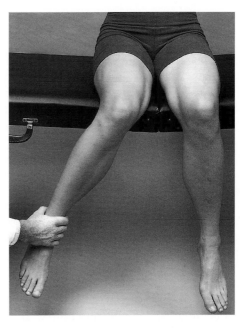

Figure 5–38. Hip rotation in flexion, seated position.

knee in one hand and foot in the other hand, flexing both the hip and the knee to 90°. The hand at the knee gently stabilizes the thigh, while the hand grasping the foot, first externally (Fig. 5–36) and then internally (Fig. 5–37), rotates the entire limb at the hip. The axis of the tibia is used to estimate the amount of rotation present. In the authors' experience, these motions average about 45° of external rotation and 30° of internal rotation, although the American Academy of Orthophaedic Surgeons handbook reports average internal rotation to be 45° in this position. If passive hip rotation is painful, pathology of the hip joint or femoral neck should be suspected.

Rotation in flexion may also be assessed with the patient in the **seated position.** Except for the fact that the patient has been rotated 90° in space, the examination in the seated position is identical to the procedure just described for the supine position. The potential advantage of the seated position is that the patient's body weight tends to stabilize the pelvis and prevent pelvic rotation from supplementing hip motion (Fig. 5–38).

It is important to note that the presence of a prosthetic hip is a contraindication to evaluating hip rotation or abduction-adduction in the flexed position. In the presence of a prosthesis, rotation is more safely assessed with the hip extended. Failure to heed this warning may result in the dislocation of a prosthetic hip, especially in the early postoperative period.

Palpation

Palpation for localized tenderness often helps to pinpoint the cause of pain around the hip and the pelvis. Often, the patient helps direct the examiner to the appropriate area by indicating the spot where the pain appears to be centered.

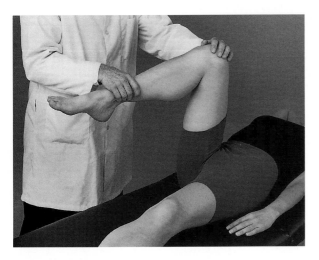

Figure 5–37. Hip internal rotation in flexion.

Anterior Aspect

ILIUM. The ASIS is an easily identifiable landmark in most patients and a good place to start palpation (see Fig. 5–1). The **ASIS,** serving as the origin of the sartorius muscle, is a common site for one of the *apophyseal avulsion fractures* that tend to occur in adolescents. Other sites include the iliac crest, the AIIS, the ischial tuberosity, and the lesser trochanter. Because these fractures are often minimally displaced and thus difficult to identify radiographically, the finding of localized tenderness over one of the typical apophyses may be the primary means of diagnosing an avulsion fracture about the hip.

Moving posteriorly from the ASIS, the examiner's fingers are able to trace the rest of the **iliac crest.** The anterior portion of the iliac crest is another common site of avulsion injury. This may present as an acute fracture or an overuse injury of insidious onset, in which case the condition is usually called *iliac apophysitis.* Exquisite tenderness over the iliac crest following a direct blow suggests the presence of a localized hematoma colloquially known as a *hip pointer,* a common injury in football and other contact sports.

Medial and inferior to the ASIS, lies the **AIIS,** a deeper and much smaller prominence that is palpable only in leaner individuals. The finding of localized tenderness at the AIIS in an adolescent suggests the possibility of an *avulsion fracture* caused by the rectus femoris origin.

About 2 cm medial to the ASIS, the **lateral femoral cutaneous nerve** passes under the inguinal ligament on its way to the anterior thigh. Compression of this nerve can produce a syndrome of dysesthesia in the anterolateral thigh known as *meralgia paresthetica.* Although the nerve itself cannot be identified by palpation, percussion of the nerve at this location may reproduce the patient's symptoms and thus confirm the suspected diagnosis. Percussion is usually performed with one or two fingertips in the same manner used to perform **Tinel's test** of other nerves.

LESSER TROCHANTER. The **lesser trochanter** is located in the floor of the femoral triangle deep to the sartorius. The prominence of the lesser trochanter cannot be distinctly felt in normal individuals, but deep palpation at this location usually yields a sense of firm resistance. Tenderness of the lesser trochanter in an adolescent suggests the possibility of an *avulsion fracture* caused by the iliopsoas muscle, which inserts here. The distal iliopsoas tendon is another common cause of the *snapping hip* syndrome. This type of snapping hip classically occurs in dancers but may be seen in many different individuals. A snapping iliopsoas tendon should be suspected if hip extension produces pain in the proximal medial thigh. Placing the lower limb in the figure-four position facilitates palpation of the lesser trochanter (Fig. 5–39). The finding of tenderness at the lesser trochanter in a patient with a snapping hip points to the iliopsoas tendon as the cause of the syndrome.

PUBIS. At the medial end of the anterior pelvis lies the superior pubic ramus and adjacent **pubic symphysis** (see Fig. 5–1). These landmarks are palpable at the superior margin of the normal area of pubic hair growth, although their definition varies greatly depending on the habitus of the patient. In a lean individual, the contours of the symphysis may be discernible at the midline, whereas in a heavier patient, only the general feeling of resistance provided by the bone is perceived. The pubic symphysis may be disrupted by acute trauma or inflamed by recurrent stress. This latter condition, known as *pubic symphysitis,* is common in soccer players owing to the forces created by the strong adductor muscles. The pubic ramus itself is a common site of fracture, particularly in elderly individuals.

NEUROVASCULAR STRUCTURES. The **femoral artery** passes under the inguinal ligament into the anterior thigh about midway between the ASIS and the pubic symphysis. Moderately firm palpation with the tips of two or three fingers at this site allows the examiner to identify the femoral artery pulse (Fig. 5–40). The femoral artery is a good point of orientation for locating other

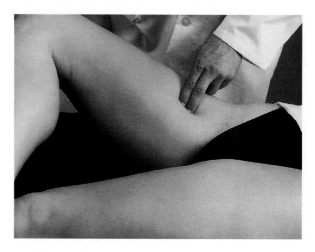

Figure 5–39. Palpation of the lesser trochanter.

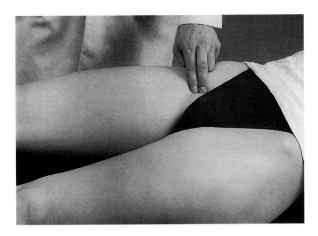

Figure 5–40. Palpation of the femoral artery.

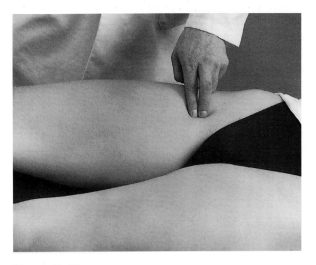

Figure 5–41. Palpation of the hip joint.

structures of the anterior hip region. The **femoral nerve** lies just lateral to the artery, and the **femoral vein** and associated lymphatics are located medial to it. Enlargement of lymph nodes in this vicinity is commonly associated with infection further distally in the lower limb.

HIP JOINT. The acetabulum and the **hip joint** are located about 2 cm lateral and 2 cm inferior to the point where the femoral pulse is palpable. This spot should be palpated for deep tenderness (Fig. 5–41). Although the outlines of the hip joint cannot be discerned, the finding of tenderness at this location suggests that the patient's pain is indeed due to a problem at the hip joint, such as arthritis, infection, slipped capital femoral epiphysis, or femoral neck fracture.

FEMORAL SHAFT. Distal to the trochanters, the **femoral shaft** is deeply enveloped in muscle until it flares out to form the femoral condyles. Because of this, palpation for bony tenderness is not as valuable for femoral shaft stress fractures as it is in the evaluation of possible stress fractures of other long bones. Palpation is, however, valuable in the evaluation of muscle injuries of the thigh.

QUADRICEPS. The large **quadriceps** muscle group is subject to two distinct types of injury: (1) muscle contusions caused by a direct blow to the muscle and (2) muscle strains or *pulls* caused by a violent eccentric contraction of the muscle itself.

In the case of a *quadriceps contusion,* careful gentle palpation allows identification of the area of injury and often delineation of an associated hematoma. When palpating these injuries, the

examiner should be alert not only for tenderness but also for warmth. When a warm firm swelling develops following a quadriceps contusion, the patient is at risk of developing the syndrome of ectopic calcification known as *myositis ossificans.*

When palpating a *quadriceps strain,* the examiner should search carefully for a divot or defect in the muscle. Such deformities are usually subtle but can occasionally be dramatic. Quadriceps strains are not typically associated with myositis ossificans. The severity of both quadriceps contusions and strains can be graded by the restriction of **prone knee flexion** that results. To do so, the examiner asks the patient to lie prone and to flex the knee as far as possible (Fig. 5–42). In severe contusions or strains, the patient is unable to flex the knee even to 90°.

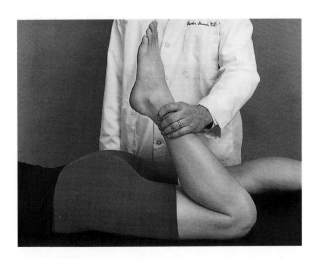

Figure 5–42. Prone assessment of knee flexion to grade the severity of quadriceps contusion or strain.

SARTORIUS. Injuries of the sartorius most commonly involve the origin near the ASIS, as already described. Identification of the proximal sartorius may be facilitated by asking the patient to place the lower limb in a figure-four position. Further distally, the sartorius is difficult to distinguish from the quadriceps in most individuals, although isolated injury to this portion of the sartorius is unusual.

Lateral Aspect

GREATER TROCHANTER. The most prominent landmark of the lateral hip and thigh is the **greater trochanter.** The **greater trochanteric bursa,** located between the bony trochanter and the overlying iliotibial tract, is a common site of painful inflammation. In obese patients, flexing and extending the hip during palpation allows the examiner to feel the trochanter moving underneath the palpating fingers and thus identify it (Fig. 5–43).

Tenderness directly over the most prominent portion of the trochanter suggests *trochanteric bursitis.* In severe cases, the examiner actually feels soft tissue crepitance as passive flexion and extension of the hip cause the trochanter to slide beneath the iliotibial tract. Trochanteric bursitis may be associated with tightness of the iliotibial tract as judged by Ober's test. Impingement of the iliotibial tract on the greater trochanter is another common cause of the *snapping hip* syndrome. In the presence of a snapping iliotibial tract, the examiner can palpate and often see the

band snap back and forth across the trochanter as the hip is passively flexed and extended in the side-lying patient. Flexing the patient's knee and adducting the hip may increase the magnitude of the snapping sensation. In contrast to trochanteric bursitis, which produces tenderness directly over the greater trochanter, *gluteus medius tendinitis* is associated with tenderness just superior to this bony prominence. Tenderness just posterior to the trochanteric prominence suggests the possibility of *piriformis tendinitis.*

Posterior Aspect

ILIUM. The **PSIS,** located at the posterior terminus of the iliac crest, is the primary landmark for orientation and palpation of the posterior pelvis and hip (Fig. 5–44; see also Fig. 5–5). Immediately deep, lateral, and inferior to the PSIS, the examiner may begin to palpate the **sacroiliac joint** (Fig. 5–44*B*). This usually is palpable as a ridge of bone that can be followed inferiorly from the PSIS. Tenderness or swelling of the sacroiliac joint may be caused by injury, infection, or an inflammatory arthritis, such as *ankylosing spondylitis.*

SCIATIC NOTCH. The **sciatic notch** lies midway between the PSIS and the ischial tuberosity (Fig. 5–45). This deep landmark is difficult to palpate with certainty, although in thin patients the examiner may appreciate a shallow groove beneath the gluteus maximus at this location. Even when the outlines of the sciatic notch cannot be felt, the finding of tenderness at this location suggests the presence of *sciatica,* a syndrome usually caused by lumbar disk disease. The sciatic nerve may also be palpated midway between the greater trochanter and the ischial tuberosity when the patient's hip is flexed.

SACRUM AND COCCYX. In the posterior midline, the firm prominence created by the sacral promontory is usually easily palpable. Tenderness of the **sacrum** may be caused by fracture, tumor, or infection. By following the sacrum distally into the natal crease, the examiner can identify and palpate the **coccyx** (Fig. 5–46). Owing to its location, the coccyx is a common site of pain, whether due to a fall on the buttocks or chronic irritation from prolonged sitting. *Coccyodynia,* or painful coccyx, may be caused by overuse, fracture, or disruption of one of the joints between the small segments that constitute the coccyx.

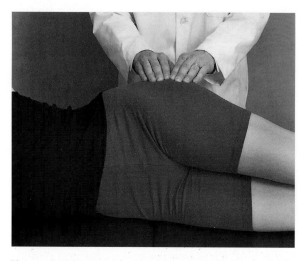

Figure 5–43. Palpation of the greater trochanteric bursa.

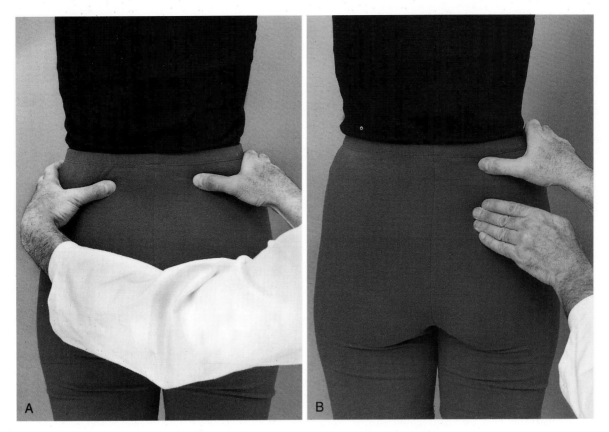

Figure 5–44. *A,* Palpation of the posterior superior iliac spine. *B,* Palpation of the sacroiliac joint.

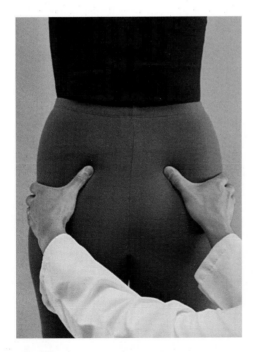

Figure 5–45. Palpation of the sciatic notch.

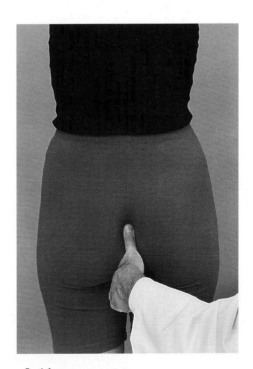

Figure 5–46. Palpation of the coccyx.

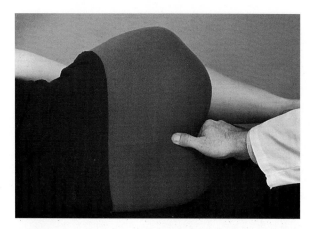

Figure 5–47. Simulated manipulation of the coccyx during rectal examination.

If any uncertainty exists, a rectal examination can be helpful in confirming the coccyx as the site of pain. In this case, the patient is placed in the decubitus position and the upper hip flexed. The examiner performs a **rectal examination** with the index finger. This allows the examiner to grasp the coccyx between the index finger, from within the rectum, and the thumb, from the outside (Fig. 5–47). The coccyx may then be manipulated back and forth to see whether pain is elicited.

ISCHIUM. The **ischial tuberosity** is located at the medial inferior margin of the gluteal prominence in the standing patient. However, palpation of the ischial tuberosity is most easily accomplished with the patient lying supine and the ipsilateral hip flexed 45° with the foot resting comfortably on the table (Fig. 5–48). Tenderness

of the ischial tuberosity may indicate an *avulsion fracture* due to the hamstrings that originate there or from a direct fall onto the buttocks. Inflammation of the bursa, which occurs over the ischial tuberosity in individuals who habitually sit on hard surfaces, is sometimes known as *weaver's bottom.*

PIRIFORMIS. Knowledge of the location of major tendon insertions of the posterior aspect of the hip helps the examiner differentiate among various sources of posterior hip pain. The **piriformis tendon** inserts into the piriformis fossa on the posterior superior aspect of the greater trochanter beneath the inferior border of the gluteus medius muscle. The piriformis fossa is not palpable directly, but lies beneath the hook of the greater trochanter, which may be palpated with the patient lying with the leg maximally internally rotated (Fig. 5–49). In this position, the most prominent posterior structure on the greater trochanter is the hook of the trochanter. Tenderness to deep palpation at this site, combined with a positive piriformis test as described in the Manipulation section, suggests the presence of *piriformis tendinitis.*

GLUTEUS MAXIMUS. The **gluteus maximus** tendon may be palpated near the gluteal fold at the inferior aspect of the gluteus maximus. Tenderness at this location, combined with a painful response to **Yeoman's test,** suggests a *gluteus maximus tendinitis.*

HAMSTRINGS. Hamstring injuries are primarily strains that occur during eccentric contraction of the muscle. They may involve almost any portion of the muscles, from their origins on

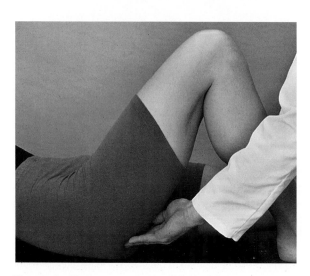

Figure 5–48. Palpation of the ischial tuberosity.

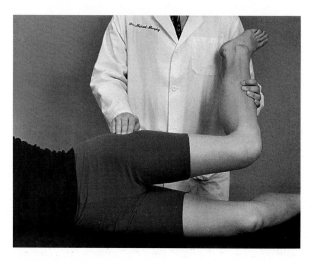

Figure 5–49. Palpation of the piriformis fossa.

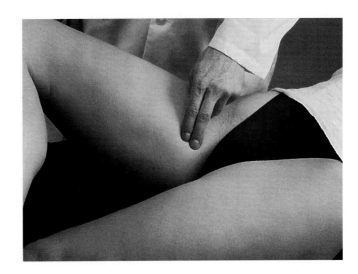

Figure 5–50. Palpation of the adductor longus.

the ischial tuberosity to just above the knee. The majority seem to occur in the proximal thigh. As with the quadriceps, hamstring injuries should be carefully palpated for defects or, rarely, complete disruption. Severe hamstring strains significantly restrict the passive straight-leg raising test and may produce a tripod sign, as described in the Manipulation section.

Medial Aspect

The adductor muscle group constitutes the primary mass of the medial thigh. The proximal portion of the **adductor longus** is the most distinctive component of the adductor group. Placing the lower limb in a figure-four position allows the examiner to easily palpate and often visualize this muscle as it originates from the pubis

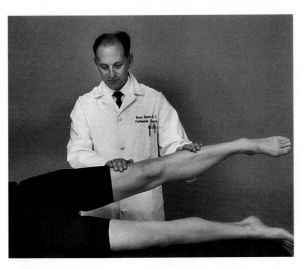

Figure 5–51. Assessing hip abduction strength.

(Fig. 5–50). The muscle mass just posterior to the adductor longus consists of the **adductor brevis, gracilis,** and **adductor magnus** muscles. Further distally, the muscles are not easily distinguished. Strains of the adductor group are often called *groin pulls*. Significant tears of the adductor longus can cause the muscle mass distal to the tear to bunch up in a prominence, which can be misconstrued as a soft tissue tumor if the history of trauma is not elicited.

Manipulation
MUSCLE TESTING

Abductors

The **gluteus medius** muscle is the principal hip abductor, with the **gluteus minimus** and **tensor fascia lata** functioning as auxiliary abductors. All three are innervated by the *superior gluteal nerve.* Hip abduction strength is best tested with the patient lying on the opposite side with the hips and knees extended. The patient is asked to abduct the limb away from the examination table. The examiner then presses downward against the limb at about the level of the knee, instructing the patient to resist the examiner's attempt to push the limb back down toward the table (Fig. 5–51). In a normal patient, it should be very difficult for the examiner to overcome the patient's abductor muscle strength. Abductor weakness is a common sequela of arthritis of the hip joint.

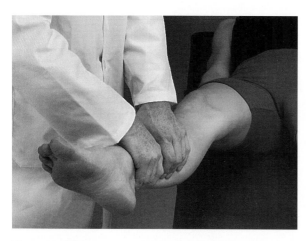

Figure 5–52. Assessing adduction strength.

Adductors

Hip adduction strength is supplied by the **adductors longus, brevis,** and **magnus,** and the **gracilis.** Innervation of these muscles is primarily via the *obturator nerve,* although the *sciatic nerve* contributes to the innervation of the adductor magnus. Testing the hip adductors against gravity is awkward because the patient must lie on the hip being tested to do so. Therefore, the adductors are usually tested with the patient lying supine on the examination table with the hips and knees fully extended. The examiner then passively abducts the limb to be tested and instructs the patient to attempt to adduct the limb back to the midline as powerfully as possible while the examiner resists (Fig. 5–52). Although the adductor muscle group is not as strong as the abductor group, the examiner should still have some difficulty resisting hip adduction in a normal patient.

Flexors

Hip flexor strength is provided primarily by the **iliopsoas** muscle, assisted by the **rectus femoris** and **sartorius.** These muscles are all innervated by the *femoral nerve,* except for the psoas portion of the iliopsoas, which is innervated directly by the second and third lumbar nerve roots.

Hip flexor strength can be tested in more than one way. To emphasize the contribution of the iliopsoas, the flexor strength is tested with the patient sitting on the side of the examination table with both the hip and the **knee flexed.** The patient is then asked to lift the thigh off the table while maintaining knee flexion. The examiner presses downward on the patient's knee while the patient tries to maximally resist the examiner's pressure (Fig. 5–53A). In normal patients, considerable resistance is noted, although the examiner should be able to overcome the strength of the iliopsoas. Hip flexor strength may also be tested with the **knee extended.** In this case, the patient lies supine on the examination table with the hip and knee fully extended.

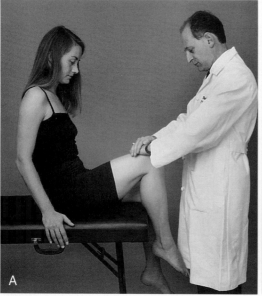
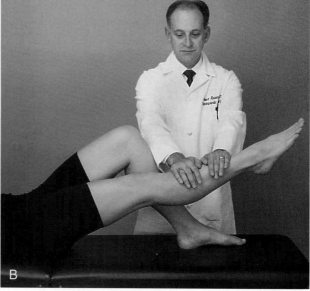

Figure 5–53. *A,* Assessing hip flexor strength, seated position. *B,* Assessing hip flexor strength, supine position (Stinchfield's test).

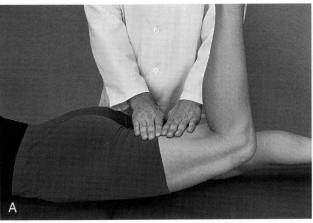
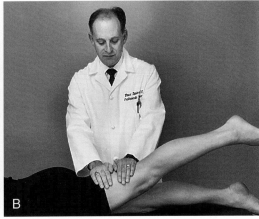

Figure 5–54. Assessing hip extensor strength. *A,* With knee flexed. *B,* With knee extended.

The patient is then asked to perform an active straight-leg raise, lifting the limb to be tested off the table while maintaining knee extension. Again, the examiner pushes downward against the patient's leg while the patient tries to resist the downward pressure (Fig. 5–53*B*). In this position, the examiner should be able to overcome the strength of a normal patient but with some difficulty. This maneuver causes significant compressive force across the hip joint, and so may elicit pain in the presence of hip pathology (see Stinchfield's test under Other Tests). If desired, the patient may flex the contralateral hip and knee to stabilize the pelvis and take stress off the lower back during this maneuver.

Extensors

The **gluteus maximus** is the principal hip extensor. Because the **hamstring** muscles cross both the hip and the knee, they also function as auxiliary hip extensors. The gluteus maximus is innervated by the *inferior gluteal nerve,* whereas the hamstrings are innervated by the *sciatic nerve.*

Hip extensor strength is tested with the patient lying prone on the examination table with the knee flexed or extended. If the patient's knee is flexed to 90°, the hamstrings are relaxed and the test tends to isolate the gluteus maximus. The patient is instructed to lift the thigh off the examination table while maintaining knee flexion. The examiner then presses downward on the patient's distal thigh, attempting to push the thigh back to the examination table while the patient maximally resists (Fig. 5–54*A*). In the normal patient, it should be difficult for the ex-

aminer to overcome the strength of the gluteus maximus. When this test is used to screen for gluteus maximus tendinitis, it is often called **Yeoman's test.** In the presence of gluteus maximus tendinitis, Yeoman's test should reproduce the patient's pain. Active hip extension may also be tested with the knee extended if greater participation of the hamstrings is desired (Fig. 5–54*B*).

SENSATION TESTING

Compression neuropathy of the **lateral femoral cutaneous nerve,** often called *meralgia paresthetica,* is a fairly common condition. The nerve is usually compressed near the ASIS. This syndrome may produce hypoesthesia or paresthesias in the nerve distribution over the anterolateral thigh. This deficit may be looked for by testing light touch or sharp/dull sensation over the proximal to middle portion of the anterolateral thigh (Fig. 5–55).

SPECIAL TESTS

Tests for Joint Contractures

THOMAS' TEST. Some of the available tests for hip joint contractures are described in the Inspection section under Range of Motion. The **Thomas test** is a valuable screening tool for loss of hip extension (flexion contracture) and flexion. Similarly, the **abduction-adduction ROM test** detects abduction or adduction contractures of the hip. Several other tests are in common use for evaluation of the hip joint.

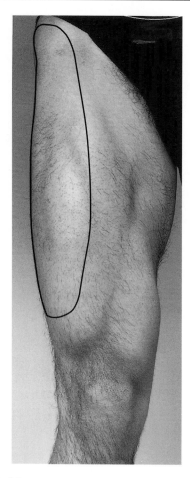

Figure 5–55. Average sensory distribution of the lateral femoral cutaneous nerve.

OBER'S TEST. The first of these is the Ober test for contractures of the *iliotibial tract.* A tight iliotibial tract may be associated with trochanteric bursitis or snapping hip syndrome proximally and iliotibial band tendinitis (iliotibial band friction syndrome) at the knee. The Ober test is performed with the patient in the lateral decubitus position with the side to be tested facing up. The patient's knee is flexed 90°, then the hip is abducted about 40° and extended to its limit (Fig. 5–56A). While the hip extension and knee flexion are maintained and the pelvis stabilized, the limb is gently adducted toward the examination table (Fig. 5–56B). In a normal patient, the hip should be able to be adducted past the midline of the body. Inability to adduct the hip past the midline indicates a contracture of the iliotibial tract.

ELY'S TEST. The **Ely test** is designed to detect contractures of the *rectus femoris* muscle. It is based on the anatomic fact that the rectus femoris originates above the hip and inserts below the knee, thus crossing both joints. To perform the Ely test, the patient is positioned prone on the examination table with the knees extended. The examiner then passively flexes the knee on the side to be tested. In the normal patient, the knee should be able to flex fully without causing any motion of the hip or pelvis (Fig. 5–57A). In

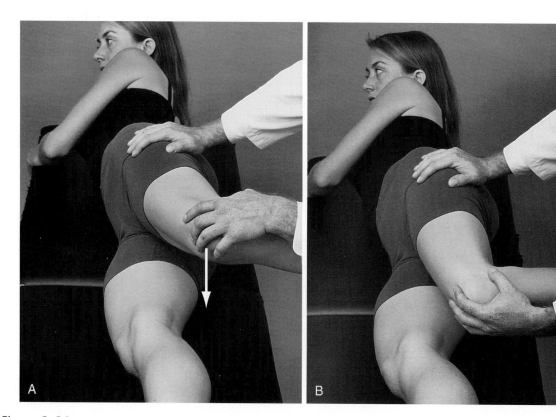

Figure 5–56. *A* and *B,* Ober's test (*arrow* in *A* indicates direction of movement).

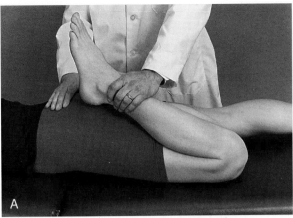
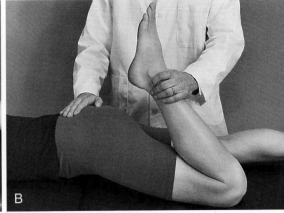

Figure 5–57. Ely's test. *A,* Normal. *B,* Abnormal (tight rectus femoris).

the presence of a tight rectus femoris, full passive knee flexion produces involuntary flexion at the hip, causing the buttocks to rise off the examination table (Fig. 5–57*B*).

TRIPOD SIGN. The tripod sign can alert the examiner to a contracture of the hamstring muscle group. This sign may occur during the performance of the seated straight-leg raising maneuver. The examiner asks the patient to sit on the side of the examining table with the knees bent to 90°. The examiner then grasps the patient's ankle on the side to be tested and passively extends the knee fully. A normal patient should be able to allow the knee to be fully extended and yet remain seated upright (Fig. 5–58*A*). In the patient with tight hamstrings, passive extension

of the knee results in involuntary extension of the ipsilateral hip. This involuntary hip extension causes the patient's trunk to fall backward, often to the point that the patient will need to support himself or herself with outstretched hands (Fig. 5–58*B*). *Sciatic nerve* irritation causes a similar response and must be considered if this test is positive. If the tripod sign is due to tight hamstrings alone, nerve root tension signs such as Lasegue's sign and the bowstring sign should be absent. Tests for sciatica are discussed in Chapter 9, Lumbar Spine.

PHELPS' TEST. The **Phelps test** is designed to detect contractures of the *gracilis* muscle, which originates from the pubis and ischium and inserts into the pes anserinus on the proximal me-

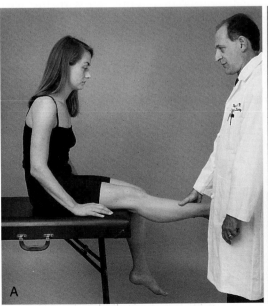
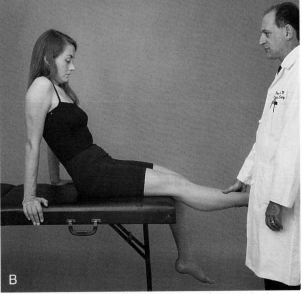

Figure 5–58. Tripod sign. *A,* Normal. *B,* Abnormal.

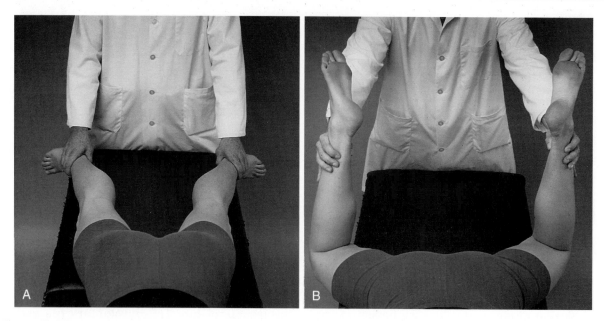

Figure 5–59. *A* and *B,* Phelps' test.

dial tibia. To perform it, the patient is placed in the prone position on the examining table with the knees fully extended. The examiner then passively abducts the patient's hips to the maximal degree possible (Fig. 5–59*A*). The patient's knees are then flexed, thereby relaxing tension in the gracilis muscles, and the examiner attempts to abduct the hips further (Fig. 5–59*B*). If the patient's hips are capable of further abduction when the knees are flexed, a significant gracilis contracture is present.

Screening Tests for Tendinitis

As in other parts of the body, two general types of tests can be used to screen for tendinitis about the hip. The *first type* of test consists of having the patient perform a **resisted contraction** of the suspected muscle-tendon unit to see if pain is elicited. The tests already described to assess the strength of the major muscle groups about the hip can be used for this purpose. For example, resisted hip extension (Yeoman's test) may be painful in the presence of gluteus maximus tendinitis. The *second type* of test consists of **stretching** the suspected muscle-tendon unit to see whether pain is elicited. The tests already described for muscle contractures about the hip may be used for this purpose. For example, Ely's test may be painful in the presence of proximal rectus femoris tendinitis.

In addition to the tests already described, the examiner should be familiar with the **piriformis test.** As already noted, the piriformis muscle exits the pelvis and inserts into the posterior superior portion of the greater trochanter, where it functions primarily as an external rotator of the hip. In most individuals, the sciatic nerve exits the pelvis just distal to the piriformis, but in about 15% of the population, the nerve actually passes through the piriformis. The tendon of the piriformis may become painful as an isolated phenomenon or in conjunction with hip pathology.

The **piriformis test** is performed with the patient in the lateral decubitus position with the side to be examined facing up. The patient's hip is flexed 45° with the knee flexed about 90°. The examiner stabilizes the patient's pelvis with one hand to prevent pelvic rotation (Fig. 5–60*A*). The examiner's other hand then pushes the flexed knee toward the floor, thus internally rotating the hip (Fig. 5–60*B*). This maneuver stretches the piriformis muscle and elicits pain when the muscle is tight or involved with tendinitis.

If the pain is not localized to the piriformis tendon but radiates in a manner suggestive of sciatica, a *piriformis syndrome* should be suspected. The piriformis syndrome is an uncommon cause of sciatica in which the radiation of pain along the course of the sciatic nerve is caused by entrapment within the piriformis muscle instead of lumbar disk disease.

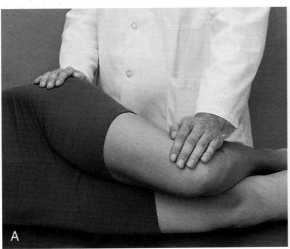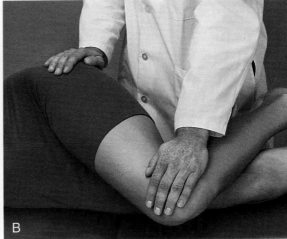

Figure 5–60. *A* and *B*, Piriformis test.

Pelvic Stress Tests

PATRICK'S TEST. Several tests are designed to screen for pain arising from the joints of the pelvis. They may be helpful in localizing pain due to pathology such as arthritis or infection of these joints. They are provocative tests designed to elicit pain by stressing an affected joint. The most well known of these is **Patrick's test** of the sacroiliac joint. Patrick's test is also known as the **FABER test,** an acronym for **F**lexion-**AB**duction **E**xternal **R**otation, the figure-four position in which the test is performed.

To perform Patrick's test, the patient is placed supine on the examination table, and the limb to be examined is guided into the figure-four position with the ipsilateral ankle resting across the contralateral thigh proximal to the knee joint. The examiner then presses downward on the ipsilateral knee with one hand while providing counterpressure with the other hand on the contralateral ASIS (Fig. 5–61). This maneuver tends to stress the sacroiliac joint on the side being tested. In the normal patient, this maneuver should not be painful. If Patrick's test produces posterior hip pain, pathology of the sacroiliac joint should be suspected. An arthritic hip may also be painful when placed in this position, but the pain is normally felt in the anterior groin. The figure-four position also places the iliopsoas muscle on stretch. Pathology of the iliopsoas, such as an intrapelvic abscess irritating the iliopsoas sheath, leads to pain in this position. This is sometimes called the **iliopsoas sign.**

Figure 5–61. Patrick's test.

GAENSLEN'S TEST. Gaenslen's test is another indirect stress test for the sacroiliac joint. To perform it, the patient is positioned supine on the examination table with the buttock of the side to be examined projecting over the side of the table. The patient is instructed to draw both knees up to the chest, as in the first step of the Thomas test (Fig. 5–62*A*). The examiner carefully stabilizes the patient while the ipsilateral thigh is allowed to drop off the side of the table, thus fully extending the hip (Fig. 5–62*B*). This maneuver stresses the ipsilateral sacroiliac joint. If it induces pain in the sacroiliac joint, then pathology of that joint is suggested.

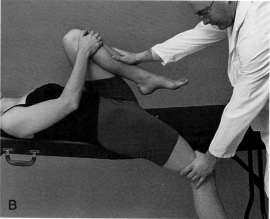
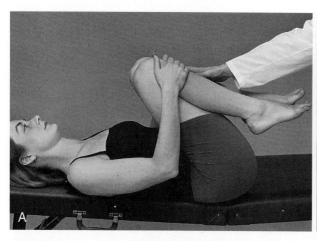

Figure 5–62. *A* and *B*, Gaenslen's test.

LATERAL PELVIC COMPRESSION TEST. The **lateral pelvic compression test** is a screening examination for pathology of the major joints of the pelvic ring. To perform it, the patient is placed in the lateral decubitus position on the examination table. The examiner presses on the iliac crest, thus compressing the pelvis against the examination table (Fig. 5–63). Pain localized by the patient to either sacroiliac joint or the pubic symphysis is indicative of pathology at that site.

ANTEROPOSTERIOR PELVIC COMPRESSION TEST. The **anteroposterior pelvic compression test** is analogous to the lateral pelvic compression test but compresses the pelvis in a different plane. In this case, the patient lies supine on the examination table, and the examiner presses downward on the pubic symphysis (Fig. 5–64). This maneuver may be slightly uncomfortable but should not be painful in a normal patient. As in the lateral pelvic compression test, pain localized to one of the major joints of the pelvis suggests pathology in that joint.

PUBIC SYMPHYSIS STRESS TEST. The **pubic symphysis stress test** is designed to detect instability or pain associated with an injured or inflamed pubic symphysis. It is performed with the patient lying supine on the examination table. The examiner places one hand on the superior aspect of one pubic bone and the other hand on the inferior aspect of the other pubic bone. The hands are then pushed toward each other, creating a shearing motion at the pubic symphysis (Fig. 5–65). The test is positive if motion or pain is produced with this maneuver. In the case of an acute fracture or major disruption, gentle palpation may be sufficient to arrive at a diagnosis.

Other Tests

STINCHFIELD'S TEST. The **Stinchfield test** is an excellent tool to screen for pathology of the hip joint. This maneuver is designed to simulate the normal walking forces across the hip joint and usually elicits pain in the presence of any significant hip pathology such as arthritis, fracture, or infection. The test is performed by asking the supine patient to perform an active straight-leg raise with the ipsilateral knee locked in extension (see Fig. 5–52*B*). This maneuver generates a force 1.8 to 2 times the patient's body

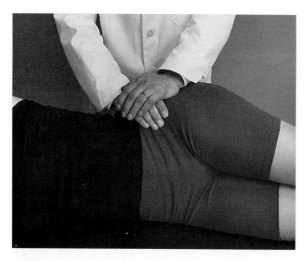

Figure 5–63. Lateral pelvic compression test.

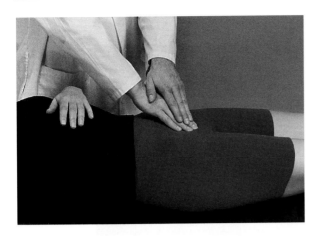

Figure 5–64. Anteroposterior pelvic compression test.

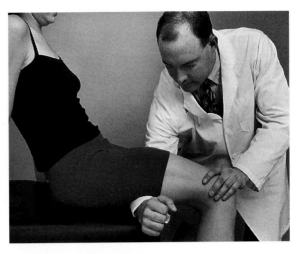

Figure 5–66. Fulcrum test.

weight across the hip joint. If attempting this maneuver produces pain, pathology of the hip joint should be suspected. If the response is equivocal, the examiner may add manual resistance to increase the compressive force. The examiner must keep in mind that pathology involving the hip flexors, such as an avulsion fracture or tendinitis, is also painful with this maneuver.

FULCRUM TEST. The **fulcrum test** helps in the detection of stress fractures of the femoral shaft. This condition may occur in the high demand athlete as well as in the nonathletic individual with metabolic bone disease, such as osteoporosis. Although the fulcrum test may be used to screen for stress fractures of other long bones, it is particularly helpful in the femur because the femoral shaft is enveloped in muscle and cannot be easily palpated. The fulcrum test is performed with the patient seated at the side

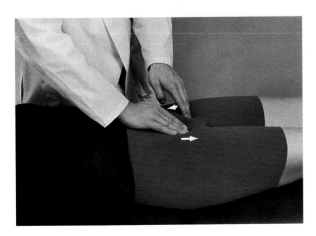

Figure 5–65. Pubic symphysis stress test (*arrows* indicate direction of applied forces).

of the examination table. The examiner places one forearm beneath the middle of the patient's thigh to serve as a fulcrum and then presses down on the ipsilateral knee (Fig. 5–66). This maneuver places a bending force along the femoral shaft. If the maneuver is painful, a stress fracture of the femoral shaft should be suspected.

TRENDELENBURG'S TEST. The **Trendelenburg test** is a screening examination for weakness of the hip abductor muscles: the gluteus medius and the gluteus minimus. The pathomechanics of Trendelenburg's test have already been delineated in the section describing Trendelenburg's gait. To perform the Trendelenburg test, the examiner stands or sits behind the standing patient (Fig. 5–67A). The patient is then asked to lift each foot off the ground in turn. When the left foot is lifted, the right abductor muscles are being tested; when the right foot is lifted, the left abductor muscles are being tested. Normally, the abductors should be strong enough to allow the pelvis to remain level when a foot is lifted off the ground (Fig. 5–67B). Frequently, the unsupported side actually rises slightly due to the normal contraction of the abductor muscles of the weight-bearing limb. If the abductors are weak, the pelvis droops toward the unsupported side when the foot is lifted from the ground (Fig. 5–67C). In cases of more severe weakness, the patient is unable to lift the opposite foot without leaning sideways over the weight-bearing limb (Fig. 5–67D). This maneuver uses the same adaptation that produces the abductor lurch during gait.

The physical findings in common conditions of the pelvis, hip, and thigh are summarized in Table 5–1.

Bruce Reider

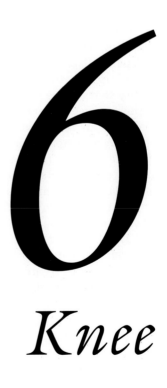

6

Knee

The largest joint in the body, the knee has been the subject of intense investigation since the late 1970s. The driving force behind this research has been a very practical one: owing to its location at the middle of the weightbearing lower extremity, the knee is subject to a great variety of traumatic and degenerative conditions.

Outwardly simple, the knee is actually quite complex. At first glance, it is a hinge joint connecting two major bones, the femur and the tibia. It is actually two interconnected joints, however, whose articular surfaces blend together: the patellofemoral and the tibiofemoral joints. It is also more than just a simple hinge. Subtle but significant amounts of rotation complicate the job of its ligaments and make their function more difficult to assess. The addition of the menisci, which serve to increase the contact area between the femur and the tibia, provides yet another site of potential injury or malfunction.

The tibiofemoral joint is inherently unstable. The rounded contours of the femoral condyles perch tenuously on the relatively flat tibial plateaus. Although the menisci do increase the contact area, this nevertheless incongruous joint is heavily dependent on its ligaments for adequate stability. Injuries to these ligaments can result in morbidity that ranges from the mild and transient to the severe and permanent.

The patella is by far the largest sesamoid bone in the body. A sesamoid bone is an ossicle that forms in a tendon, in this case the quadriceps tendon. The patella acts as a fulcrum, greatly increasing the mechanical advantage of the quadriceps and, thus, its effective strength. The patella's exposed position on the front of the knee puts it at great risk for direct trauma. In addition, the sesamoid nature of the patella renders it subject to potentially unbalanced muscular forces that can lead to instability, pain, or degeneration.

Inspection

Owing to its exposed position in the middle of the lower extremity, the knee is probably more amenable to visual examination than any other major joint in the body. Because it is crossed by very little muscle tissue, except posteriorly, its bony prominences, tendons, and subcutaneous ligaments usually are more visible than the corresponding structures of other major joints. Although this is particularly true in lean individuals, many abnormalities can be detected even in obese patients if the examiner knows where to look.

SURFACE ANATOMY

Anterior Aspect

PATELLA. Whether viewed from the front or the sides, the **patella** forms the visual focal point of the knee (Fig. 6–1). Normally, only a thin layer of tendon, bursa, and subcutaneous tissue lies between the patella and the skin. Even in obese patients, subcutaneous fat tends to be relatively sparse over the patella. In such patients, the patella often appears as a depression amid the billows of the surrounding limb (Fig. 6–2). The prominence of the patella is normally accentuated by the presence of a depression or sulcus on both sides. In these areas, the patellar retinaculum and the underlying synovium are stretched from the patella to the adjacent femoral condyles. When excess fluid is present in the knee, whether from a hemarthrosis, a pyarthrosis, or a synovial effusion, these sulci fill up, and the prominence of the patella is reduced, although the bone remains subcutaneous.

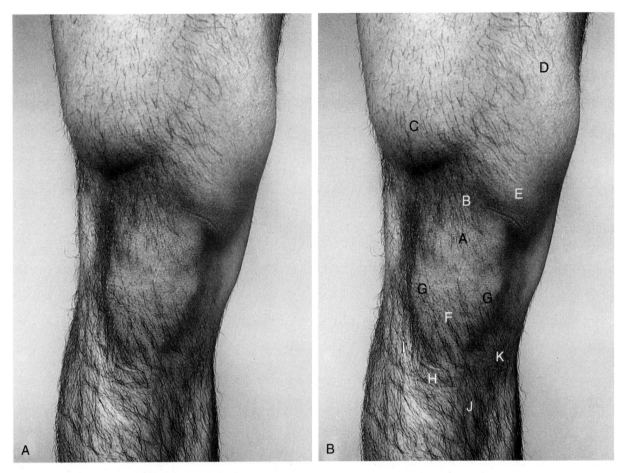

Figure 6–1. *A* and *B*, Anterior aspect of the knee. A, patella; B, quadriceps tendon; C, vastus lateralis; D, vastus medialis; E, vastus medialis obliquus; F, patellar tendon; G, Hoffa's fat pad; H, tibial tubercle; I, tubercle of Gerdy; J, pes anserinus; K, medial tibial plateau.

The patella normally appears oval. In the presence of **bipartite patella,** distortion of this shape may be visible. Most commonly, this is manifested as a protruding prominence at the supralateral aspect of the patella (Fig. 6–3). The

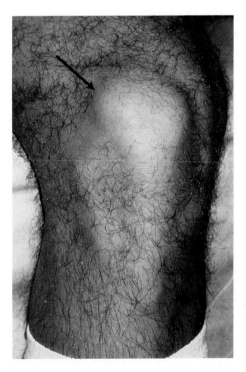

Figure 6–3. Bipartite patella. The *arrow* indicates the location of the supralateral accessory fragment.

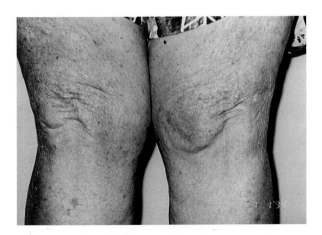

Figure 6–2. Knees of an obese individual.

203

accretion of osteophytes around the edges of the patella can create an enlarged appearance known as **patella magna** (Fig. 6–4).

PREPATELLAR BURSA. *Prepatellar bursitis* presents with a very characteristic clinical appearance: a subcutaneous egg-like swelling anterior to the patella. This swelling is usually fairly soft and fluid-filled. An average prepatellar bursa measures about 5 cm in diameter, but it may be several times that size in individuals who have spent a lot of time on their knees, such as wrestlers, roofers, or carpet layers (Fig. 6–5). This predisposing factor often is reflected in the rough, thickened skin overlying the bursa. If the bursa is infected, the overlying skin is erythematous and hot. Chronic thickening or nodule formation can sometimes be seen or palpated in a prepatellar bursa that has been inflamed in the past.

EXTENSOR MECHANISM. Along with the patella, the distal quadriceps muscles and the associated tendinous structures are sometimes collectively referred to as the *extensor mechanism* of the knee. These structures complement the patella in giving the anterior aspect of the knee its typical appearance. The **quadriceps complex** is formed by the central rectus femoris muscle, flanked medially by the vastus medialis and laterally by the vastus lateralis. The fourth component, the vastus intermedius, lies deep to the rectus femoris.

The anatomy of the distal quadriceps is best appreciated with the knee in full extension, especially when the muscles are set (Fig. 6–6). The

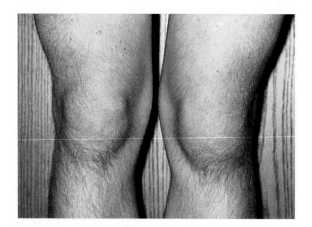

Figure 6–5. Appearance of a knee with prepatellar bursitis (left knee).

quadriceps tendon is the common tendon of insertion of the **rectus femoris** and the **vastus intermedius,** with additional contributions from the two other vasti. Because the muscular portions of the **vastus medialis** and the **vastus lateralis** extend much more distally than those of the rectus femoris, the quadriceps tendon is usually visible as a distinct hollow between the bulges created by these two muscle bellies. The vastus lateralis muscle belly usually terminates

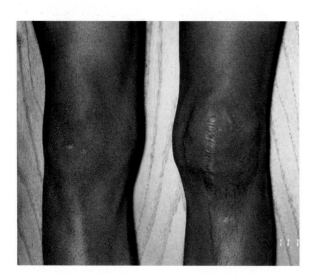

Figure 6–4. Patella magna in the left knee due to osteophytes.

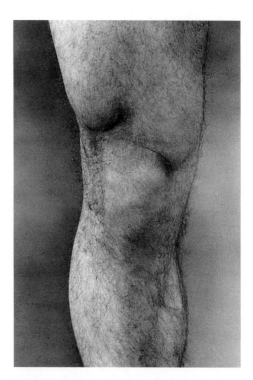

Figure 6–6. Appearance of the anterior aspect of the knee with the quadriceps set.

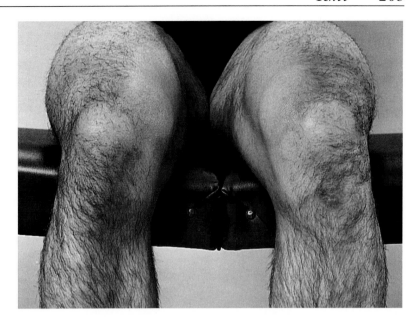

Figure 6–7. Appearance of the knee in flexion.

about 2 cm proximal to the patella, and the muscle fibers of the vastus medialis extend even further distally, almost inserting into the supero-medial aspect of the patella. The distal prominence of the vastus medialis muscle is formed by oblique fibers whose direction tends much more toward the transverse than the majority of the vastus medialis muscle fibers. This portion is called the **vastus medialis obliquus** and is thought to stabilize the patella against lateral subluxation. In some individuals with recurrent patellar instability, the quadriceps mechanism is dysplastic, and the normal prominence of the vastus medialis obliquus may be reduced or entirely absent.

PATELLAR TENDON AND INFRAPATELLAR FAT PAD. Distal to the patella is the **patellar tendon** or patellar ligament, the broad flat band that connects the patella to the tibia. The **infrapatellar fat pad,** or **Hoffa's fat pad,** bulges forward on both sides of the patellar tendon and may obscure it. Flexing the knee causes the fat pad to retract and increase the visibility of the patellar tendon (Fig. 6–7). *Ganglion cysts* are occasionally found in or around the fat pad, where they appear as firm nodular or multilobulated masses.

PROXIMAL TIBIA. The patellar tendon inserts on a bony prominence of the anterior tibia called the **tibial tubercle,** or **tibial tuberosity.** This prominence may be enlarged if the patient has had *Osgood-Schlatter disease* (Fig. 6–8). The enlargement is formed by abnormal bone accretion

at the tibial tubercle and by ossicle formation in the distal patellar tendon. A similar, subtler swelling at the distal tip of the patella may be seen in patellar tendinitis, or *jumper's knee,* and *Sinding-Larsen-Johansson disease.* Lateral and slightly proximal to the tibial tubercle is another prominence known as the **tubercle of Gerdy,** which serves as the insertion point of the iliotibial tract. Medial to the tibial tubercle, the curved contour of the **medial tibial plateau** usually can be seen. The **pes anserinus,** a structure formed by the confluence of the sartorius, the gracilis, and the semitendinosus tendons, inserts on the tibia in this region. The pes anserinus is not usually visible.

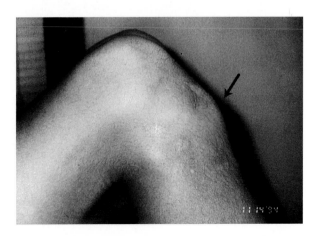

Figure 6–8. Enlarged tibial tubercle in Osgood-Schlatter disease *(arrow).*

Medial Aspect

MEDIAL EPICONDYLE AND MEDIAL COLLATERAL LIGAMENT. Much less prominent than the patella, the **medial epicondyle** is, nevertheless, often detectable in the normal knee (Fig. 6–9). The medial epicondyle is a small promontory located at the superior edge of the medial femoral condyle. The insertion of the adductor muscles terminates at the superior portion of this prominence; the term **adductor tubercle** is thus often used interchangeably with the term *medial epicondyle*.

With regard to knee anatomy, the medial epicondyle is most important as the origin of the superficial fibers of the **medial collateral ligament** (MCL), also known as the **tibial collat-**

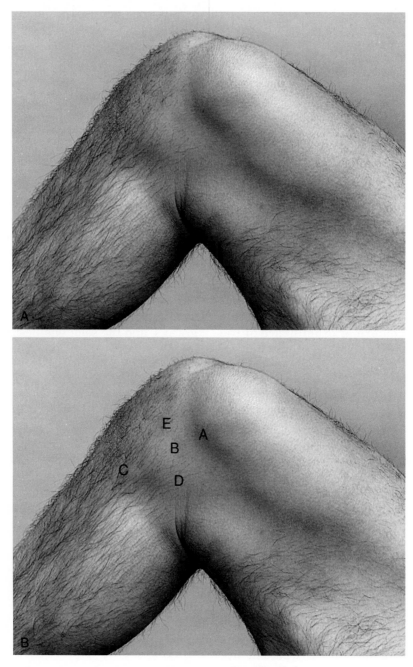

Figure 6–9. *A* and *B*, Medial aspect of the knee. A, medial epicondyle; B, medial collateral ligament; C, pes anserinus; D, semimembranosus insertion; E, medial joint line.

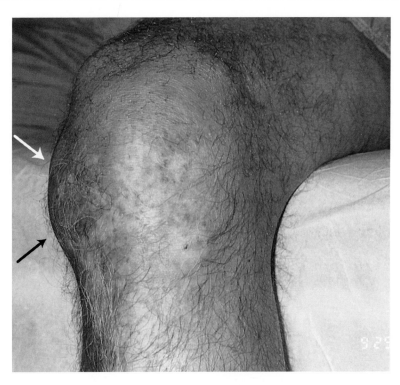

Figure 6–10. Visible osteophytes in an osteoarthritic knee *(arrows)*.

eral ligament. These fibers course obliquely across the medial joint line in an anterioinferior direction, inserting broadly on the tibia underneath the **pes anserinus.** This latter structure, formed by the confluence of the tendons of the sartorius, the semitendinosus, and the gracilis muscles, is not directly visible. However, its characteristic location on the flare of the medial tibial plateau can usually be identified.

Because it is the proximal attachment of the MCL, the prominence of the medial epicondyle may be increased in the face of sprains involving the proximal fibers of this ligament. In the acute case, the increased prominence may be due to localized hemorrhage and edema. In the chronic case, a calcific deposit may form; this occurrence is identified radiographicly as the *Pelligrini-Stieda sign.* On physical examination, the existence of this calcification may manifest itself as an enlargement of the prominence of the medial epicondyle.

MEDIAL JOINT LINE. The anterior border of the MCL can occasionally be seen and usually palpated in leaner individuals. It is most easily visualized in the flexed knee. In lean subjects, the anterior portion of the **medial femorotibial joint line** is visible as a subtle depression. The point where the line disappears is the anterior edge of the MCL. In the presence of osteoarthritis, *periarticular osteophytes* may create a visible ridge along the medial joint line (Fig. 6–10). *Medial meniscus cysts,* which are quite rare, can produce a round firm swelling at the middle or posterior portions of the medial joint line.

SEMIMEMBRANOSUS TENDON. The **semimembranosus** tendon has its own insertion on the posteromedial aspect of the tibia; it is quite distinct from the insertion of the pes anserinus tendons. This tendon can normally be visualized only in the leanest individuals; however, in most patients, the tendon can be palpated behind the knee. The insertion of the semimembranosus is an anatomist's delight, with seven distinct components. Most of these can be distinguished only by dissection. However, if the semimembranosus tendon is followed distally to the tibia, the direct insertion into the posteromedial tibia just inferior to the joint line can usually be distinctly appreciated.

Lateral Aspect

LATERAL EPICONDYLE. The prominence of the **lateral epicondyle** is more difficult to see than that of its medial counterpart. It is best visualized with the knee in 90° of flexion (Fig. 6–11). The lateral epicondyle is a very small prominence on the lateral femoral condyle that serves as the proximal point of attachment of the **lateral collateral ligament** (LCL), also known as the **fibular collateral ligament.**

LATERAL COLLATERAL LIGAMENT. The distal attachment of the LCL is at a small tubercle on the fibular head. The **fibular head** itself is located more posteriorly than often appreciated, and it is also best visualized with the knee flexed 90°. The LCL courses distally across the joint in a posterolateral direction, opposite in direction to the course of the MCL. In lean individuals, the LCL is more likely to be visible than its medial counterpart. Having the subject cross the legs in a so-called figure-four position places a varus stress on the knee that pulls the LCL taut and

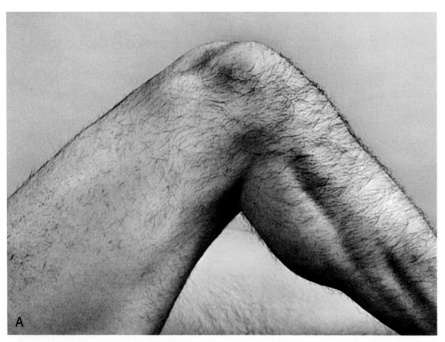

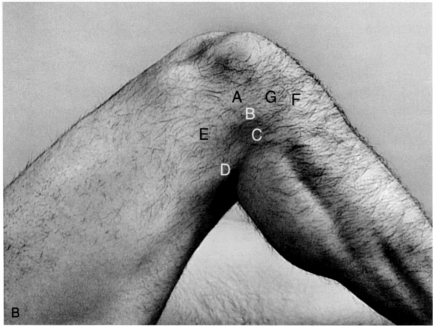

Figure 6–11. *A* and *B*, Lateral aspect of the knee. A, lateral epicondyle; B, lateral collateral ligament; C, fibular head; D, biceps tendon; E, iliotibial tract; F, tubercle of Gerdy; G, lateral joint line.

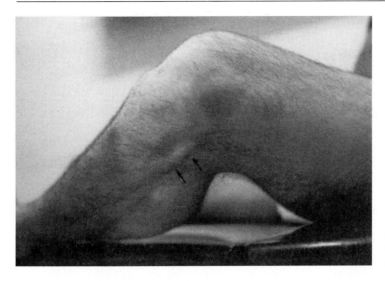

Figure 6–12. Lateral collateral ligament seen with the knee in the figure-four position *(arrows)*. (From Reider B: Sports Medicine: The School-Age Athlete. Philadelphia, WB Saunders, 1996, p 325.)

increases its prominence (Fig. 6–12). The **biceps tendon,** the sole hamstring on the lateral aspect of the knee, also inserts into the fibular head, approaching it from the posterior aspect and inserting around the distal LCL. It is also visible in the flexed knee of many individuals.

ILIOTIBIAL TRACT. Proceeding anteriorly from the biceps tendon, one encounters a small depression and then another prominent longitudinal band, the **iliotibial tract.** The iliotibial tract is a thickening of the *fascia lata,* or the deep investing fascia of the thigh, which runs from the pelvis to the proximal tibia. Because it inserts both proximal and distal to the lateral joint line, it contributes to the stability of the lateral side of the knee. Its most visible point of insertion is

the **tubercle of Gerdy** on the proximal tibia. This prominent tubercle is located anterior to the fibular head and may sometimes be mistaken for it.

LATERAL JOINT LINE. The **lateral joint line** is less visible than the medial joint line because much of it is covered by the iliotibial tract. In the presence of a chronic *lateral meniscus tear,* a localized band of synovitis may occur along the lateral joint line and create a characteristic bulge (Fig. 6–13). A *lateral meniscus cyst* creates a rounder, firmer prominence at the midlateral joint line that can vary from a few millimeters to marble-sized (Fig. 6–14). Lateral compartment degenerative arthritis can produce a ridge of visible osteophytes at the lateral joint line.

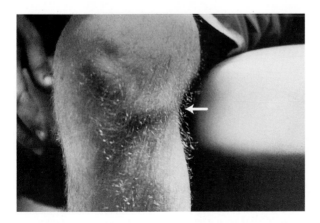

Figure 6–13. Localized swelling associated with lateral meniscus tear *(arrow).*

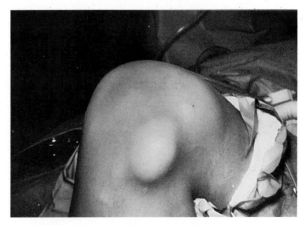

Figure 6–14. Very large lateral meniscus cyst.

Posterior Aspect

SEMIMEMBRANOSUS, SEMITENDINOSUS, AND BICEPS FEMORIS. The posterior aspect of the knee can be inspected with the patient standing, although it is usually more comfortable and convenient for both the examiner and the patient if it is done with the patient lying in the prone position. The focal point of the posterior knee is the **popliteal fossa,** a gap between the inferior hamstring and the superior calf muscles that is roughly diamond-shaped (Fig. 6–15). The superior limbs of this diamond are formed by the semimembranosus and semitendinosus muscles medially and the biceps femoris laterally as they separate and course distally to their insertions below the knee joint. Asking the prone patient to flex the knee enough to raise the foot off the table should increase the prominence of these muscles, which are either visible or palpable depending on the leanness of the patient (Fig. 6–16). The **semitendinosus,** true to its name, is the more

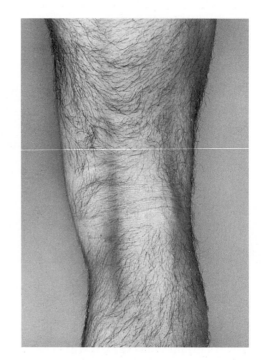

Figure 6–15. Posterior aspect of the knee.

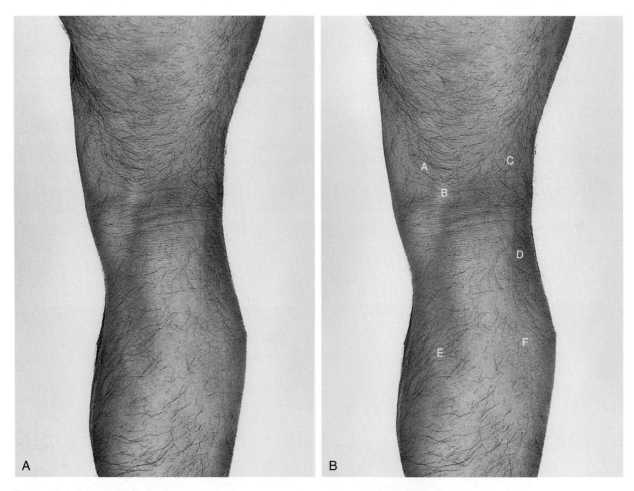

Figure 6–16. *A* and *B*, Posterior aspect of the knee during active flexion. A, semimembranosus; B, semitendinosus; C, biceps femoris; D, common peroneal nerve; E, medial head gastrocnemius; F, lateral head gastrocnemius.

tendinous and, therefore, the more clearly visible of the two medial hamstrings. It is more superficial than the **semimembranosus** and stands out as a distinct bowstring when the patient is asked to flex the knee. On the lateral side, the posterior edge of the **biceps** is usually visible or at least palpable. The **common peroneal nerve** can sometimes be identified just medial to the biceps tendon as it emerges from the posterior thigh to course around the neck of the fibula.

GASTROCNEMIUS. The distal limbs of the diamond-shaped popliteal fossa are composed of the medial and lateral heads of the **gastrocnemius.** The prominence of these tendons, which are rather broad and fleshy, can be increased by asking the patient to plantar flex the foot against manual resistance. The gastrocnemius tendons originate on the distal femur above the femoral condyles and they are each located closer to the midline of the limb than their respective hamstrings.

POPLITEAL CYSTS. A popliteal cyst, or *Baker's cyst,* is a well-known knee phenomenon. These swellings may be isolated anomalies in children but in adults they are usually secondary to intraarticular pathology, such as a meniscus tear or arthritis. They are not always visible. When they are, they may appear as a generalized fullness of the popliteal fossa or a small spherical mass. They are best seen with the patient prone and relaxed. Smaller cysts may be palpable but not visible and are most likely to be located toward the medial side of the popliteal fossa.

ALIGNMENT

To be able to arrive at a meaningful assessment of knee alignment, the examiner should habitually assess it with the patient in a standardized position. The examiner should bear in mind that malalignment is not a diagnosis per se but an indication of forces that may potentially produce symptoms.

Standing Limb Alignment

Standing knee alignment is probably more properly referred to as standing limb alignment because the relationship of the axis of the thigh to the axis of the lower leg is included in this assessment. The patient is asked to stand facing the examiner with the feet together and pointing straight ahead (Fig. 6–17). If the thighs or knees come together first and prevent the feet from touching, the patient is asked to bring the thighs comfortably together and to stand with the inner borders of the feet parallel and facing forward. When ideal alignment is present, the patient is able to stand with the knees and feet touching simultaneously. To allow this to occur, the femur and the tibia must actually be in mild valgus because the hip joints are farther apart than the knees. This relationship is known as *physiologic valgus alignment* and averages about 7° in women and 5° in men when measured on a radiograph.

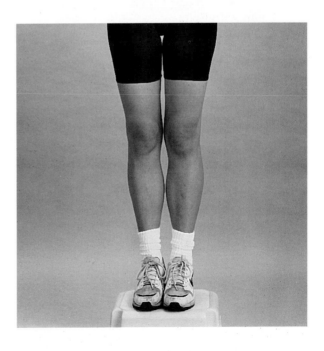

Figure 6–17. Position for examining knee alignment.

GENU VALGUM. When pathologic valgus, or **genu valgum**, alignment is present, the patient's ankles are still apart when the knees have been brought together (Fig. 6–18). Pathologic valgus means that there is more than the normal amount of valgus present. Possible causes are congenital or developmental variations, angular deformity following a fracture of the femur or the tibia, or arthritic erosion and collapse of the lateral compartment of the knee. It is important to keep in mind that corpulent thighs limit the patient's ability to bring the legs together and thus may give the false appearance of excessive valgus.

GENU VARUM. In the case of varus alignment, or **genu varum**, the patient's knees are still separated once the feet or ankles have made contact (Fig. 6–19). If the separation between the knees is small, the femur and the tibia actually are in valgus alignment but less than the usual amount. In more severe varus, the angle formed by the femur and tibia in the coronal plane is actually reversed from the normal valgus configuration. Abnormal varus alignment is more common than pathologic valgus alignment. Possible causes include congenital or developmental abnormalities, angular deformity from old frac-

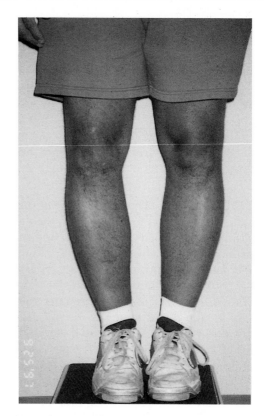

Figure 6–19. Genu varum.

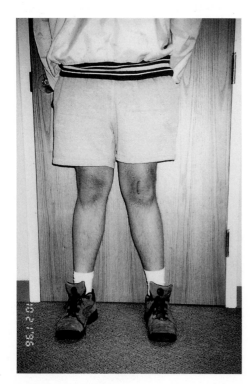

Figure 6–18. Genu valgum.

tures, severe lateral ligament injuries, and arthritic erosion and collapse of the medial compartment of the knee.

WINDSWEPT DEFORMITY. In osteoarthritis, the most common cause of angular knee deformity, loss of medial joint space is much more common than loss of lateral joint space. Thus, pathologic genu varum from osteoarthritis is much more common than pathologic genu valgum. Occasionally, one knee is in varus and the other knee is in excess valgus. This situation has been whimsically described as a **windswept deformity** because the knees appear to have been swept to the right or to the left.

Patellar Alignment

Examining the orientation of the patella gives an indication of the presence of rotational malalignment in the limb. To assess rotational variations, the patient must be examined in a standardized position. Again, this is best done by asking the patient to stand with the feet together. A line formed by the inner borders of the feet should

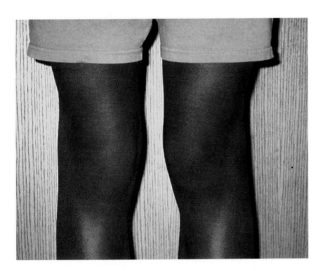

Figure 6–20. Squinting patellae.

OUT-FACING PATELLAE. Out-facing patellae is a less common variation in alignment because the reverse of the deformities that can produce in-facing seldom occur. Out-facing patellae can be seen in individuals with habitual subluxation or dislocation of the kneecaps. In such persons, the patellae sublux outward whenever the knees are fully extended, producing the out-facing configuration.

Q ANGLE. The **Q angle** is a measurement of overall patellar alignment. Technically speaking, it is the angle between a line from the anterior superior iliac spine to the center of the patella and a line from the center of the patella through the center of the tibial tubercle (Fig. 6–21). It averages 15° in normal individuals: 14° in men, 17° in women. An increased Q angle may be caused by anatomic variants that produce either in-facing patellae or lateral displacement of the tibial tubercle. The term *Q angle* is short for quadriceps angle, and it was conceived as an indication of the lateral force vector produced by the quadriceps on the patella. An increased Q angle may be associated with a tendency toward patellofemoral pain. In habitual subluxation of the patellae, as described previously, the chronic lateral subluxation of the patellae actually results in a decreased Q angle.

face directly toward the examiner. When generous thighs or valgus knees prevent the feet being brought together, the patient is asked to bring the limbs together until the knees meet and stand with the inner borders of the feet parallel to each other and pointing toward the examiner. When ideal coronal patellar alignment is present, the kneecaps face directly forward when the patient stands in this position.

SQUINTING PATELLAE. If the kneecaps are angled toward each other, the patient is said to have **in-facing,** or **squinting, patellae** (Fig. 6–20). (This latter description recalls the ophthalmologic meaning of *squint,* indicating strabismus.) This deformity may be associated with patellofemoral pain.

One common cause of squinting patellae is increased femoral anteversion with compensatory increased external tibial torsion: the femur and the patella are internally rotated, whereas the compensatory external rotation of the tibia allows the feet to still point forward. An isolated increase in external tibial torsion may also produce squinting patellae. This may not seem to be intuitively correct. An individual with normal femoral anteversion but increased external tibial torsion might be expected to stand and walk with the femora and the patellae facing forward but the ankles and feet facing outward in what is sometimes called a *duck-footed* or *slew-footed* manner. However, such an individual may try to disguise this deformity by internally rotating the lower limbs at the hips so that the feet face forward. This results in in-facing patella even though normal femoral anteversion is present.

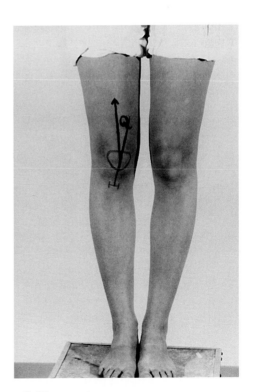

Figure 6–21. Q angle.

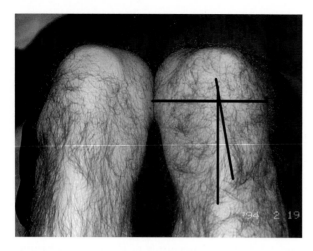

Figure 6–22. Tubercle-sulcus angle.

TUBERCLE-SULCUS ANGLE. The **tubercle-sulcus angle** is a variation on the Q angle, designed to eliminate the effect of femoral rotation and to detect abnormal lateral displacement of the tibial tubercle. For this measurement, the patient sits on the end or the side of the examination table with the knees flexed 90°. In this position, the patellae are well seated in the trochlear sulcus of the distal femur. One line is drawn from the center of the patella through the center of the tibial tubercle, and another line is drawn from the center of the patella perpendicular to a line parallel to the examination table and the floor (Fig. 6–22). This angle is normally less than 8° in women and 5° in men. An increase in this angle reflects relative lateral displacement of the tibial tubercle and may be associated with patellofemoral pain or instability.

Patellar Height

Patellar height is a parameter that is definitively assessed radiographically, but it may be estimated by physical examination. **Patella alta**, or high riding patella, is produced by a relatively long patellar tendon that allows the patella to rise more proximally on the femur than it would normally. This variation in development is associated with an increased risk of patellar instability. Patellar tendon rupture can produce an acute patella alta (Fig. 6–23). **Patella baja**, also known as **patella infra**, is a low riding patella. Patella baja is usually a sequela of trauma or surgery and may lead to patellofemoral pain and restricted flexion.

To assess patellar height, the patient is asked to sit with the knees flexed to 90° over the end or side of the table. In the average patient, the patellae should face directly forward in this position (Fig. 6–24A). In patella alta, the high riding patella faces at an angle upward toward the ceiling (Fig. 6–24B). Patella baja is more difficult to detect unless it is very severe. Because patella baja is usually unilateral, however, comparison with the normal knee is helpful: the low riding patella is subtly lower than the normal one and may seem somewhat drawn into the sulcus between the femoral condyles (Fig. 6–24C).

GAIT

Anterior and Posterior Perspectives

Observation of the knee during ambulation helps delineate abnormalities related to pain, weakness, alignment, or instability. Examination of the anterior and posterior aspects of the knee during ambulation is most easily accomplished because this can be done in a narrow hall or corridor. This perspective is most valuable for detecting abnormalities that occur in the coronal plane. The evaluation is easier if the examiner squats or sits on a low stool so that his or her eyes are positioned at the same level as the patient's knees. The patient is asked to walk away from the examiner at a normal pace and then to turn and walk directly toward the examiner. This process may need to be repeated several times to allow the examiner to observe a sufficient number of gait cycles. As the patient lifts each foot off the floor, all the patient's body weight is transmitted across the opposite knee for a brief moment. This allows the examiner to observe abnormalities of alignment that may be reduced or masked when the patient's weight is distributed between the two limbs (Fig. 6–25A).

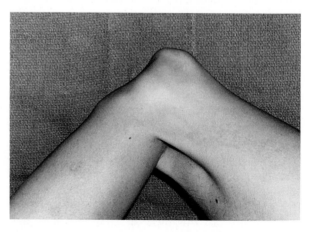

Figure 6–23. Acute patella alta due to patellar tendon rupture.

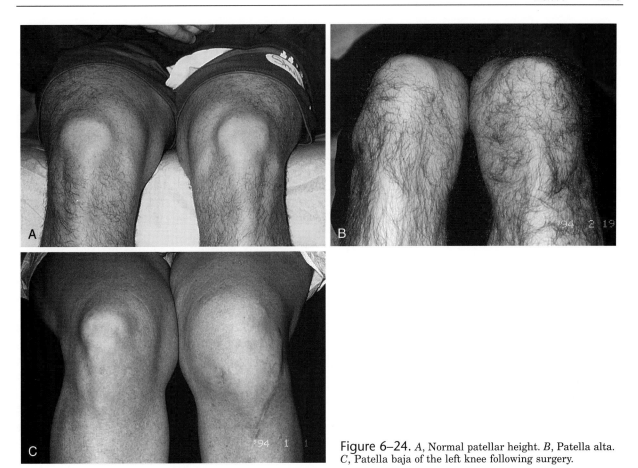

Figure 6–24. *A*, Normal patellar height. *B*, Patella alta. *C*, Patella baja of the left knee following surgery.

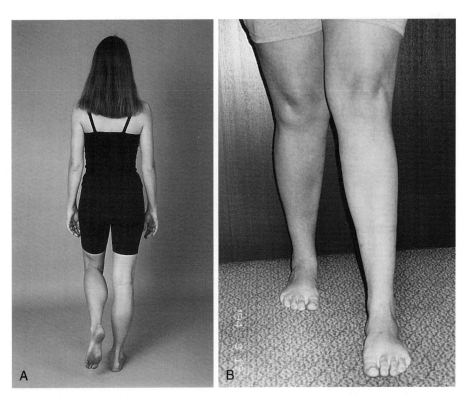

Figure 6–25. *A*, Single leg stance during normal gait. *B*, Gait in a patient with valgus knees.

VARUS THRUST. The principal abnormalities visible from this perspective are varus and valgus thrusts. In the case of a **varus thrust,** the knee collapses into a position of increased varus as the opposite foot is lifted off the ground. As the knee collapses into varus, its lateral border is noted to thrust laterally away from the patient's midline. By far the most common cause of a lateral thrust is advanced osteoarthritis with erosion of the medial joint space. A similar deformity occurring after a tibial plateau fracture could also result in a varus thrust.

An injury to the lateral ligament complex can also cause a varus thrust in the absence of medial compartment wear or deformity. However, because such abnormal lateral ligamentous laxity is usually associated with abnormal posterolateral laxity, the resulting abnormality is more likely to be a **varus recurvatum thrust** than a pure varus thrust. Varus recurvatum thrust is observed as the patient pushes himself or herself forward on the involved limb, when the knee is thrust into both varus and hyperextension. The recurvatum component of the abnormality is best seen from the lateral perspective.

VALGUS THRUST. The valgus thrust is the opposite of the varus thrust. In the **valgus thrust,** the knee collapses into pathologic valgus as the opposite foot is lifted off the ground and the medial aspect of the knee is seen to thrust further medially toward the midline. Because this tends to cause the patient's knees to butt against each other, in more severe cases the patient must also circumduct the opposite limb to avoid hitting the involved knee. This circumduction is particularly evident if both knees are affected (see Fig. 6–25*B*). Valgus thrusts are much less common than varus thrusts. The most common causes are lateral compartment erosion owing to osteoarthritis or uncorrected deformity following a lateral tibial plateau fracture.

Lateral Perspective

ANTALGIC GAIT. Observing gait from a lateral perspective is ideal for detecting several other knee abnormalities. This requires a large area to accomplish easily. If such an area is not available, the examiner may be positioned inside the examination room looking out while the patient walks past the open door of the examination room.

The most common and nonspecific gait abnormality that can be observed from this perspective is the painful or **antalgic gait.** In the antalgic gait, the patient whose knee pain is caused or increased by weightbearing is seen to hurry through the stance phase on the affected limb. Thus, the patient is observed to take alternating slow and quick steps, with the quick ones corresponding to the stance phase of the painful knee.

STIFF KNEE GAIT. Pain that only occurs when the knee is flexed is one of the possible causes of a **stiff knee gait.** This may occur because the portions of the patellofemoral and tibiofemoral articular surfaces that are in contact change according to the amount of knee flexion present. Thus, a patient whose knee pain is caused or exacerbated by weightbearing with the knee flexed may consciously or instinctively keep the knee in full extension while walking. Because this causes the involved limb to be functionally longer than the normal one, the patient may walk with a stilted or vaulting type of motion.

A stiff knee gait is also one of the abnormalities that can occur in the presence of a weak quadriceps. Because more quadriceps strength is required to support the patient's body weight when the knee is flexed than when it is locked into full extension, some patients with a weak quadriceps overcome their deficiency by walking with the knee held stiff in full extension. Patients with more severe quadriceps weakness, such as that seen after poliomyelitis, may actually thrust the knee into hyperextension or *recurvatum* to prevent it from collapsing as they propel themselves forward. In the most severe cases, the patient actually uses the ipsilateral hand to push the involved knee into recurvatum during ambulation.

FLEXED KNEE GAIT. Loss of knee motion can also produce a characteristic limp. Loss of extension (flexion contracture) is much more likely to result in a limp than loss of flexion because the greater ranges of knee flexion are not used in normal walking. Flexion contractures as mild as 5° may be associated with a limp. Flexion contractures of 10° or more almost always produce a gait abnormality. The limp associated with a flexion contracture may be described as a **flexed knee gait.** It is also best observed from the side.

In the presence of a flexion contracture, the length of the stride taken with the affected limb is shorter than the stride taken by the normal opposite limb. The shortened stride and flexed knee make it difficult for the foot on the involved side to strike the ground heel first, as seen in normal gait. Instead, the foot tends to strike the ground closer to a foot flat position. The flexion contracture also effectively shortens the limb, contributing a somewhat jerky up-and-down motion to the usually smooth gait pattern.

RANGE OF MOTION

Assessing **range of motion** in the knee is simpler than in most other joints because it is usually limited to the measurement of flexion and extension. In truth, the knee is not a simple hinge joint and some internal and external rotation is present, particularly when the knee is flexed. However, this rotation is not normally assessed unless the examiner is concerned about the possibility of abnormal laxity due to ligamentous injury. The examination for abnormal laxity is described in the Manipulation section.

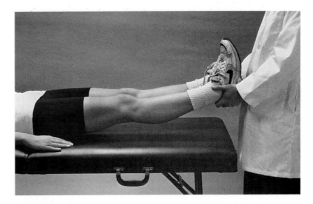

Figure 6–26. Assessing passive knee extension in the supine position.

Extension

Extension is first assessed with the patient supine (Fig. 6–26). The examiner raises both of the patient's feet in the air, holding the medial malleoli together. Because extension is normally symmetric, the knees should fall to the same level. This is an indication of the patient's **passive extension.** Normally, the knees should extend at least to neutral, so that the thigh and the lower leg are in a straight line. Many individuals' knees extend past neutral to a mildly hyperextended position. This is usually 10° or less, but it may be even greater in some loose-jointed individuals. Hyperextension at the knee is often referred to as **genu recurvatum.**

If one knee does not passively extend as far as the other, a **flexion contracture** is said to be present. This loss of extension may be due to pain, swelling, arthritic change, or a mechanical block, such as produced by a displaced meniscus tear. Impingement of the stump of a torn anterior cruciate ligament or postoperative scar tissue (especially after anterior cruciate ligament reconstruction) may also inhibit full extension.

If the less extended knee extends at least to neutral, however, the hyperextended knee may actually be the abnormal one. This pathologic hyperextension may be due to posttraumatic bony deformity or posterior ligamentous injury. If the hyperextension is due to ligament injury, other signs of pathologic ligament laxity should be present.

PRONE HANGING TEST. An excellent way to assess and measure loss of extension is the prone hanging test. The patient is asked to lie prone with the lower limbs from the knee downward projecting beyond the end of the examination table. The patient is encouraged to relax fully, both through talking and by massaging the hamstrings, if necessary. A knee flexion contracture causes the ipsilateral heel to come to rest higher than its counterpart (Fig. 6–27). Measuring the **heel height difference** can provide a fairly accurate estimate of the amount of flexion contracture present. In an individual of average build, each centimeter of heel height difference corresponds to 1° of knee flexion. Thus, a heel height difference of 8 cm reflects a flexion contracture of about 8°. This method is particularly useful for following up patients with pathologic flexion contractures because small degrees of improvement can be reliably detected.

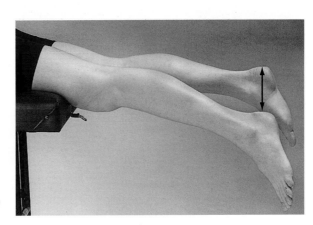

Figure 6–27. Prone hanging test to assess passive knee extension. The *arrow* indicates heel height difference.

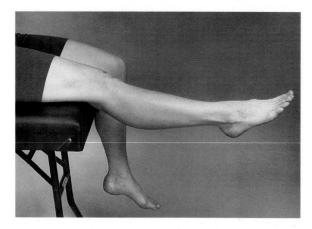

Figure 6–28. Active knee extension.

plete inability to extend the knee against gravity suggests an *extensor mechanism disruption* such as a quadriceps tendon rupture, patellar fracture, or patellar tendon rupture.

Flexion

Flexion is usually assessed by asking the supine patient to flex the knee as far as possible. Normally, a patient should be able to get the heel close to the ipsilateral buttock, or even touching it (Fig. 6–29A). This usually corresponds to a measured angle of 130° to 150°, depending on the patient's build. Flexion to 110° is usually sufficient to allow patients to descend stairs and complete other daily activities. Measuring and comparing the **heel-to-buttock distance** is a good way to assess small amounts of loss of flexion (Fig. 6–29B). Loss of flexion is commonly due to effusion, arthritic change, or patellofemoral pain. Assessment of passive flexion is not always done because it is of limited clinical significance and may often produce pain. If **passive flexion** produces pain localized to one joint line, however, it may signify a tear of the respective meniscus. Flexion may also be assessed with the patient lying supine. In this position, however, the obligate hip extension tightens the rectus femoris, which originates above the knee, and this may limit knee flexion to less than would be possible with the hip flexed.

ACTIVE EXTENSION. Active extension should also be assessed. The patient is seated on the side of the examination table and asked to extend the knee fully (Fig. 6–28). If active extension does not seem full, the examiner may lift the heel to see whether greater passive extension is possible. When active extension is less than passive extension, an **extension lag** is said to be present. This is usually due to an extensor mechanism problem, such as quadriceps weakness or patellofemoral pain. It should be remembered, however, that patients with sciatica or tight hamstrings may also have difficulty fully extending the knee in the seated position. Com-

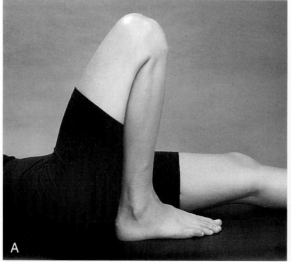
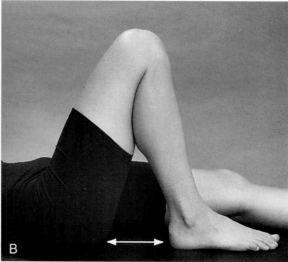

Figure 6–29. Active knee flexion. *A,* Full. *B,* Restricted (*arrow* indicates heel-to-buttock distance).

Palpation

Palpation of the knee has several uses. First, it allows the examiner to become oriented with the joint by identifying structures that are fairly superficial but not quite visible. This is particularly important in the presence of obesity or edema, when landmarks that might be visible in other patients are obscured. Second, it allows the examiner to verify the integrity of certain structures, such as the patellar tendon and LCL. Finally, it may allow the examiner to make a presumptive diagnosis by documenting point tenderness on a specific anatomic structure. Palpation flows naturally from inspection. Any of the normal structures or abnormal prominences already described may be palpated for identification or to elicit tenderness. The areas of palpation described next are only those in which palpation is most commonly useful.

Anterior Aspect

PATELLA. The extensor mechanism is one of the most fruitful venues for palpation. Because the **patella** is such a frequent source of pain, its palpation should be part of virtually every knee examination. **Patellar facet tenderness** is a common finding in cases of patellofemoral pain. To elicit it, the examiner should ask the patient to lie supine with the legs fully extended and relaxed. If the quadriceps is adequately relaxed, it should feel flaccid and the patella should feel loose when the examiner shifts it from side to side. First, the examiner gently shifts the patella medially with one hand to expose as much of the medial facet as possible (Fig. 6–30A). While the patella is in this position, the index finger or thumb of the other hand is worked under the medial facet as far as possible and pressed upward. The patient is observed for visible or verbal expressions of discomfort (Fig. 6–30B). Then the examiner reverses the process, shifting the patella laterally with one hand and palpating the exposed lateral facet with the

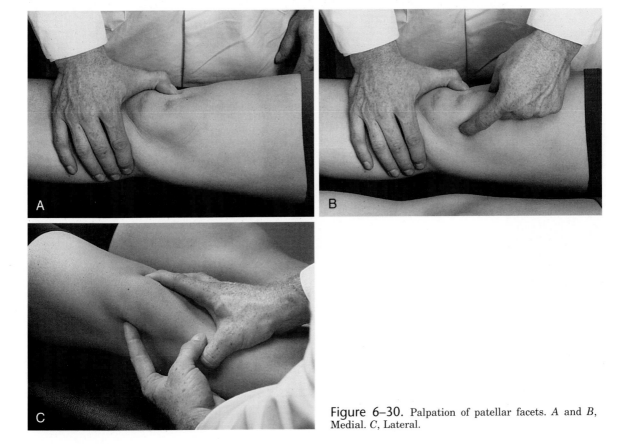

Figure 6–30. Palpation of patellar facets. *A* and *B*, Medial. *C*, Lateral.

other (Fig. 6–30C). Most of the time, pain elicited in this manner reflects sensitivity of the patella itself. However, it has been suggested that the lateral retinaculum itself may sometimes be the true source of pain.

In the presence of the uncommon condition known as *excessive lateral pressure syndrome,* very little lateral play or glide is possible (see Patellofemoral Joint in the Manipulation section). Careful palpation in this case reveals that tenderness is localized to the *lateral patellofemoral ligament,* a tight band about 1 cm wide connecting the lateral border of the patella to the lateral epicondyle.

Anteromedial knee pain may occasionally be attributable to an inflamed **medial patellar plica.** This can sometimes be palpated as a palpable fibrous band running longitudinally between the patella and the medial femoral condyle. Flexion of the knee may tighten the plica over the medial femoral condyle and make it more prominent.

Tenderness of the anterior patella itself may be due to a nondisplaced *fracture*. In the case of a displaced fracture, a gap in the patella may be palpable if not too much hematoma has accumulated to obscure it.

EXTENSOR MECHANISM. Palpation of other portions of the extensor mechanism is indicated if the history or inspection raise the question of localized pathology. Figure 6–31 shows the common sites of tenderness in *Osgood-Schlatter disease, Sinding-Larsen-Johansson disease, patellar tendinitis,* and *quadriceps tendinitis.* In the presence of **quadriceps tendon** rupture, the examiner may be able to palpate a gap as well as tenderness when the patient attempts to perform a straight-leg raise. Palpating the **patellar tendon** during an attempted straight-leg raise is also a good way to check for rupture of this structure. Normally, the patellar tendon can be easily felt to tense during this maneuver. If the tendon is ruptured, it remains flaccid, and a gap, usually just distal to the patella, may be palpable (see Fig. 6–23).

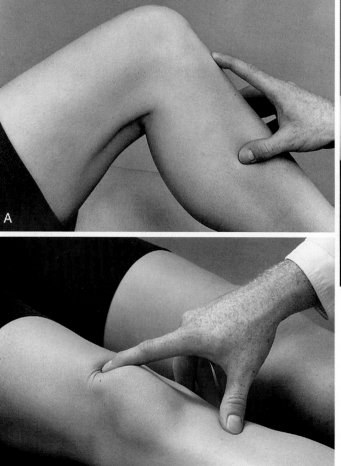

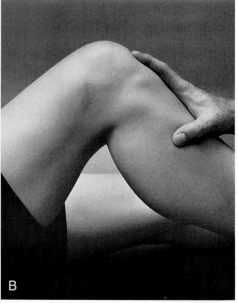

Figure 6–31. The examiner's index fingertip indicates the sites of tenderness in various conditions. *A,* Osgood-Schlatter disease. *B,* Sinding-Larsen-Johansson disease and patellar tendinitis. *C,* Quadriceps tendinitis.

Jumper's knee is the general term that includes proximal patellar tendinitis, distal patellar tendinitis, and quadriceps tendinitis. By far the most common location is in the proximal patellar tendon just distal to the inferior tip of the patella. In addition to eliciting pain, the examiner should feel a spongy crepitant sensation when firmly palpating this area with a fingertip. Palpable or visible swelling of the tendon is present in more severe cases of patellar tendinitis.

Medial Aspect

MEDIAL JOINT LINE. Palpation for tibiofemoral joint line tenderness is another important part of a basic knee examination. The joint lines are most easily identified by asking the patient to flex the knee to 90°. This may be done in either the seated or the supine position (see Fig. 6–9). As mentioned elsewhere, flexion causes the femur to roll posteriorly on the tibia and makes the anterior joint line more visible. The examiner identifies the anterior portion of the **medial joint line** with an index finger and then repeatedly presses with the tip of the finger while progressing posteriorly around the side of the joint (Fig. 6–32). The finding of tenderness at the middle to the posterior portions of either joint line is highly suspicious for pathology localized to the tibiofemoral compartment, most commonly a meniscus tear or osteoarthritis.

Tenderness that is elicited only at the **anterior portion of the joint line** is usually nonspecific. An exception to this statement is found in the knee that is locked, or unable to fully extend, owing to a displaced bucket handle fragment of a torn medial meniscus. In this condition, a longi-

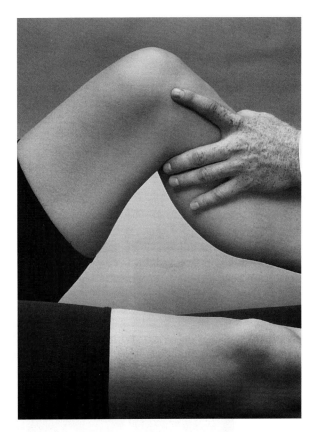

Figure 6–32. Palpation of the medial joint line.

tudinal tear allows a long strip of meniscus to displace anterior to the medial femoral condyle and prevent extension. In the presence of such an injury, exquisite tenderness usually is found at the point where the curvature of the medial femoral condyle meets the medial joint line (Fig. 6–33). Bucket handle tears also occur in the lateral meniscus, although much less often, but such a characteristic point of tenderness is found less frequently than in medial meniscus tears.

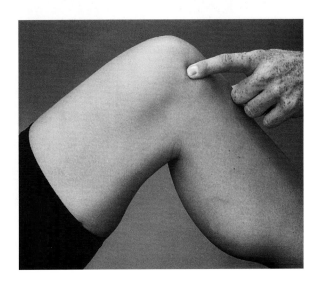

Figure 6–33. Palpation of the typical point of maximal tenderness in a patient with a locked knee due to a displaced bucket handle tear of the medial meniscus.

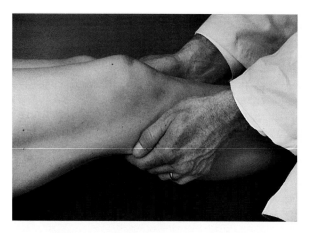

Figure 6–37. Palpation of popliteal artery pulse in the supine position.

POSTERIOR ASPECT

The palpation of the posterior aspect of the knee follows the pattern of inspection. Careful search should be made for the presence of a **popliteal cyst,** also called a Baker's cyst. The examiner may perceive a general fullness in the popliteal fossa or a more discrete rounded mass in the medial portion of the fossa (see Fig. 6–16).

The central diamond of the popliteal fossa contains the major *neurovascular bundle* leading to the leg. These structures are covered with enough fat that their outlines are not normally visible or even palpable. The pulsations of the **popliteal artery,** however, can usually be felt, especially when the knee is flexed and the surrounding muscles are relaxed. The popliteal pulse may be palpated with the patient in the prone position by flexing the knee with the lower leg supported. The examiner's fingers, lined up with the longitudinal axis of the limb, are pressed progressively deeper in the midline of the popliteal fossa until the pulsations are appreciated. The popliteal artery can also be located by feel and palpated with the patient in the supine position (Fig. 6–37).

Manipulation

MUSCLE TESTING

Muscle testing for the knee is relatively straightforward, because only two major muscle groups are involved. The quadriceps femoris provides the primary extensor force, and the hamstrings—the semitendinosus, the semimembranosus, and the biceps femoris—supply the vast majority of flexion force.

Quadriceps

To assess the **quadriceps,** the patient is seated on the end or the side of the examination table so that the posterior flexion crease of the knee just clears the edge of the table. The patient is instructed to maximally extend the knee and to maintain this position against the examiner's attempt to force the knee into flexion. The examiner then pushes downward on the anterior surface of the patient's lower leg with one hand (Fig. 6–38). In a normal patient, the examiner is unable or just barely able to overcome the strength of the patient's quadriceps and initiate flexion at the knee. In strong patients, the quadriceps may be so powerful that the patient's trunk is raised off the table while the knee remains fully extended. Patellofemoral pain can produce the impression of a weak quadriceps complex in the absence of a true muscular deficit. Quadriceps atrophy is a common nonspecific sequela of a painful knee injury. Injury to the *femoral nerve* or herniation of the L3 to L4 disk can also lead to quadriceps weakness.

Quadriceps function has also been traditionally assessed by measuring decreases in **thigh circumference.** Such a measurement does not truly distinguish between quadriceps and hamstring atrophy, but quadriceps atrophy is much more common than hamstring atrophy. To mea-

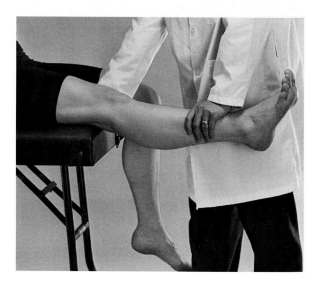

Figure 6–38. Assessing quadriceps strength.

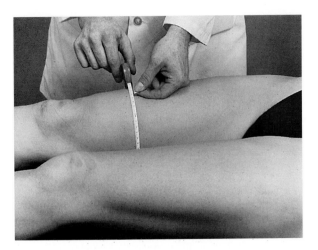

Figure 6–39. Measuring thigh circumference.

sure thigh circumference, the examiner picks a point in the distal thigh where muscle bulk seems maximal, usually about 10 cm to 15 cm proximal to the patella. Using a landmark that appears symmetric and easily identifiable in both knees, such as the proximal pole of the patella or the tibial tubercle, the examiner uses a tape measure to place a pen mark on the anterior thigh at the desired spot in both thighs. The examiner then measures the circumference of each thigh at the point of the mark using the tape measure (Fig. 6–39). These measurements may be made with the thigh muscles relaxed or set, as long as the same method is used for both thighs. Differences of 1 cm or more are usually indicative of significant muscle atrophy, most often involving the quadriceps.

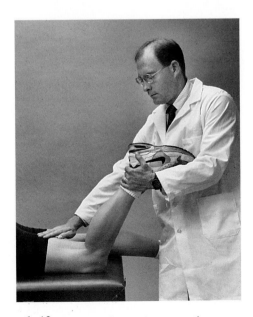

Figure 6–40. Assessing hamstring strength.

Hamstrings

Hamstring strength is usually measured with the patient in the prone position. The patient is instructed to flex the knee and to maintain this position against the examiner's attempts to passively extend it (Fig. 6–40). In most normal patients, the examiner is able to slowly overcome the strength of the hamstrings but with considerable difficulty. Although it is difficult to test the individual hamstrings, the examiner should inspect and, if necessary, palpate the three individual muscles to verify that they are all firing. The hamstrings are innervated by the *sciatic nerve.*

SENSATION TESTING

The most common sensory nerve about the knee to be injured is the **infrapatellar branch of the saphenous nerve,** also known as the **infrapatellar nerve.** Although the exact course of this nerve is highly variable, it runs across the knee just inferior to the patella in a medial to lateral direction, supplying the skin along its course. Its primary clinical significance lies in the fact that almost any longitudinal incision on the anterior knee usually transects it, leaving the area immediately lateral to the incision anesthetic (Fig. 6–41). The infrapatellar nerve can also be injured by a direct blow to or a fall on the knee.

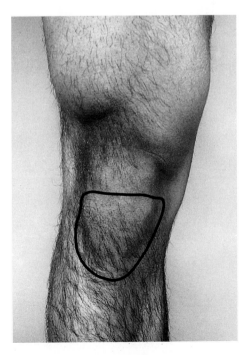

Figure 6–41. Average sensory distribution of the infrapatellar nerve.

SPECIAL TESTS

Effusion

The lack of muscle tissue overlying the front of the knee makes detection of an **effusion** easier than in most other joints. Effusion is a general term for increased intraarticular fluid: it may be caused by excess synovial fluid, blood, or occasionally, pus. The detection of an effusion is important diagnostically because it establishes that an intraarticular process is present.

VISIBLE FLUID WAVE. Several techniques are useful for detecting an effusion. The choice generally depends on its size. All of these tests are best performed with the patient supine, knees relaxed and extended. The **appearance** of the knee usually gives the examiner the first clue that an effusion is present. As noted earlier, a hollow or sulcus is normally present on both sides of the patella in patients of lean or average build. When this hollow appears filled in (Fig. 6–42), the examiner should suspect an effusion.

If a mild effusion is suspected, the examiner may be able to demonstrate a **visible fluid**

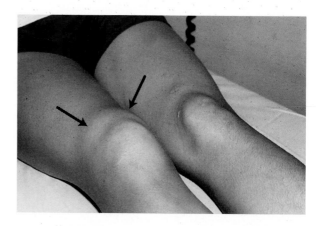

Figure 6–42. Effusion of the right knee. The *arrows* indicate bulging of fluid in the suprapatellar pouch.

wave. In this technique, the examiner compresses the hollows on both sides of the kneecap simultaneously, with the thumb on one side and the index and the long finger on the other (Fig. 6–43A). This maneuver is designed to force the fluid from these hollows into the suprapatellar pouch. The examiner then lifts the first hand away (Fig. 6–43B) and quickly compresses the suprapatellar pouch with the palm and fingers of

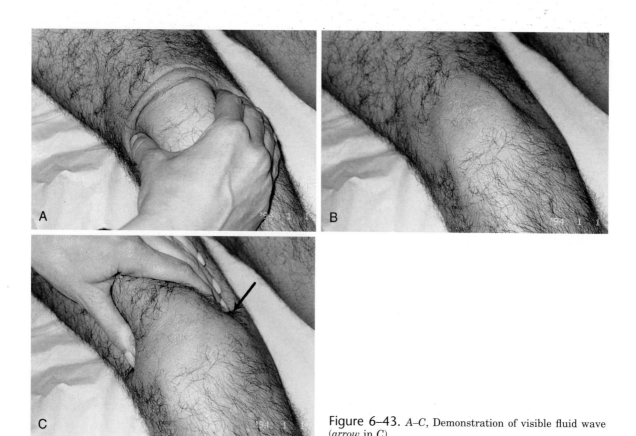

Figure 6–43. *A–C,* Demonstration of visible fluid wave (*arrow* in *C*).

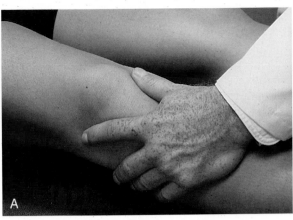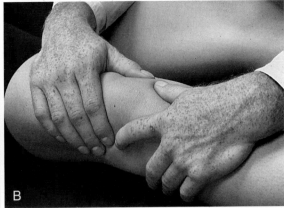

Figure 6–44. *A* and *B*, Demonstration of palpable fluid wave.

the other hand while looking at the hollows. In the presence of a small effusion, compression of the suprapatellar pouch forces the fluid back into the hollows, usually resulting in a visible fluid wave (Fig. 6–43*C*). This maneuver should be repeated several times, as the fluid wave may not always be visible. This sign is not useful in the obese patient because the adipose tissue hides the normal hollows even when no effusion is present.

PALPABLE FLUID WAVE. If a slightly larger effusion is present, a variation of this technique must be used because the fluid returns to the hollows too quickly for the examiner to see a fluid wave. This may be thought of as the **palpable fluid wave.** In this variation, the examiner compresses the hollows on both sides of the patella with one hand but does not lift it from the knee, instead maintaining gentle compression (Fig. 6–44*A*). The examiner then compresses the suprapatellar pouch firmly with the other hand (Fig. 6–44*B*). This forces the fluid back distally beneath the first hand. In the presence of an effusion, the examiner should be able to feel the fluid pushing the thumb and fingers of the first hand outward. This technique is very useful in obese patients. Although the hollows cannot be seen in these patients, the examiner compresses on the sides of the kneecap where the hollows should be and is able to feel the fluid wave when the suprapatellar pouch is compressed.

GROSS SWELLING. When gross knee swelling is present, it is diagnostically important to distinguish between intraarticular fluid and extraarticular soft tissue swelling caused by hematoma or edema. The test described earlier for a palpable fluid wave can usually make this distinction. The

appearance of the swelling can also be helpful. A large effusion tensely fills the suprapatellar pouch, creating a characteristic bulge under the distal quadriceps (see Fig. 6–42). Extraarticular soft tissue swelling tends to be more diffuse and fusiform. Of course, both types of swelling may be present simultaneously. A hematoma, especially one caused by a direct blow, may appear as a localized asymmetric bulge at the point of contact.

When an effusion is large, a **ballotable patella sign** may be present. This is also looked for in the supine, extended knee. In this position, a large effusion distends the knee so much that the patella is lifted off the femoral trochlea. To ballot the patella, the examiner pushes the patient's patella posteriorly with two or three fingers using a quick, sharp motion (Fig. 6–45). In the presence of a large effusion, the patella descends to the trochlea and is felt to strike it with a distinct impact. An extremely large, tense effusion may sometimes prevent this impact from being felt.

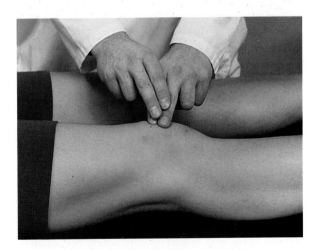

Figure 6–45. Technique of patellar ballottement.

Stability Tests

Valgus and Varus Laxity

The first two stability tests are the **valgus** and **varus stress tests.** In the valgus stress test, a force directed at the midline is applied at the knee while an opposing force directed away from the midline is applied at the foot or ankle. The varus stress test is exactly the opposite: a force directed away from the midline is applied at the knee while an opposing force directed toward the midline is applied at the foot or ankle.

VALGUS STRESS TEST. The valgus stress test assesses the integrity of the *MCL complex.* The superficial MCL is the primary restraint to valgus stress at the knee. The deep fibers of the MCL (meniscofemoral ligament and meniscotibial ligament) act as secondary restraints to valgus stress. The posteromedial capsule is an important restraint to valgus stress when the knee is in full extension; when the knee is in flexion, the posteromedial capsule is relaxed and therefore ineffective in resisting valgus stress. Finally, the cruciate ligaments come into play as tertiary restraints against extreme valgus stress once the medial structures have failed.

To perform the **valgus stress test,** have the patient lie supine and relaxed on a flat examining table (Fig. 6–46*A* and *B*). The examiner raises the patient's lower limb off the examining table by grasping it gently at the ankle. The patient's muscles should be fully relaxed so that the knee falls into complete extension. When the patient is properly relaxed, the lower limb feels like a dead weight. If the examiner senses that the patient is assisting in raising the leg, it is important to encourage the patient to relax fully before proceeding with the rest of the examination. If the patient finds relaxation difficult, the test may be performed without raising the limb by abducting it until the knee is at the edge of the table so that the patient's thigh is still supported by the table (Fig. 6–46*C*).

With the patient's knee in full extension, the examiner applies a gentle inward force at the knee and a reciprocating outward force at the ankle (see Fig. 6–46*A*). The force is then relaxed. The examiner both looks and feels for a separation of the femur and the tibia on the medial side of the knee in response to the valgus stress. In the normal knee, virtually no separation of the medial tibia and femur is felt when the knee is in full extension. In the abnormal case, the femur and the tibia are felt to separate when the valgus stress is applied and to clunk back together when the stress is relaxed. The same test should be conducted on the opposite, presumably normal, knee for comparison.

Increased laxity to valgus stress with the knee in full extension signifies damage not only to the superficial and the deep MCL fibers but also to the posteromedial capsule. In such a knee, the incidence of concomitant injury to one or both cruciate ligaments is extremely high. If valgus stability in full extension is normal, the examiner then flexes the patient's knee about 10° or 15° and repeats the test (see Fig. 6–46*B*). Flexing the knee relaxes the posteromedial capsule and concentrates the force on the MCL. (If the examiner flexes the knee too much, the limb tends to internally rotate at the hip when a valgus force is applied.) Again, the examiner looks and feels for abnormal separation of the medial tibia and the femur in response to the valgus stress and the feeling of the two bones clunking back together when the stress is relaxed. The combination of normal valgus stability when the knee is fully extended and abnormally increased valgus laxity when the knee is flexed suggests more isolated damage to the MCL with an intact posteromedial capsule.

GRADING ABNORMAL LAXITY. MCL injuries are often divided into three grades according to the physical findings. The most widely accepted grading system is based on the general anatomic classification of ligament injuries, in which grade I signifies injury without any elongation of the ligament, grade II signifies a ligament that is elongated but not completely disrupted, and grade III signifies a ligament that has lost all structural integrity. In this system, a **grade I** injury is one in which the MCL is tender and swollen but exhibits no increased laxity. In **grade II** injuries, there is the additional finding of increased laxity to the valgus stress test but with a firm endpoint. This means that the medial joint separates more than in the other knee when a valgus stress is applied, but a firm resistance is eventually felt when the injured ligament pulls taut. In **grade III** injuries, there is increased valgus laxity with an indefinite endpoint. In other words, the examiner feels no resistance no matter how far the medial joint surfaces are separated. Although this is the most widely accepted system of classification, it does have some

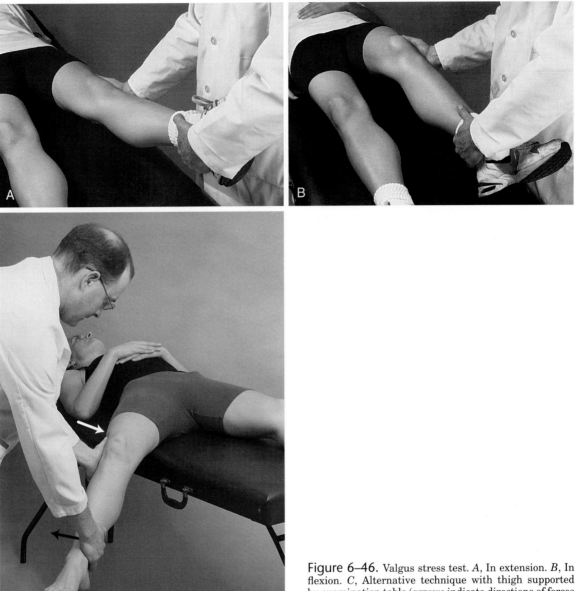

Figure 6–46. Valgus stress test. *A*, In extension. *B*, In flexion. *C*, Alternative technique with thigh supported by examination table (*arrows* indicate directions of forces applied at the knee and the ankle).

problems. The distinction between grade II and grade III injuries is somewhat arbitrary. Identical injuries may be classified as either grade II or grade III depending on whether or not the patient is able to relax enough to allow the examiner to feel an endpoint.

The **alternative system** of classification, proposed years ago by Fetto and Marshall, distinguishes between grade II and grade III injuries depending on whether or not there is increased valgus laxity in full extension, instead of on the endpoint. In this classification, **grade II** injuries include all those in which there is increased valgus laxity in flexion but normal valgus laxity in full extension. In **grade III** injuries, there is increased valgus laxity in both flexion and extension. Not only is the distinction between grade II and grade III injuries easier to make with this classification but also it carries greater prognostic significance. As noted earlier, increased valgus laxity in full extension implies not only damage to the MCL but also concomitant injury to the posteromedial capsule and usually one or both of the cruciate ligaments.

VARUS STRESS TEST. The varus stress test is the counterpart of the valgus stress test for detecting injury to the *LCL complex.* Again, the patient lies supine and fully relaxed. The examiner raises the patient's lower limb off the examining table by grasping it at the ankle. As in the valgus stress test, the knee is first tested in full extension and then in about 10° or 15° of flexion. This time, the examiner applies an outward force at the knee and a reciprocating inward force at the ankle (Fig. 6–47A). Again, the examiner both looks and feels for abnormal separation of the femur and the tibia, this time on the lateral side of the knee, in response to the varus stress. In the normal knee, virtually no separation of the lateral tibia and the femur are felt when the knee is in full extension. When the lateral ligamentous structures are torn, the femur and the tibia are felt to separate abnormally when the stress is applied and to clunk back together when the stress is relaxed.

The major difference between the varus and the valgus stress tests is that most patients have more natural laxity of the lateral ligaments than the medial ligaments. This natural laxity is evident when the varus stress test is repeated with the knee in flexion (see Fig. 6–47B): when the varus stress is applied, a definite separation is felt, and when the stress is relaxed, the femur and the tibia clunk back together. This separation is probably about 3 mm to 5 mm in the average normal knee. Thus, it is extremely important to compare the two limbs to verify that the varus laxity felt is increased compared with the other side and not just a consequence of the patient's physiologic varus laxity. As in the valgus stress test, increased varus laxity in full extension implies more extensive injury, usually involving the posterolateral ligament complex and one or both cruciate ligaments.

Anterior Laxity

The next set of tests are those designed to detect abnormal anterior knee laxity. This is conventionally defined as the ability to translate the tibia anteriorly an abnormal amount in relation to the femur. It has been shown that increased anterior laxity is a sign of injury to the *anterior cruciate ligament* (ACL), although concomitant injury to other ligaments can increase the magnitude of the abnormal anterior translation. The two most basic tests for abnormal anterior knee laxity are the anterior drawer and Lachman tests.

ANTERIOR DRAWER TEST. In the **anterior drawer test,** the patient lies supine with the involved knee bent to a 90° angle. The examiner sits at the end of the examination table with his or her thigh against the patient's toes to restrain the foot (Fig. 6–48A). The examiner then grasps the tibia just below the joint line and asks the patient to relax. If the patient is properly relaxed, the lower limb should feel as if it would fall over to the side if the examiner released it. The examiner then pulls forward with both hands (Fig. 6–48B) and assesses both the amount of anterior translation of the tibia with respect to the femur and the quality of the endpoint.

In most patients, the tibia can be felt to move forward at least a few millimeters and then stop suddenly with a hard endpoint. As in the other stability tests, comparison to the other side is important. In the case of ACL injury, the tibia is felt to translate forward more than on the uninvolved side, and the endpoint feels soft (see Fig. 6–48C).

Although the anterior drawer test is the most well known test for abnormal anterior knee lax-

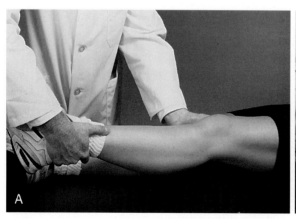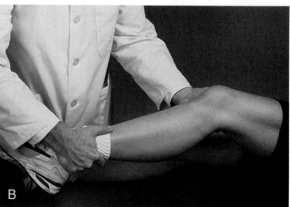

Figure 6–47. Varus stress test. *A,* In extension. *B,* In flexion.

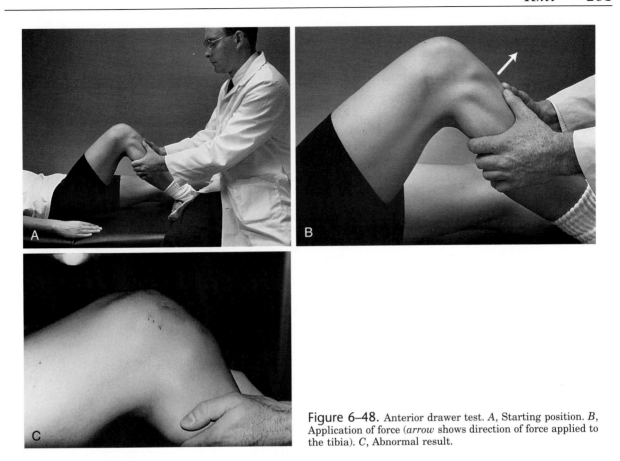

Figure 6–48. Anterior drawer test. *A,* Starting position. *B,* Application of force (*arrow* shows direction of force applied to the tibia). *C,* Abnormal result.

ity, it has some problems and limitations. First, many patients have considerable normal laxity in the 90° flexed position, making it more difficult to distinguish between abnormal and normal. Second, it may be difficult for the patient to flex the knee to 90° if the knee is acutely injured and painful. Finally, when the knee is flexed 90°, the hamstrings are in an excellent position to mask abnormal anterior translation in the patient who is unable to relax fully.

LACHMAN'S TEST. For these reasons, the **Lachman test** has surpassed the anterior drawer test as a basic screening examination for abnormal anterior knee laxity. This test was first described by Torg and attributed to his mentor, Lachman. The Lachman test is similar in concept to the anterior drawer test but is performed with the knee in 20° to 30° of flexion.

Again, the patient lies supine on the examination table (Fig. 6–49A). The examiner stands at

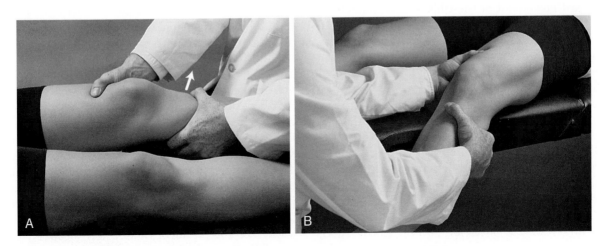

Figure 6–49. Lachman's test. *A,* Standard position (*arrow* shows direction of force applied to the tibia). *B,* Alternative technique with the thigh supported by the exam table.

the side of the table near the knee and grasps the lower leg with one hand. Usually, the examiner's thumb is placed just over the tibial tubercle and the other fingers are wrapped around the rest of the calf. The other hand is used to grasp the thigh just above the patella. The thumb of this upper hand presses against the femur through the quadriceps tendon while the other fingers wrap around the posterior thigh. If the patient is properly relaxed, the limb should feel like a dead weight. The fingers of the examiner's upper hand, which are supporting the thigh, are also able to sense any tightening in the hamstrings. If any of the hamstrings are felt to be tight, identifying the tight muscle to the patient and massaging it a bit often allows the patient to relax.

As with the valgus stress test, better relaxation may sometimes be obtained by abducting the lower limb and allowing the thigh to rest on the examination table (see Fig. 6–49B). In this case, the knee is flexed over the side of the table and the foot rests on the lap of the seated examiner. Once the patient is adequately relaxed, the examiner pulls forward on the tibia with one hand while simultaneously pushing backward on the femur with the other hand in a reciprocating manner. As in the anterior drawer test, the amount of anterior excursion and the quality of the endpoint are assessed.

One of the differences that makes the Lachman test easier to assess than the anterior drawer test is that in most normal patients, there is little or no excursion of the tibia when the Lachman test is performed. Either no translation at all or 1 mm to 2 mm of translation with a very firm endpoint is appreciated. In the presence of ACL tear, the translation is increased and the endpoint indefinite. Often, this increased translation can be visibly appreciated by focusing on the forward movement of the tibia at the tubercle of Gerdy or over the medial tibial plateau. In subtly abnormal cases, the examiner may not be sure that increased excursion is present, but he or she may sense a soft feel that differs from the uninjured knee.

A special case is the *incomplete ACL injury,* in which the ACL is elongated but not totally disrupted. In these cases, increased anterior laxity is present but a firm endpoint is still noted. This endpoint is usually easier to appreciate after the swelling and stiffness of the acute injury have subsided.

Theoretically, the Lachman test is more specific for injury to the posterior portion of the ACL, and the anterior drawer test is more specific for injury to the anterior fibers. This distinction would only be important, however, in the relatively unusual case in which some of the ACL fibers are torn but the others are relatively intact.

Pivot Shift Phenomenon

The **pivot shift test** and its variations are dynamic tests that demonstrate the subluxation that can occur when the ACL is nonfunctional. Thus, they are indirect tests of ACL injury. An abnormal result usually indicates complete rupture of the ACL but may also be present when the ligament is excessively elongated but still in continuity. In addition, some patients with greater than average anterior knee laxity may demonstrate a mild *physiologic pivot shift* in the absence of any knee injury. Many patients whose knees hyperextend can be expected to demonstrate this physiologic pivot shift. In laboratory studies, sectioning the ACL has been shown to be sufficient to produce a positive pivot shift, although sectioning the lateral ligament complex usually increases the magnitude of the pivot shift.

CLASSIC PIVOT SHIFT TEST. The classic pivot shift test was described by Galway and McIntosh. With the patient supine and relaxed, the examiner lifts the lower limb off the table by the foot and internally rotates it (Fig. 6–50A).

(Although the classic description of the pivot shift test is performed with internal rotation of the lower limb, some researchers recommend a neutral or even externally rotated position.)

If the patient is properly relaxed, the limb feels like a dead weight and the knee naturally falls into full extension. This may be a straight position or hyperextension, depending on what is normal for that particular patient. If the knee does not fall into full extension, whether due to pain, swelling, or a displaced meniscus tear, the pivot shift test may not be accurate.

In a patient with a nonfunctional ACL, gravity causes the femur to fall posteriorly when the limb is held in this manner, resulting in an anterior subluxation of the tibia with respect to the femur. The examiner then places the palm of the other hand on the lateral aspect of the proximal leg, just below the knee, and gently applies a force that results in valgus stress as well as flexes the knee (see Fig. 6–50B). Somewhere between 20° and 30°, the anteriorly subluxed tibia spontaneously reduces into its normal position with re-

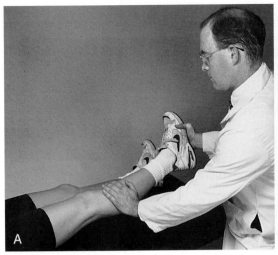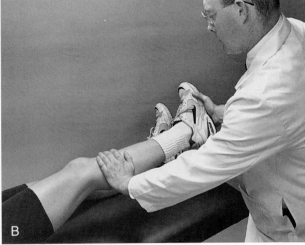

Figure 6–50. *A* and *B*, Pivot shift test.

spect to the femur, resulting in a sudden visible jump or shift. The best place to watch for this jump is at the tubercle of Gerdy. In most normal individuals, the knee bends smoothly with no such shift. As mentioned, some loose-jointed individuals exhibit a mild pivot shift in their uninjured knees.

Because the pivot shift is a dynamic phenomenon, it is difficult to grade. Some clinicians distinguish a *trace pivot shift* or *pivot glide* in which the tibia can be seen to move smoothly into a reduced position as the knee flexes, without the sudden jump of the frank pivot shift. In most patients with a physiologic pivot shift, such a pivot glide is present. At the severe end of the spectrum, the tibia subluxes so far anteriorly when the knee is extended that a spontaneous reduction does not occur as the knee flexes. In these cases, the knee appears to be stuck between 20° and 30° of flexion and does not flex past the sticking point until the examiner manually pushes the tibia posteriorly into a reduced position.

JERK TEST. Several variants of the pivot shift test have been described. In the **jerk test,** described by Hughston, the procedure is the reverse of the pivot shift test: the examiner begins with the knee flexed and the tibia reduced and watches the tibia sublux as the knee is passively extended.

FLEXION-ROTATION DRAWER TEST. The **flexion-rotation drawer test** is a gentler version of the pivot shift test that has become quite popular. In the flexion-rotation drawer test, the examiner grasps the patient's leg at the ankle with both hands (Fig. 6–51*A*). The internal rotation, valgus, and flexion forces are applied indirectly at the ankle (Fig. 6–51*B*). This usually produces a less violent reduction than the classic pivot shift and is less threatening to the patient with significant abnormal anterior laxity. A good method is to begin with the flexion-rotation drawer test and to proceed to the classic pivot shift technique if the results of the flexion-rotation drawer are equivocal.

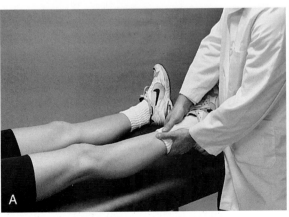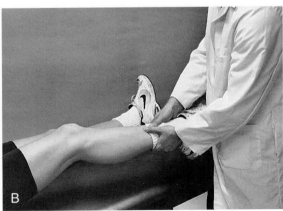

Figure 6–51. *A* and *B*, Flexion-rotation drawer test.

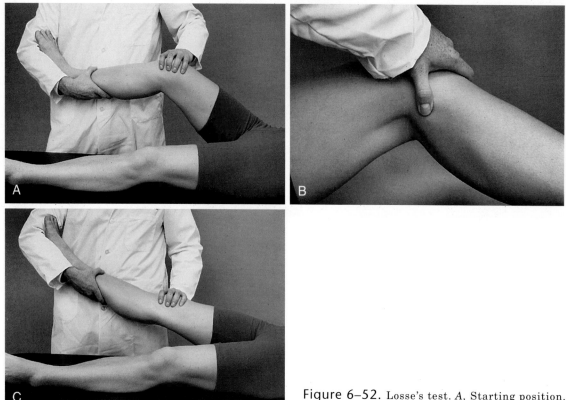

Figure 6–52. Losse's test. *A,* Starting position.
B, Close-up of left hand position. *C,* Finishing position.

LOSSE'S TEST. The **Losse test** is another technique for demonstrating the pivot shift phenomenon. To perform the Losse test, the examiner stands facing the supine patient from the side of the examination table. To examine the right knee, the examiner's right hand supports the patient's right foot and ankle in an externally rotated position braced against the examiner's abdomen. The patient's knee is then pushed into 30° of flexion to relax the hamstrings (Fig. 6–52*A*). The examiner's left hand is placed on the knee with the fingers over the patella and the thumb behind the head of the fibula, and a valgus stress is applied (Fig. 6–52*B*). As the knee is slowly extended, the head of the fibula is pushed forward with the thumb of the left hand, using the fingers placed over the patella to provide counterpressure.

If the test is positive, the lateral tibial plateau is felt to sublux anteriorly as the knee approaches full extension (see Fig. 6–52*C*). Losse and colleagues emphasized that the patient must identify the subluxation maneuver as his or her chief complaint for the test to be considered positive.

Posterior Laxity

The next group of tests are those for abnormal posterior laxity of the knee. Rupture of the *poste-*

rior cruciate ligament (PCL) is necessary for a detectable increase in straight posterior laxity, although damage to the posterolateral structures further increases the magnitude of the abnormal posterior laxity.

Laboratory research has shown that sectioning the PCL produces the greatest increase in posterior laxity when the knee is flexed between 70° and 90°. Therefore, the most sensitive way to test for PCL injury is with the knee flexed between 70° and 90°.

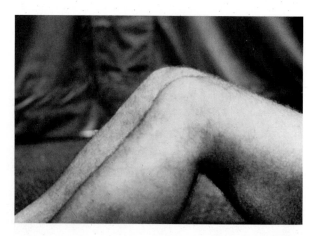

Figure 6–53. Dropback phenomenon in the left knee. Note subtle concavity of left knee profile (in foreground).

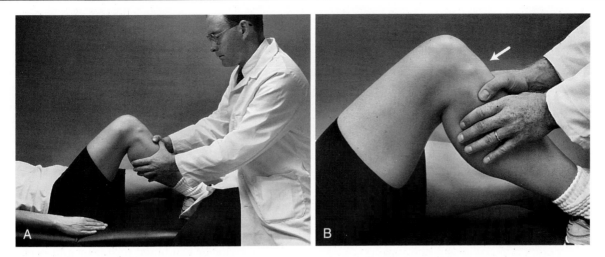

Figure 6–54. Posterior drawer test. *A,* Starting position. *B,* Application of force (*arrow* indicates direction of force applied to the tibia).

POSTERIOR DRAWER TEST. The most basic test for PCL injury is the **posterior drawer test.** The starting position is essentially the same as that for the anterior drawer test; the patient's knee is flexed 90° and the foot stabilized. In a patient with a torn PCL, a **dropback phenomenon** usually occurs in this position: gravity causes the tibia to sublux posteriorly with respect to the femur, resulting in an abnormal appearance that is best appreciated when both knees are viewed in profile (Fig. 6–53). When such a dropback phenomenon occurs, the tibial tubercle appears less prominent than usual, and the patella appears more prominent than usual. Subtle changes may often be detected by comparing the injured with the normal knee. In the acute injury situation, the dropback is less likely to occur or may be masked by acute swelling.

The posterior drawer test is completed by pushing posteriorly on the proximal tibia with both hands (Fig. 6–54). In the abnormal case, the tibia is felt or seen to sublux further posteriorly with respect to the femur. If considerable dropback has already occurred, the application of a posterior force may not sublux the tibia much further. Unlike the anterior drawer test, a fairly firm endpoint is usually felt once the abnormal posterior laxity has been taken up, even in the case of complete PCL rupture.

GODFREY'S TEST. The **Godfrey test** is another way of looking for the dropback phenomenon. In Godfrey's test, the examiner or an assistant holds the patient's legs in the 90/90 position with both the knees and the hips flexed to 90° (Fig. 6–55). Again, in this position gravity causes

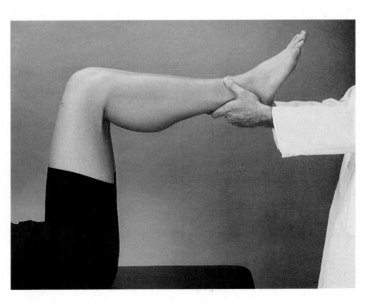

Figure 6–55. Godfrey's test.

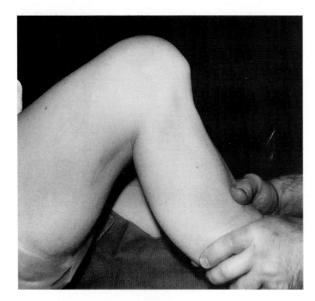

Figure 6–56. Grade 3 posterior drawer.

the tibia to sublux posteriorly in a knee with an injured PCL.

GRADING POSTERIOR LAXITY. The results of the posterior drawer and dropback tests are usually graded by the relationship of the proximal tibia to the distal end of the femoral condyles. Normally, the anterior cortex of the proximal tibia sits about 10 mm anterior to the distal end of the femoral condyles when the knee is flexed about 90°. Every 5 mm of posterior dropback or posterior drawer is considered a grade of abnormal laxity. Thus, in a **grade 1** posterior drawer, the normal 10 mm of prominence of the anterior tibia with respect to the femoral condyles is reduced to 5 mm. In a **grade 2** posterior drawer or dropback, the proximal tibial cortex is flush with the femoral condyles. In the **grade 3** or **grade 4** posterior drawer or dropback, the anterior tibial cortex is respectively displaced 5 mm or 10 mm posterior to the femoral condyles (Fig. 6–56).

QUADRICEPS ACTIVE DRAWER TEST. The **quadriceps active drawer test,** described by Daniel and colleagues, is very helpful for confirming the presence of posterior subluxation when the dropback is equivocal. With the patient's knee flexed 90°, the examiner elicits an isometric contraction of the patient's quadriceps by asking the patient to attempt to slide the ipsilateral foot distally while the examiner secures it in place and resists such movement (Fig. 6–57). (It is important to confirm, either visually or by palpation, that such a quadriceps contraction actually occurs.) The examiner focuses his or her attention on the proximal tibia. In the

normal case, the relationship between the proximal tibia and the distal femur remains constant as the quadriceps contracts. In the abnormal case, the posteriorly subluxed tibia is seen to shift anteriorly into a reduced position as the quadriceps contracts. Comparison with the other knee helps to detect subtly abnormal cases. Occasionally, a small physiologic shift may be observed, but this should be symmetric with the uninjured knee.

DYNAMIC POSTERIOR SHIFT TEST. The **dynamic posterior shift test** is an adjunctive test that may be abnormal in the presence of abnormal posterior or combined posterior and posterolateral laxity. In this test, the examiner passively raises the patient's thigh until the hip is flexed 90°. The patient's foot is supported with the examiner's other hand so that the knee is flexed 90° as well. In this position, the hip flexion tightens the patient's hamstrings and thus may sublux the tibia posteriorly (Fig. 6–58A). The examiner then passively extends the patient's knee while keeping the hip flexed 90° (Fig. 6–58B). Although such extension further tightens the hamstrings, the passive extension causes the subluxed tibia to reduce, sometimes with a sudden noticeable shift.

Posterolateral Laxity

Recently, further attention has been directed at tests for abnormal **posterolateral laxity.** Such laxity reflects injury to the *LCL, popliteus tendon,* and associated structures of the *posterolateral ligament complex* such as the fabellofibular

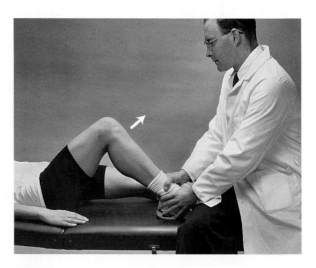

Figure 6–57. Quadriceps active drawer test. The *arrow* shows the direction of abnormal tibial movement, when present.

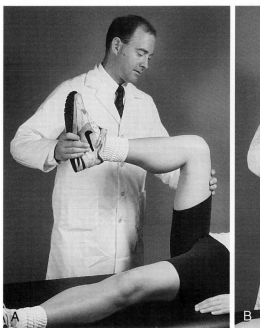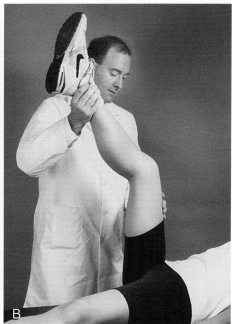

Figure 6–58. *A* and *B*, Dynamic posterior shift test.

ligament. Abnormal posterolateral laxity is occasionally present as an isolated finding, but it is much more commonly found in association with abnormal posterior or anterior laxity. When abnormal posterolateral laxity is present, the tibia rotates externally an abnormal amount with respect to the femur, and the lateral tibial plateau subluxes posteriorly with respect to the lateral femoral condyle. This can be observed most directly by flexing the patient's knee to 90° and

observing the relationship of the tubercle of Gerdy and fibular head to the lateral femoral epicondyle as the tibia is rotated externally (Fig. 6–59). Patients with physiologically lax knees demonstrate considerable external rotation with this maneuver, therefore, comparison with the contralateral side is important. In such a patient, distinguishing the increased posterolateral rotation compared with the lax normal side may be difficult.

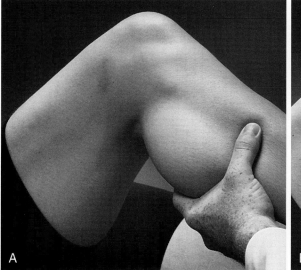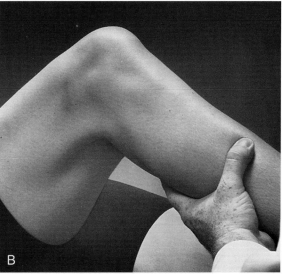

Figure 6–59. Direct observation of posterolateral laxity. *A,* Tibia is internally rotated. *B,* Tibia is externally rotated.

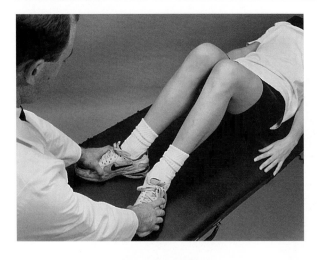

Figure 6–60. External rotation test.

EXTERNAL ROTATION TEST. Another technique for demonstrating increased posterolateral laxity is to use the position of the foot as an indirect indicator of the amount of external rotation of the tibia present. In this technique, which may be called the **external rotation test,** the supine patient is asked to flex the knees while keeping the knees and ankles together. The examiner then passively externally rotates the feet and compares the amount of external rotation of the involved limb with the normal one (Fig. 6–60). Classically, this test is performed with the knees flexed 30° and again with the knees flexed 90°. In the rare case of isolated posterolateral laxity, increased external rotation is noted at 30° but not at 90°. When combined posterior and posterolateral laxity are present, increased external rotation is noted in both positions.

VARUS RECURVATUM TEST. Other tests for abnormal posterolateral laxity include the varus recurvatum test, the posterolateral drawer sign, and the reverse pivot shift test. In the **varus recurvatum test,** first described by Hughston and Norwood, the patient lies supine and relaxed with the legs extended. The examiner grasps one of the patient's great toes in each hand and lifts them straight up about a foot off the examination table (Fig. 6–61). In the abnormal case, the knee falls into recurvatum (hyperextension) and varus compared with the uninjured contralateral knee. This requires a complex injury involving the PCL, the posterolateral ligament complex, and the LCL. The patient with a positive varus recurvatum test usually exhibits a varus recurvatum gait and is significantly disabled.

POSTEROLATERAL DRAWER SIGN. Hughston and Norwood also described the **posterolateral drawer sign.** This is elicited by performing the

posterior drawer test with the patient's foot in external rotation, neutral position, and internal rotation. An increase of the magnitude of the posterior drawer in external rotation suggests abnormal posterolateral laxity.

REVERSE PIVOT SHIFT TEST. The **reverse pivot shift test,** described by Jakob, begins with the patient in the same supine, relaxed position. To test the right knee, the examiner faces the patient and rests the patient's right foot on the right side of the examiner's pelvis with the foot in external rotation. The palm of the examiner's left hand supports the lateral side of the calf at the level of the proximal fibula. The examiner

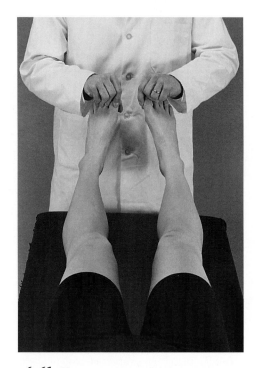

Figure 6–61. Varus recurvatum test.

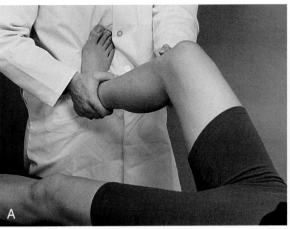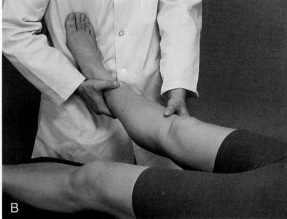

Figure 6–62. *A* and *B*, Reverse pivot shift test.

then bends the knee to 70° or 80° (Fig. 6–62A). In patients with posterolateral rotatory instability, external rotation in this position causes the lateral tibial plateau to sublux posteriorly in relation to the lateral femoral condyle. This is perceived as a posterior sag of the proximal tibia. The examiner now allows the knee to extend, leaning slightly against the foot to transmit an axial and valgus load to the knee. As the knee approaches 20° of flexion, the lateral tibial plateau reduces from its posterior subluxed position and a jerk-like shift is appreciated (Fig. 6–62B).

The test can also be done in the opposite direction. If the test is begun with the tibia in the reduced position of full extension and neutral rotation, rapid flexion produces the jerk-like phenomenon as the tibia subluxes with external rotation posteriorly in relation to the lateral femoral condyle.

Patellofemoral Joint

Besides the observations of patellar malalignment and facet tenderness already described, the specific patellofemoral joint examination includes tests for patellofemoral crepitus and instability.

PASSIVE PATELLAR GRIND TEST. The **passive patellar grind test** is probably the most well known test for patellofemoral crepitus. With the patient supine and relaxed, the examiner presses the patella against the femur with the palm of one hand while passively flexing the knee with the other (Fig. 6–63). When degeneration or traumatic irregularity of the articular surface of the patella or the femoral trochlea is present, the examiner feels a distinctive crunching sensation transmitted through the patella. Pressure should be light.

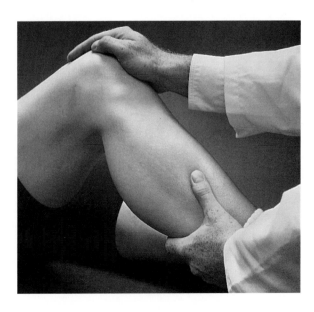

Figure 6–63. Passive patellar grind test.

This test can be uncomfortable even in the normal knee, and it is very painful in the abnormal one. Because of this, the **active patellar grind test** is recommended for routine use. In this variation, the patient sits with the knee flexed over the end or side of the examination table. The examiner gently places a hand on the patient's patella, asks the patient to actively extend the knee, and again feels for crepitus (Fig. 6–64). In this case, the patient's own quadriceps contraction provides the compressive force and the patient can voluntarily stop the process if it is too painful. The *degree of flexion* in which the crepitus is felt may also be a clue to the area of articular cartilage damage. Because the contact pattern of the patellofemoral joint varies with the position of the knee, crepitus that occurs near extension tends to be associated with lesions of the inferior portion of the patella or the superior femoral trochlea, whereas crepitus that occurs deeper into flexion usually represents injury to the superior patella or inferior trochlea.

STEP-UP–STEP-DOWN TEST. The most sensitive test for patellofemoral crepitus is the **step-up–step-down test.** In this test, the examiner asks the patient to step up onto a low stool as if climbing a stair, then to step back down again (Fig. 6–65). Again, the examiner lightly feels for crepitus during the process. This procedure loads the patellofemoral joint with a multiple of the patient's body weight and brings out crepitus not detected by the active patellar compression test. In more severe cases of articular cartilage damage, this crepitus is audible. While performing

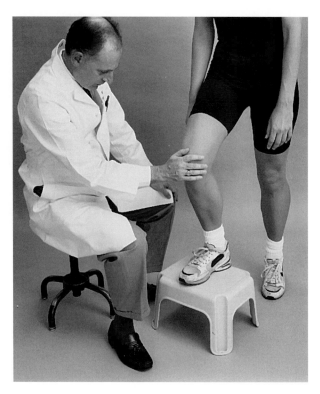

Figure 6–65. Step-up–step-down test.

any of these tests for patellofemoral crepitus, the examiner should keep in mind that normal or hypertrophied synovial folds or fronds may produce a much softer popping sensation, which needs to be distinguished from true cartilaginous crepitus.

DYNAMIC PATELLAR TRACKING. The next group of patellofemoral tests is for patellar mobility and functional instability. To assess dynamic **patellar tracking,** the examiner asks the seated patient to actively extend the knee from 90° to full extension while observing the movement pattern of the patella from the front (Fig. 6–66). Lightly placing the thumb and the index finger of one hand on either side of the patella may help the examiner follow the tracking pattern. In most individuals, the patella appears to move straight proximally, then it often shifts and tilts a bit laterally near terminal extension. When this lateral shift and tilt are more marked, the patient is at risk for symptomatic patellar instability. In the unusually extreme case, termed *habitual patellar dislocation,* the patella dislocates off the lateral edge of the femoral trochlea with every active extension.

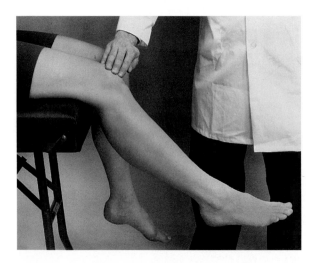

Figure 6–64. Active patellar grind test.

PATELLAR GLIDE TEST. The **patellar glide test** measures passive patellar mobility. In this test, the patient lies supine with the knees extended and the quadriceps relaxed. (Some authors recommend that the knees be slightly flexed.) The examiner pushes the patella first medially, then laterally, each time estimating the excursion of the patella with respect to the distal femur (Fig. 6–67). This excursion may be estimated in absolute terms (centimeters) or relative terms (quadrants of the patient's patella). Although the absolute amount of excursion varies widely, the average is about 1 cm in each direction. In *excessive lateral pressure syndrome,* lateral glide is extremely limited. However, not all individuals with diminished lateral glide have excessive lateral pressure syndrome. Conversely, patients with increased passive patellar mobility are at increased risk for symptomatic patellar instability, although, again, not all individuals with passive patellar hypermobility develop clinical symptoms of patellar instability.

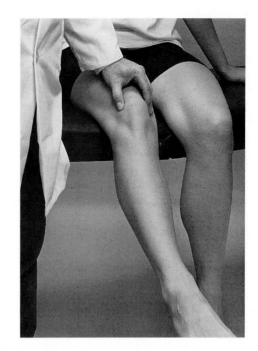

Figure 6–66. Assessing patellar tracking.

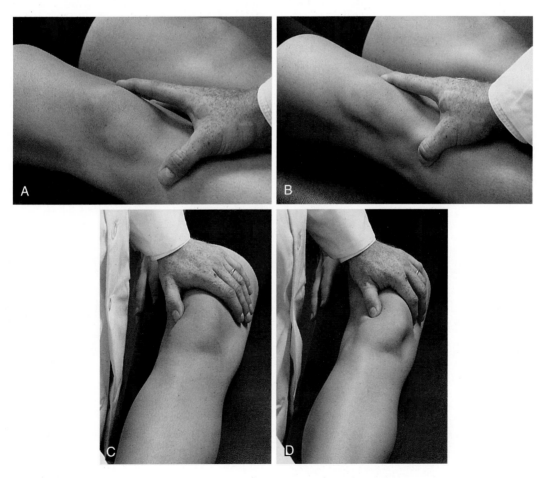

Figure 6–67. Passive patellar glide. *A,* Lateral glide, starting position. *B,* Lateral glide, displaced position. *C,* Medial glide, starting position. *D,* Medial glide, displaced position.

PATELLAR APPREHENSION TEST. A test that is more suggestive of clinically symptomatic patellar instability (recurrent subluxation or dislocation) is the **patellar apprehension test,** sometimes called the **Fairbanks apprehension test.** This test is designed to simulate an episode of patellar instability under controlled circumstances. With the patient supine and relaxed, the examiner grasps the symptomatic limb at the ankle and abducts it sufficiently to allow the knee to be flexed over the side of the table. With the thumb or fingers of the other hand, the examiner performs a lateral patellar glide, pushing the patient's patella as far laterally as possible (Fig. 6–68A). The examiner then slowly flexes the patient's knee with the other hand (Fig. 6–68B). In the patient with a history of patellar subluxation or dislocation, this maneuver usually creates an apprehension that another episode of instability is imminent. This apprehension manifests itself with behavior ranging from verbal expressions of anxiety to an involuntary quadriceps contraction that prevents further knee flexion. The test is conducted slowly enough so that it can be terminated once the anticipated response is elicited but before causing the patient undue discomfort.

Meniscal Tests

A number of manipulative tests have been developed over the years to diagnose tears of the menisci. They are variable in their sensitivity and should be thought of as adjuncts to the finding of joint line tenderness. They are all based on two facts: (1) most meniscal tears occur in the posterior third of the menisci and (2) as the knee flexes, the femur rolls posteriorly on the tibial plateau, increasing the contact between the femoral condyles and the posterior portions of the menisci. All these tests place the knee in a flexed or hyperflexed position and then compress it, resulting in pain and sometimes clicking localized to the symptomatic meniscus.

CHILDRESS' TEST. In the **Childress test,** the patient is asked to duck walk, that is, to walk in a deep squat. As the patient lifts the uninvolved limb to step forward, all the body weight momentarily compresses the symptomatic knee (Fig. 6–69). If a meniscus tear is present, this maneuver usually causes pain localized to the joint line of the involved meniscus. This localization is important because other conditions can produce pain with the Childress test. For example, patellofemoral pain usually is induced or aggravated by the duck walk, but the patient localizes the pain to the retropatellar region. When an effusion is present in the knee, whatever the cause, the patient usually feels pain or discomfort in the popliteal fossa during the duck walk.

McMURRAY'S TEST. For the **McMurray test,** the supine patient is asked to flex the involved knee as far as possible. To test the **medial meniscus,** the examiner grasps the patient's hindfoot and externally rotates the foot while placing a varus stress at the knee to compress the medial meniscus (Fig. 6–70A). The knee is then pas-

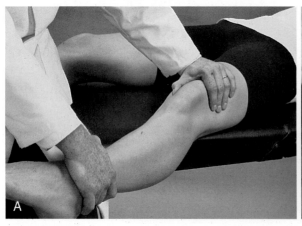
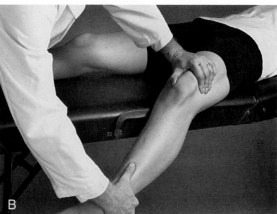

Figure 6–68. *A* and *B,* Patellar apprehension test.

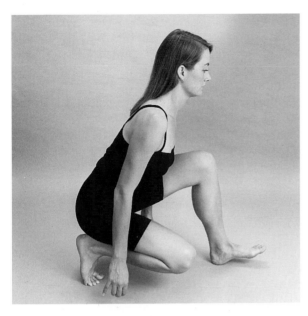

Figure 6–69. Childress' test.

sively extended while the examiner palpates the medial joint line with the index finger of the other hand (Fig. 6–70*B*).

In McMurray's original description, the test is positive if the patient complains of pain localized to the medial joint line and the examiner feels a click in this location. In our experience, the true McMurray click is only occasionally felt, although joint line pain is commonly elicited in the absence of such a click and often indicates a meniscus tear. The pain of osteoarthritis can sometimes also be elicited by the McMurray test.

To test for a **lateral meniscus** tear, the examiner applies an internal rotation–valgus force to the hyperflexed knee (see Fig. 6–70*C*). In the presence of a lateral meniscus tear, the patient reports pain localized to the lateral joint line as the knee is passively extended (see Fig. 6–70*D*). A click is only rarely felt with the lateral McMurray test.

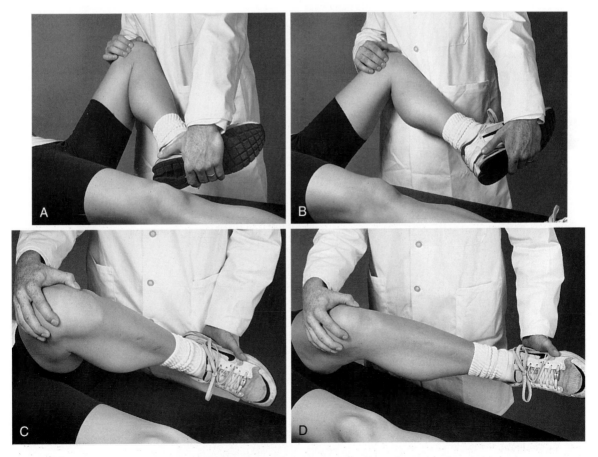

Figure 6–70. McMurray's test. *A* and *B*, Medial meniscus. *C* and *D*, Lateral meniscus.

APLEY'S TEST. The **Apley test** for posterior meniscus tears has two parts. In both portions, the patient is asked to be prone and to flex the knee to 90°. The examiner then grasps the foot and asks the patient to relax. For the control or **distraction** portion of the test, the examiner stabilizes the patient's thigh using downward pressure from the examiner's own knee while pulling the patient's foot upward to distract the patient's knee. The examiner then alternately externally and internally rotates the patient's foot (Fig. 6–71A and B). The patient should not have pain with the distraction portion of the test. If pain is experienced during distraction, the test is not considered reliable (although the patient may still have a meniscus tear) and is abandoned.

If the distraction test causes no pain, the examiner proceeds to the **compression** test, pushing downward on the patient's foot to compress the knee while alternately externally and internally rotating the foot (see Fig. 6–71C and D). Pain localized to the medial joint line (usually produced by external rotation) suggests a medial

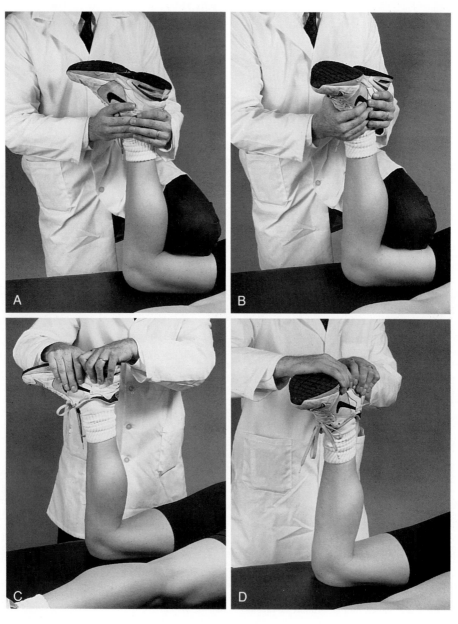

Figure 6–71. Apley's test. *A* and *B*, Distraction. *C* and *D*, Compression.

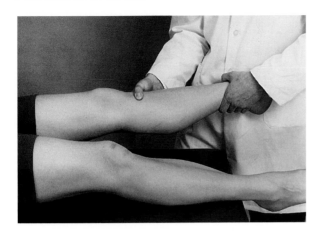

Figure 6–72. Passive extension test.

meniscus tear, whereas pain localized to the lateral joint line (usually produced by internal rotation) suggests a lateral meniscus tear.

PASSIVE EXTENSION TEST. The final manipulative meniscus test is designed specifically to detect displaced bucket handle tears, which occur primarily on the medial side. As already mentioned, this condition should be suspected when the patient is unable to extend the involved knee and tenderness is localized to the junction of the medial femoral condyle and medial tibial plateau. In the **passive extension test,** sometimes known as the **bounce home test,** the examiner asks the patient to actively extend the knee as far as possible. The examiner then gently and slowly extends the knee a bit further.

In the presence of a displaced bucket handle

tear of the *medial meniscus,* the patient usually indicates a sharp pain at the junction of the medial femoral condyle and the medial tibial plateau (Fig. 6–72).

A displaced bucket handle tear of the *lateral meniscus* will also cause pain when this test is performed, but the pain is not usually as well localized as with medial meniscus tears.

If a torn *ACL stump* is preventing extension, the patient usually describes the pain as central and deep. In the presence of less specific causes of flexion contracture, such as effusion and hamstring spasm, pain may also be produced by this maneuver, but it will not be localized.

Osteochondritis Dissecans

The **Wilson test** was described as a physical sign of osteochondritis dissecans. It is not frequently used. For the test, the supine patient is asked to flex the knee. The examiner then passively internally rotates the foot (Fig. 6–73A) and then extends the knee completely (Fig. 6–73B). This maneuver is meant to impinge the ACL against the classic osteochondritis dissecans lesion located adjacent to the intercondylar notch on the lateral aspect of the medial femoral condyle. In an abnormal test, the patient experiences pain when the internally rotated knee reaches full extension, and the pain should subside when the internal rotation force is relaxed.

The physical findings in common conditions of the knee are summarized in Table 6–1.

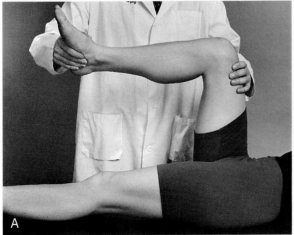 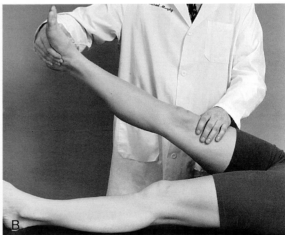

Figure 6–73. *A* and *B,* Wilson's test.

TABLE 6–1.
PHYSICAL FINDINGS IN COMMON CONDITIONS OF THE KNEE

Osteoarthritis

Tibiofemoral joint line tenderness (medial more common than lateral)
Patellofemoral joint tenderness (if involved)
Patellofemoral crepitus (if involved)
Angular deformity (varus more common than valgus)
Effusion (variable)
Visible osteophytes (variable)

Anterior Cruciate Ligament Injury

Effusion (acutely or after recurrent injury)
Lachman's test abnormal
Anterior drawer test abnormal
Pivot shift test (flexion rotation drawer test, jerk test, Losse's test) abnormal
Loss of full extension (if the stump of the ligament is impinged)
Signs of associated injuries (other ligament tears, meniscal tears)

Meniscus Tear

Joint line tenderness
Effusion (variable)
McMurray's test abnormal (variable)
Apley's test abnormal (variable)
Childress' test abnormal (variable)
Pain reproduced by passive knee flexion (variable)
Flexion contracture (if a displaced bucket handle fragment is present)
Bounce home test painful (if a displaced bucket handle fragment is present)

Medial Collateral Ligament Injury

Tenderness over the injured portion of the ligament
Swelling over the injured portion of the ligament
Effusion (usually mild)
Valgus stress test abnormal (grade II and grade III injuries)
Signs of associated injuries (if present)

Patellofemoral Chondrosis or Pain Syndrome

Patellar facet tenderness
Patellar crepitus (grind test, step-up–step-down test) (variable)
Decreased patellar glide (variable)
Effusion (more severe cases)
Stigmata of malalignment (variable) (in-facing patella, increased Q angle, increased tubercle-sulcus angle)
Patella baja (some postsurgical cases)
Lateral patellofemoral ligament tenderness (excessive lateral pressure syndrome)

Patellofemoral Instability

Increased patellar glide (especially lateral)
Dysplastic quadriceps mechanism (variable)
Apprehension test abnormal
Patellar facet tenderness and crepitus (variable)
Patella alta (variable)
Lateral patellar tracking (variable)
Increased tubercle-sulcus angle (variable)

Posterior Cruciate Ligament Injury

Dropback sign
Quadriceps active drawer test abnormal
Posterior drawer test abnormal
Effusion (acute)
Dynamic posterior shift test abnormal (variable)
Signs of other ligament injuries (if present)

Posterolateral Ligament Injury

Increased external tibial rotation
Varus stress test abnormal
Varus recurvatum test abnormal (frequently)
Posterolateral drawer test abnormal
Reverse pivot shift test abnormal (variable)
Signs of posterior cruciate ligament injury (frequently)
Signs of other associated ligament injuries (when present)

Osgood-Schlatter Disease

Increased prominence of tibial tubercle
Tender tibial tubercle

Patellar Tendon Rupture

Inability to extend knee against gravity
Swelling
Ecchymosis
Palpable gap in the patellar tendon (frequent), usually at the inferior pole of the patella
Patella alta

Quadriceps Tendon Rupture

Inability to extend the knee against gravity
Swelling
Ecchymosis
Palpable gap in the quadriceps tendon (variable), usually at the superior pole of the patella

Bibliography

Anderson AF, Lipscomb AB: Clinical diagnosis of meniscal tears. Description of a new manipulative test. Am J Sports Med. 1986;14:291–293.

Apley G: The diagnosis of meniscus injuries. J Bone Joint Surg. 1947;29:78–84.

Bach BR Jr, Warren RF, Wickiewicz TL: The pivot shift phenomenon: results and description of a modified clinical test for anterior cruciate ligament insufficiency. Am J Sports Med. 1988;16:571–576.

Baker CL Jr, Norwood LA, Hughston JC: Acute posterolateral rotatory instability of the knee. J Bone Joint Surg Am. 1983;65:614–618.

Blazina ME, Kerlan RK, Jobe FW, Carter VS, Carlson GJ: Jumper's knee. Orthop Clin North Am. 1973;4:665–678.

Bousquet G: Laxites post-traumatiques du genou. Les lésions grave récentes. Classification et principle du traitement. Rev Chir Orthop Reparatrice Appar Mot. 1972;58(suppl 1):49–56.

Broom MJ, Fulkerson JP: The plica syndrome: a new perspective. Orthop Clin North Am. 1986;17:279–281.

Butler DL, Noyes FR, Grood ES: Ligamentous restraints to anterior-posterior drawer in the human knee. A biomechanical study. J Bone Joint Surg Am. 1980;62:259–270.

Carson WG Jr, James SL, Larson RL, Singer KM, Winternitz WW: Patellofemoral disorders: physical and radiographic evaluation. Part I: Physical examination. Clin Orthop. 1984;185:165–177.

Chambers GH: The prepatellar nerve. A cause of suboptimal results in knee arthrotomy. Clin Orthop. 1972;82:157–159.

Childress HM: Popliteal cysts associated with undiagnosed posterior lesions of the medial meniscus. J Bone Joint Surg Am. 1954;36:1233–1240.

Clancy WG Jr, Shelbourne KD, Zoellner GB, Keene JS, Reider B, Rosenberg TD: Treatment of knee joint instability secondary to rupture of the posterior cruciate ligament. Report of a new procedure. J Bone Joint Surg Am. 1983;65:310–312.

Cooper DE, Warren RF, Warner JJP: The posterior cruciate ligament and posterolateral structures of the knee: anatomy, function and patterns of injury. Instr Course Lect. 1991;40:249–270.

Dandy DJ: Recurrent subluxation of the patella on extension of the knee. J Bone Joint Surg Br. 1971;53:483–487.

Daniel DM, Stone ML, Sachs R, Malcom L: Instrumented measurement of anterior knee laxity in patients with acute anterior cruciate ligament disruption. Am J Sports Med. 1985;13:401–407.

Daniel DM, Stone ML, Barnett P, Sachs R: Use of the quadriceps active test to diagnose posterior cruciate ligament disruption and measure posterior laxity of the knee. J Bone Joint Surg Am. 1988;70:386–391.

DeLee JC, Riley MB, Rockwood CA Jr: Acute posterolateral rotatory instability of the knee. Am J Sports Med. 1983;11:199–207.

Fetto JF, Marshall JL: Medial collateral ligament injuries of the knee: a rationale for treatment. Clin Orthop. 1978;132:206–218.

Fetto JF, Marshall JL: Injury to the anterior cruciate ligament producing the pivot-shift sign. An experimental study in cadaver specimens. J Bone Joint Surg Am. 1979;61:710–714.

Fetto JF, Marshall JL: The natural history and diagnosis of anterior cruciate ligament insufficiency. Clin Orthop. 1980;147:29–38.

Fowler PJ: The classification and early diagnosis of knee joint instability. Clin Orthop. 1980;147:15–21.

Fukubayashi T, Torzilli PA, Sherman ME: An in vitro biomechanical evaluation of antero-posterior motion of the knee. J Bone Joint Surg Am. 1982;64:258–264.

Fulkerson JP, Gossling HR: Anatomy of the knee joint lateral retinaculum. Clin Orthop. 1980;153:183–188.

Galway HR, McIntosh DL: The lateral pivot shift: a symptom and sign of anterior cruciate ligament insufficiency. Clin Orthop. 1980;147:45–50.

Galway RD: Pivot-shift syndrome. J Bone Joint Surg Br. 1972;54:558.

Galway RD, Beaupre A, McIntosh DL: Pivot shift: a clinical sign of symptomatic anterior cruciate insufficiency. J Bone Joint Surg Br. 1972;54:763–774.

Girgis FG, Marshall JL, Al Monajem ARS: The cruciate ligaments of the knee joint: anatomical, functional and experimental analysis. Clin Orthop. 1975;106:216–231.

Gollehon DL, Torzilli PA, Warren RJ: The role of the posterolateral and cruciate ligaments in the stability of the human knee: a biomechanical study. J Bone Joint Surg Am. 1987;69:233–242.

Grood ES, Noyes FR, Butler DL, Suntay WJ: Ligamentous and capsular restraints preventing medial and lateral laxity in intact human cadaver knees. J Bone Joint Surg Am. 1981;63:1257–1269.

Grood ES, Stowers SF, Noyes FR: Limits of movement in the human knee: effect of sectioning the posterior cruciate ligament and posterolateral structures. J Bone Joint Surg Am. 1988;70:88–97.

Gruel JB: Isolated avulsion of the popliteus tendon. Arthroscopy. 1990;6:94–95.

Helfet AJ: Disorders of the Knee. Philadelphia, JB Lippincott, 1982.

Hughston JC, Andres JR, Cross MJ, Moschi A: Classification of knee ligament instabilities: Part I. The medial compartment and cruciate ligaments. J Bone Joint Surg Am. 1976;58:159–172.

Hughston JC, Bowden JA, Andrews JR, Norwood LA: Acute tears of the posterior cruciate ligament. Results of operative treatment. J Bone Joint Surg Am. 1980;62:438–450.

Hughston JC, Norwood LA: The posterolateral drawer test and the external rotational recurvatum test for posterolateral rotatory instability of the knee. Clin Orthop. 1980;147:82–87.

Hughston JD, Deese J: Medial subluxation of the patella as a complication of lateral retinacular release. Am J Sports Med. 1988;16:383–388.

Inoue M, McGurk-Burleson E, Hollis JM, Woo SL: Treatment of the medial collateral ligament injury: I. The importance of anterior cruciate on varus-valgus knee laxity. Am J Sports Med. 1987;15:15–21.

Insall J, Goldberg V, Salvati E: Recurrent dislocation and the high-riding patella. Clin Orthop. 1972;88:67–69.

Insall J: "Chondromalacia patellaeu": patellar malalignment syndrome. Orthop Clin North Am. 1979;10:117–127.

Jakob RP, Hassler H, Staeubli HU: Observations on rotary instability of the lateral compartment of the knee. Acta Orthop Scand Suppl. 1981;191:6–27.

Jakob RP, Staeubli HU, Deland JT: Grading the pivot shift: objective tests with implications for treatment. J Bone Joint Surg Br. 1987;69:294–299.

Jonsson T, Althoff B, Peterson L, Renstrom P: Clinical diagnosis of ruptures of the anterior cruciate ligament: a comparative study of the Lachman test and the anterior drawer sign. Am J Sports Med. 1982;10:100–102.

Kennedy JC, Fowler PJ: Medial and anterior instability of the knee. An anatomical and clinical study using stress machines. J Bone Joint Surg Am. 1971;53:1257–1270.

Kolowich PA, Paulos LE, Rosenberg TD, Farnsworth S: Lateral release of the patella: indications and contraindications. Am J Sports Med. 1990;18:359–365.

Kozin F, McCaarty DJ, Sims J, Genanth K: The reflex sympathetic dystrophy syndrome. Am J Med. 1976;60:321–331.

Lancourt JE, Cristini JA: Patella alta and patella infera. J Bone Joint Surg. 1975;57:1112–1115.

Lemaire M: Ruptures anciennes du ligament croise anterieur du genou. J Chir (Paris). 1967;93:311–320.

Losee RE, Johnson E, Southwick WO: Anterior subluxation of the lateral tibial plateau. J Bone Joint Surg Am. 1978;60:1015–1030.

Mariani PP, Caruso I: An electromyographic investigation of subluxation of the patella. J Bone Joint Surg Br. 1979;61:169–171.

Martens M, Libbrect P, Burssens A: Surgical treatment of the iliotibial band friction syndrome. Am J Sports Med. 1989;17:651–654.

McConnell J: The management of chondromalacia patellae: a long term solution. Aust J Physiother. 1986;2:215–223.

McMurray TP: The semilunar cartilages. Br J Surg. 1942;29:407–414.

Metheny JA, Mayor MD: Hoffa disease. Chronic impingement of the infrapatellar fat pad. Am J Knee Surg. 1988;1:134–139.

Mital MA, Matza RA, Cohen J: The so-called unresolved Osgood-Schlatter lesion. J Bone Joint Surg Am. 1980;62:732–739.

Murphy SB, Simon SR, Kijewski PK, Wilkinson RH, Griscom NT: Femoral anteversion. J Bone Joint Surg Am. 1987;69:1169–1176.

Mysnyk MC, Wroble RR, Foster DT, Albright JP: Prepatellar bursitis in wrestlers. Am J Sports Med. 1986;44:46–54.

Noble CA: Iliotibial band friction syndrome in runners. Am J Sports Med. 1980;8:232–234.

Noyes FR, Bassett RW, Grood E, Butler DL: Arthroscopy in acute traumatic hemarthrosis of the knee. Incidence of anterior cruciate tears and other injuries. J Bone Joint Surg Am. 1980;62:687–695.

Noyes FR, Grood E, Stowers SA: A biomechanical analysis of knee ligament injuries producing posterolateral subluxation. Proceedings of the International Society of the Knee. Am J Sports Med. 1986;12:440.

Noyes FR, Grood ES, Tarzill PA: The definitions of terms for motion and position of the knee and injuries of the ligaments. J Bone Joint Surg Am. 1989;71:465–472.

Ogata K, McCarthy JA, Dunlap J, Manske PR: Pathomechanics of posterior sag of the tibia in posterior cruciate deficient knees. Am J Sports Med. 1988;16:630–636.

Ogden JA, Southwick WO: Osgood-Schlatter's disease and tibial tuberosity development. Clin Orthop. 1976;116:180–189.

Ogden JA, McCarthy SM, Jokl P: The painful bipartite patella. J Pediatr Orthop. 1982;2:263–269.

Osgood RB: Lesions of tibial tubercle occurring during adolescence. Boston Med Surg J. 1903;148:114.

Reider B, Marshall JL, Koslin B, Ring B, Girgis FG: The anterior aspect of the knee joint: an anatomical study. J Bone Joint Surg. Am. 1981;63:351–356.

Reider B, Marshall JL, Warren RF: Clinical characteristics of patellar disorders in young athletes. Am J Sports Med. 1981;9:270–274.

Roels J, Martens M, Mulier JC, Burssens A: Patellar tendinitis (jumper's knee). Am J Sports Med. 1978;6:362–368.

Seebacher JR, Inglis AE, Marshall JL, Warren RF: The structures of the posterolateral aspect of the knee. J Bone Joint Surg Am. 1982;64:53.

Shakespeare DT, Rigby HS: The bucket-handle tear of the meniscus. A clinical and arthrographic study. J Bone Joint Surg Br. 1983;65:383–387.

Shelbourne RD, Benedict F, McCarroll JR, Rettig AC: Dynamic posterior shift test. Am J Sports Med. 1988;17:275–277.

Shoemaker SC, Daniel DM: The limits of knee motion: in vitro studies. In Daniel DM, Akeson WH, O'Connor JJ, eds. Knee Ligaments: Structure, Function, Injury, and Repair. New York, Raven, 1990, pp 153–161.

Sinding-Larsen MF: A hitherto unknown affliction of the patella in children. Acta Radiol. 1921;1:171–173.

Torg JS, Conrad W, Kalen V: Clinical diagnosis of anterior cruciate ligament instability in the athlete. Am J Sports Med. 1976;4:84–93.

Warren LF, Marshall JL, Girgis F: The prime static stabilizer of the medial side of the knee. J Bone Joint Surg Am. 1974;56:665–674.

Wilson JN: A diagnostic sign in osteochondritis dissecans of the knee. J Bone Joint Surg Am. 1967;49:477–480.

Michael E. Brage
Bruce Reider

7

Lower Leg, Foot, and Ankle

The foot and ankle are the foundation of the human body. They provide the necessary stability for our distinctive upright posture and function as the focal point through which total body weight is transmitted during ambulation. With 28 bones and 57 articulations, the foot is uniquely adapted to provide flexibility on uneven terrain and to absorb shock. The faultless function of this complex mechanism is often taken for granted until a breakdown occurs.

The lower leg contains the major motors that power the foot and the ankle. It is streamlined and lightweight, increasing the length and leverage of the lower limb, while adding minimal bulk and weight. This composition, unfortunately, leaves the tibia exposed to external trauma. The structure of the lower leg is simplified compared with the forearm, so that the elegant mechanism of rotation found in the latter structure is absent.

The magnitude of forces concentrated in the lower leg, the foot, and the ankle puts them at risk for a variety of acute and overuse injuries. Finally, the external stresses that people impose on their feet by sometimes illogical choices in footwear lead to another array of potential problems.

Inspection

Observation of the foot is often critical to understanding the patient's complaints of pain or dysfunction. The patient should remove socks and shoes from both feet. If pants are worn, they should be rolled up to the knees. The foot is inspected during gait, while standing, and while in a nonweightbearing position. The leg, the foot, and the ankle should be viewed from the front, the sides, and behind. Initially, the overall bony and soft tissue contours should be noted. Later, a closer inspection allows callosities, scars, and ulcers to be recorded.

SURFACE ANATOMY

Anterior Aspect

Inspecting the patient from the front allows the examiner to assess the dorsum of the foot and the anterior aspect of the ankle and the leg. At least part of the inspection should be done with the patient standing because this is the normal functioning position of the lower limb.

TOES. The toes are the most detailed and recognizable portion of the foot (Fig. 7–1). The skeleton of the great toe is composed of a **proximal phalanx** and a **distal phalanx,** which articulate with each other at the **interphalangeal joint.** Each of the other four toes has three **phalanges (proximal, middle,** and **distal),** and consequently each has both a **distal interphalangeal joint** and a **proximal interphalangeal joint.** A subtle **transverse skin crease** is often identifiable over the dorsum of the interphalangeal joint of the great toe and the distal interphalangeal joint of the second through fourth toes, due to the passive hyperextension that occurs at these joints during normal gait. The examiner should note any areas of thickened cornified skin over the dorsum of any of the interphalangeal joints. These lesions usually reflect friction between the toe and the top of the shoe, and they tend to occur in conjunction with toe deformities. They may be called **heloma durum** or *hard corns* (Fig. 7–2).

The dorsum of the distal phalanx of each toe is protected by a **toenail,** which grows from a **nail fold** near the base of each distal phalanx. The rich capillary supply of the nailbeds usually gives the toenails a bright pink color, although the exact shade varies among individuals depending on their overall coloration. A white crescent or **lunula** may be observed at the base of the toenails, particularly in the great toe.

Deformities of the toenails and surrounding tissue are common and may reflect local trauma, infection, or systemic illness. A *subungual hematoma* is the common sequela of a direct blow to

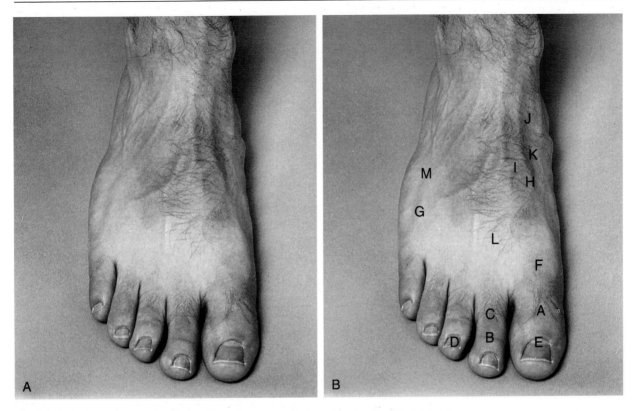

Figure 7–1. *A* and *B*, The dorsum of the foot. A, interphalangeal joint; B, distal interphalangeal joint (note transverse skin crease); C, proximal interphalangeal joint; D, toenail; E, lunula; F, first metatarsophalangeal joint; G, fifth metatarsal; H, first metatarsal-cuneiform joint; I, dorsalis pedis artery; J, tarsal navicular; K, medial cuneiform; L, typical site of second metatarsal stress fracture; M, typical site of Jones fracture.

the toe or recurrent pressure from an activity, such as running. It appears as a maroon to black discoloration that is visible through the base of the toenail and sometimes involves the entire nail. *Malignant melanoma* may produce a dark discoloration beneath the nail as well, initially

appearing innocuous but becoming aggressive with time. Chronic *fungal infections* may produce deformities of the toenails including ridging, thickening, and yellow to orange discoloration (Fig. 7–3). Injury to the matrix at the base of the toenail may subsequently cause the nail to split

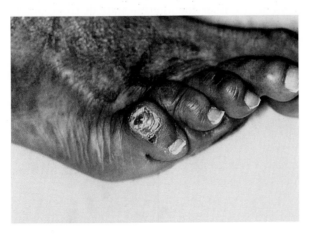

Figure 7–2. Heloma durum of the fifth toe.

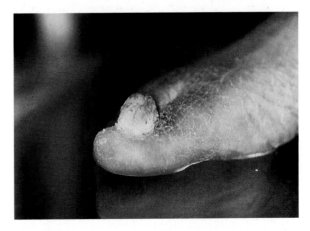

Figure 7–3. Chronic fungal infection of the great toenail.

or to be deformed. A *paronychia* is an infection around the base or sides of the toenail, manifested by swelling and erythema of the soft tissue in this area (Fig. 7–4). Paronychia may be associated with an *ingrown toenail*, a condition in which the edge of the toenail curves inward, irritating the underlying soft tissue. In a longstanding ingrown toenail, abundant hypertrophic granulation tissue is visible protruding around the side of the nail. The adjacent paronychial tissue may be swollen, erythematous, and tender.

Contractures and alignment deformities of the interphalangeal joints of the toes are common and are described later.

FOOT. The base of the proximal phalanx of each of the toes is linked to the head of one of the five corresponding metatarsals at the **metatarsophalangeal joint.** The web spaces between the toes are located approximately at the midpoints of the proximal phalanges of the adjacent toes; consequently, the metatarsophalangeal joints are located quite proximal to the visible web spaces. Passively plantar flexing a toe should produce a visible prominence on the dorsum of the foot corresponding to the metatarsophalangeal joint of that toe. The metatarsophalangeal joints of the great and fifth toes may also be identifiable by subtle flaring convexities visible on the medial and lateral borders of the foot, respectively.

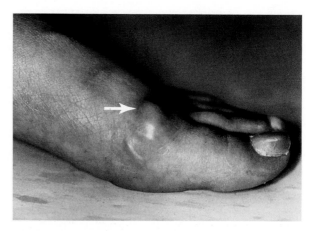

Figure 7–5. Dorsal osteophytes of the first metatarsophalangeal joint *(arrow)*.

Osteoarthritis of the first metatarsophalangeal joint is common and may be associated with a visible ridge of osteophytes on the dorsum of the foot (Fig. 7–5). A **bunion** is a large bump on the medial aspect of the first metatarsophalangeal joint. It is produced by the accretion of bone on the medial aspect of the head of the first metatarsal and the thickening of the overlying soft tissue. An adventitial bursa, which may intermittently become inflamed or even infected, constitutes a significant portion of the bunion deformity (Fig. 7–6A). Bunions are usually associated with **hallux valgus,** which is described in the Alignment section.

A similar prominence over the lateral aspect of the head of the fifth metatarsal is known as a **bunionette** or **tailor's bunion** (see Fig. 7–6B). In times past, tailors traditionally acquired such deformities by sitting with their legs crossed and with the lateral borders of their feet pressed against the floor for long periods of time; nowadays, such deformities are primarily related to tight footwear.

The proximal ends of the five metatarsals articulate with the three cuneiforms medially and the cuboid laterally at the **tarsometatarsal joint,** also known as **Lisfranc's joint.** The tarsometarsal joint is not normally visible unless periarticular osteophytes have formed that accentuate it. Such osteophytes frequently form a visible ridge at the **first metatarsal–medial cuneiform joint.**

The tendons of the long toe extensors are usually visible in the metatarsal region. If they are not visible at rest, asking the patient to actively extend the toes should increase their prominence (Fig. 7–7). The tendon of the **extensor hallucis longus** roughly parallels the shaft of the first

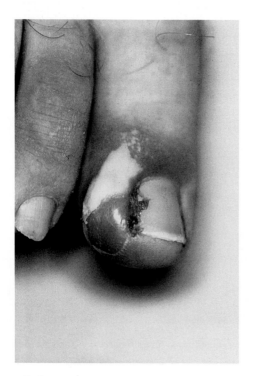

Figure 7–4. Paronychia.

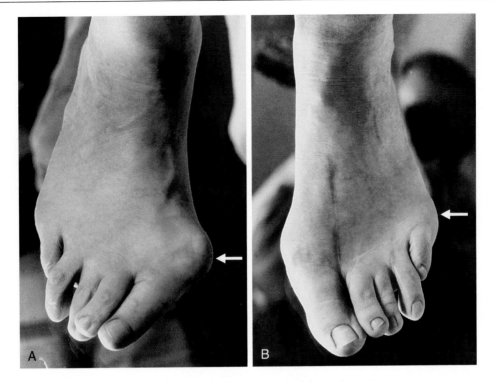

Figure 7–6. *A*, Bunion deformity *(arrow)*. *B*, Tailor's bunion (bunionette) *(arrow)*.

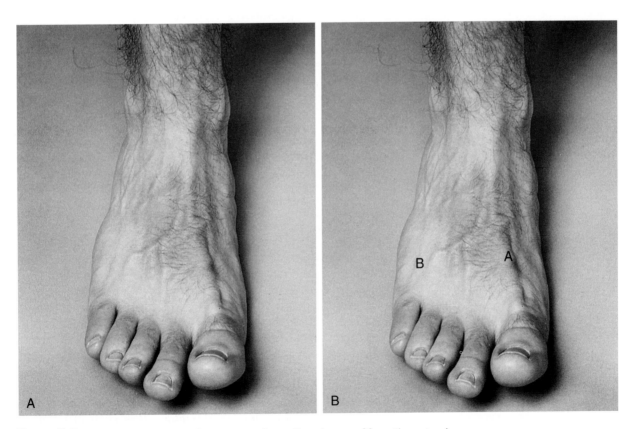

Figure 7–7. *A* and *B*, Prominence of extensor tendons of toes increased by active extension. A, extensor hallucis longus; B, extensor digitorum longus to fifth toe.

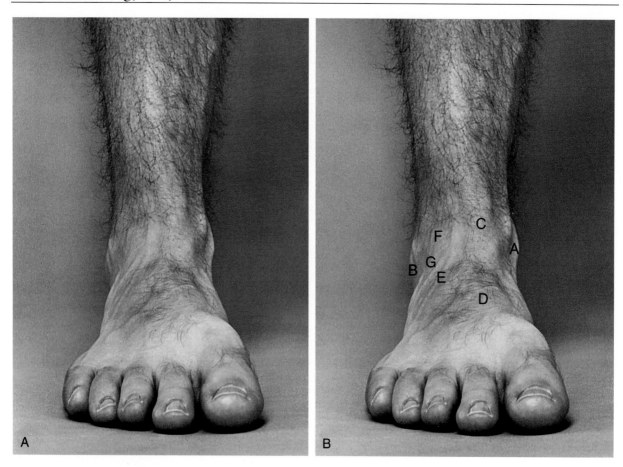

Figure 7–8. *A* and *B*, Anterior aspect of the ankle joint. A, medial malleolus; B, lateral malleolus; C, tibialis anterior tendon; D, extensor hallucis longus; E, extensor digitorum longus; F, anterior inferior tibiofibular ligament; G, peroneus tertius.

metatarsal and is the most visible. It serves as a landmark for locating the **dorsalis pedis artery,** which is situated just lateral to it. The **extensor digitorum longus** tendons to the lateral four toes fan out from a common sheath in the inferior extensor retinaculum located just distal to the ankle.

ANKLE. Proceeding proximally on the limb, the examiner encounters the **ankle** joint. The ankle joint is framed by the **medial** and **lateral malleoli,** the bony prominences of the distal tibia and fibula, respectively (Fig. 7–8). The examiner notes that the lateral malleolus is normally posterior to the medial malleolus because the plane of the ankle joint is externally rotated about 15° to the true coronal plane. Conditions such as fractures, sprains, tendinitis, and osteoarthritis can deform the normal contours of the malleoli (Fig. 7–9). Between the malleoli, several tendons can be seen crossing the ankle joint. The **tibialis anterior** (anterior tibial) is the largest

and most medial of these. It should be visible in almost all individuals, especially if the subject is asked to dorsiflex the ankle actively. Lateral to the tibialis anterior, the **extensor hallucis longus** and **extensor digitorum longus** tendons can be seen in leaner individuals. The **peroneus tertius** tendon runs along the lateral border of the extensor digitorum longus tendons.

LOWER LEG. Above the ankle, the anterior crest of the tibia is seen as a subtle longitudinal ridge that arises above the ankle joint and runs proximally to blend with the tibial tubercle (Fig. 7–10). Medial to the tibial crest lies the flat subcutaneous border of the tibia. Because this portion of the tibia is so superficial, deformities due to acute fractures or malunions of prior fractures are usually quite obvious. The uncommon type of tibial stress fracture that occurs at the midpoint of the anterior tibial crest is often visible as a small lump arising along this ridge. Lateral to the tibial crest lie the **anterior compartment**

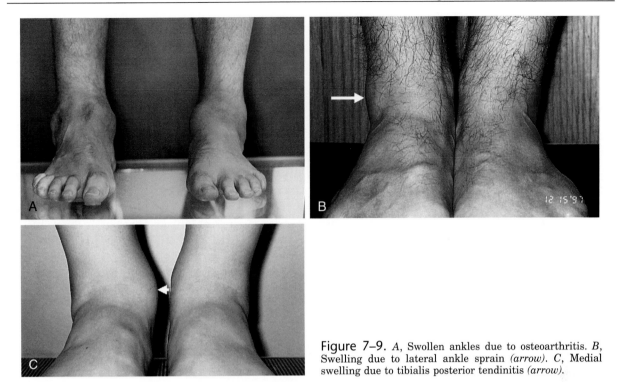

Figure 7–9. *A,* Swollen ankles due to osteoarthritis. *B,* Swelling due to lateral ankle sprain *(arrow).* *C,* Medial swelling due to tibialis posterior tendinitis *(arrow).*

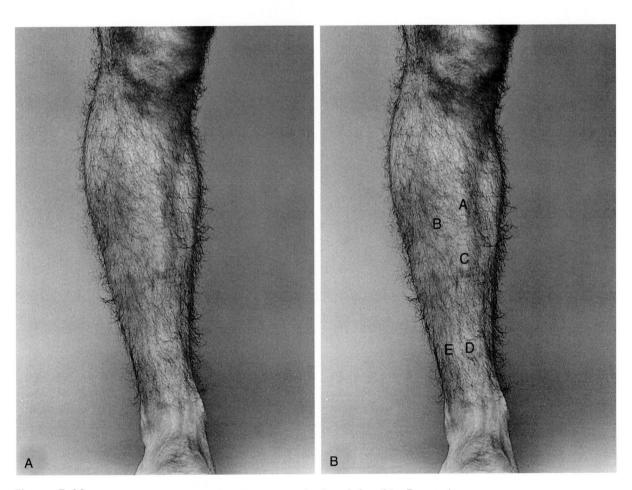

Figure 7–10. *A* and *B,* Anterior leg. A, subcutaneous border of the tibia; B, anterior compartment muscles; C, typical site of anterior crest stress fracture; D, site of tibialis anterior peritendinitis; E, site of possible superficial peroneal nerve compression.

muscles, the tibialis anterior and the toe extensors. Active use of these muscles causes them to become visible in a lean individual.

Lateral Aspect

FOOT AND ANKLE. Viewing the foot from the lateral position allows the examiner to reinspect many of the structures already seen and to visualize some new ones (Fig. 7–11). From this viewpoint, the base of the **fifth metatarsal** and the **lateral malleolus** are seen bulging toward the examiner. Distal to the lateral malleolus, a soft fleshy mound is seen in most individuals. The mound is formed by a fat pad that lies over the

sinus tarsae of the subtalar joint and **extensor digitorum brevis** muscle belly. The tendon of the **peroneus brevis** muscle can usually be seen as it curves around the posterior border of the lateral malleolus and courses toward the base of the fifth metatarsal. Asking the patient to evert the foot against resistance increases the prominence of this tendon (Fig. 7–12). The **peroneus longus** tendon courses deeper than the peroneus brevis and cannot normally be distinguished from it.

The **Achilles tendon** constitutes the posterior border of the ankle from this perspective. In the presence of chronic Achilles tendinitis, a fusiform swelling of the Achilles may be visible several centimeters proximal to the tuberosity of the cal-

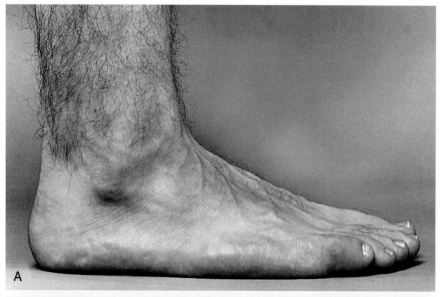

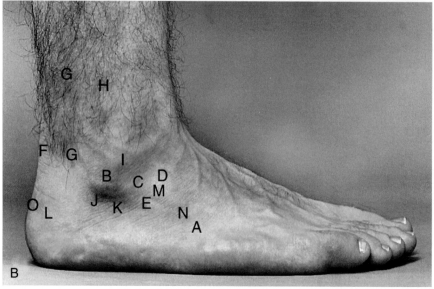

Figure 7–11. *A* and *B*, Lateral aspect of the foot and ankle. A, base of the fifth metatarsal; B, lateral malleolus; C, sinus tarsae; D, extensor digitorum brevis; E, peroneus brevis tendon; F, Achilles' tendon; G, sural nerve; H, typical site of fibular stress fracture; I, anterior talofibular ligament; J, calcaneofibular ligament; K, peroneal tubercle; L, tuberosity of the calcaneus; M, anterior process of the calcaneus; N, cuboid; O, subcutaneous bursa.

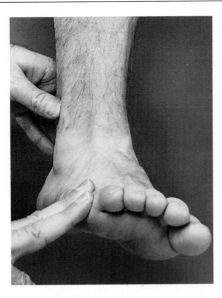

Figure 7–12. Everting the foot increases the prominence of the peroneal tendons.

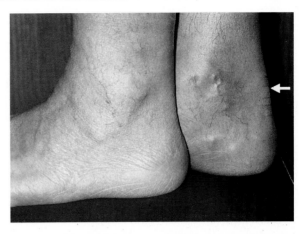

Figure 7–13. Achilles' tendinitis of the right ankle *(arrow)*.

caneus (Fig. 7–13). The lateral malleolus and Achilles are landmarks for the **sural nerve,** which courses distally in the leg along the lateral border of the Achilles tendon and curves around the lateral malleolus into the foot.

LOWER LEG. As the examiner's gaze moves proximal from the lateral malleolus, the **fibula** disappears from view deep to the muscle bellies of the **peroneal muscles** of the lateral compartment of the leg (Fig. 7–14). The posterior contour of the calf is made up of the **gastrocnemius** and **soleus** muscles of the posterior compartment. In lean individuals, the transition between the contours of the peroneal muscles and the gastrocsoleus complex is visible.

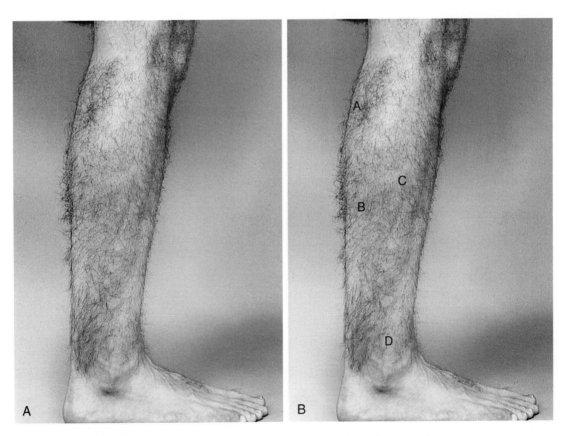

Figure 7–14. *A* and *B*, Lateral aspect of the leg. A, gastrocnemius; B, soleus; C, peroneal muscles; *D*, fibula.

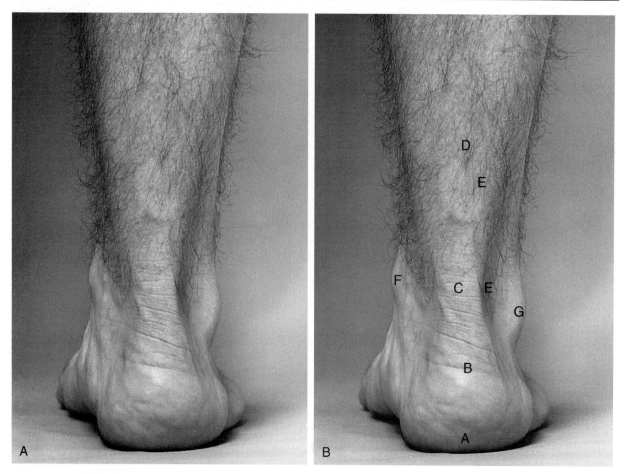

Figure 7–15. *A* and *B*, Posterior aspect of the foot and ankle. A, plantar fat pad; B, calcaneal tuberosity; C, Achilles' tendon; D, soleus; E, sural nerve; F, medial malleolus; G, lateral malleolus.

Posterior Aspect

FOOT. When the foot is viewed from the posterior position, the rounded contour of the **plantar fat pad,** which cushions the calcaneus during weightbearing, is seen bulging toward the examiner (Fig. 7–15). More superiorly, the posterior aspect of the **calcaneal tuberosity** is almost subcutaneous; therefore, its outlines are usually clearly visible. Abnormally increased prominence of the superior aspect of the calcaneal tuberosity is known as *Haglund's deformity.* This deformity is manifested by a large visible bump, especially over the supralateral corner of the calcaneal tuberosity (Fig. 7–16). Thickened skin and subcutaneous bursal enlargement may further increase the prominence of this deformity. Because it is thought to be caused, or at least exacerbated, by shoe pressure over the calcaneal tuberosity, this deformity is often popularly described as a *pump bump.* The **retrocalcaneal bursa** lies between the distal Achilles tendon and the superior portion of the calcaneal tuberosity. In the presence of retrocalcaneal bursitis, chronic thickening of

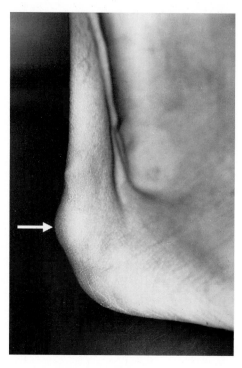

Figure 7–16. Haglund's deformity *(arrow).*

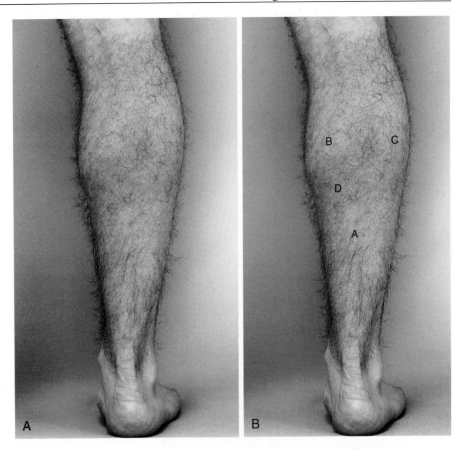

Figure 7–17. *A* and *B*, Posterior aspect of the leg. A, soleus; B, medial gastrocnemius; C, lateral gastrocnemius; D, usual site of gastrocnemius tear.

this bursa also adds to the apparent prominence of the calcaneal tuberosity.

ANKLE. More proximally, the **Achilles tendon** can be seen coursing between the **medial** and the **lateral malleoli** to its insertion on the calcaneal tuberosity. This subcutaneous tendon should be visible in virtually all individuals. Achilles tendinitis (tendinosis) and rupture usually occur about 2 cm to 3 cm proximal to the tendon's insertion. More severe cases of Achilles tendinitis can be diagnosed by the presence of a visible bulbous enlargement of the tendon at about the level of the malleoli (see Fig. 7–13). In the case of a rupture, the examiner notes more diffuse swelling throughout the visible length of the tendon owing to the accumulation of hemorrhage and edema.

CALF. More proximally, the Achilles tendon fans out into a flat aponeurosis over the posterior aspect of the **soleus** muscle belly (Fig. 7–17). Still higher on the leg, the two distinct heads of the **gastrocnemius** insert into this common aponeurosis. The outlines of the medial and the lateral heads of the gastrocnemius are visible in many individuals, especially if the patient is asked to perform a toe raise (Fig. 7–18). Calf atrophy should be looked for. Because the normal

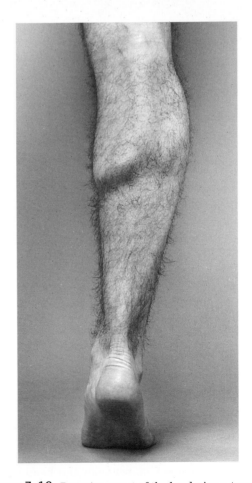

Figure 7–18. Posterior aspect of the leg during a toe raise.

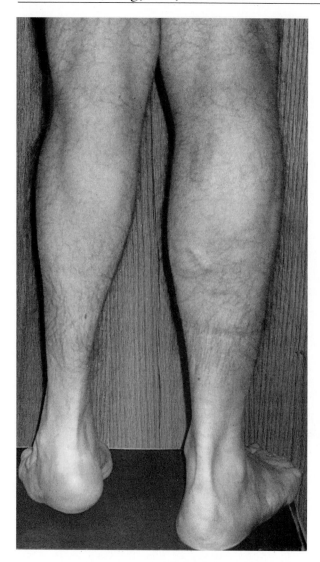

Figure 7–19. Residual left calf atrophy following clubfoot.

bulk of the calf muscles can vary tremendously from one individual to another, a lack of symmetry is the key finding that should suggest abnormality. Calf atrophy may be the residuum of an otherwise corrected clubfoot deformity (Fig. 7–19) or prior Achilles' tendon rupture, or the nonspecific consequence of immobilization.

Medial Aspect

FOOT AND ANKLE. The medial viewpoint gives the examiner a direct view of the arch and the vicinity of the major neurovascular bundle (Fig. 7–20). In the standing individual, the medial border of the foot between the head of the first metatarsal and the calcaneal tuberosity should arch away from the floor. The concavity thus created is called the **medial longitudinal arch.** An abnormally high arch is known as **pes cavus** (Fig. 7–21A), whereas an abnormally low arch is known as **pes planus** (Fig. 7–21B).

Bony contours that are visible from the medial perspective include the head of the **first metatarsal,** the **calcaneal tuberosity,** and the **medial malleolus.** This latter landmark usually appears as a pointed prominence. Distal and anterior to the medial malleolus, the examiner often can see the much smaller prominence created by the **navicular tuberosity.** When an **accessory navicular** or **cornuate navicular** is present, the prominence of the navicular tuberosity may be increased until it rivals that of the medial malleolus in size. Patients with such anomalies often describe themselves as having two ankle bones.

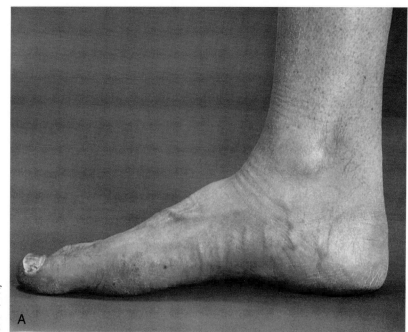

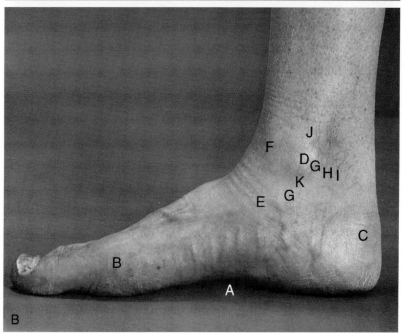

Figure 7–20. *A* and *B*, Medial aspect of the foot and ankle. A, medial longitudinal arch; B, head of the first metatarsal; C, calcaneal tuberosity; D, medial malleolus; E, navicular tuberosity; F, saphenous vein; G, posterior tibial tendon; H, flexor digitorum longus tendon; I, posterior tibial artery; J, typical site of stress fracture of the medial malleolus; K, deltoid ligament.

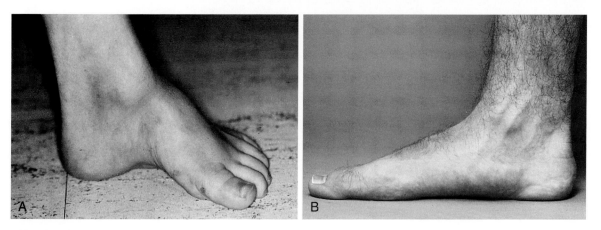

Figure 7–21. *A*, Pes cavus. *B*, Pes planus.

The **saphenous vein** is usually large and superficial at the ankle and can often be seen as it passes anterior to the medial malleolus.

Proceeding immediately posteriorly from the medial malleolus one encounters, in order, the **tibialis posterior** (posterior tibial) and **flexor digitorum longus** tendons, the **posterior tibial artery** and **nerve,** and the **flexor hallucis longus** tendon. Of all these structures, only the tibialis posterior is normally visible, and resisted inversion and plantar flexion are usually necessary to make it stand out distinctly (Fig. 7–22). When this resistance is applied, the tibialis posterior tendon is most easily seen between the posterior edge of the lateral malleolus and its insertion on the navicular tuberosity.

LOWER LEG. The surface anatomy of the medial leg is quite straightforward (Fig. 7–23). From this perspective, the anterior portion of the leg is defined by the straight margin of the subcutaneous border of the **tibia,** whereas the

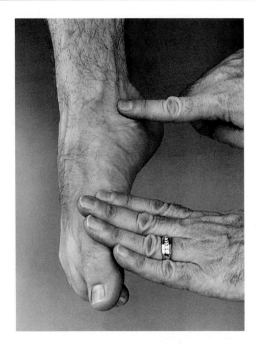

Figure 7–22. Inverting the foot against resistance to demonstrate the posterior tibial tendon.

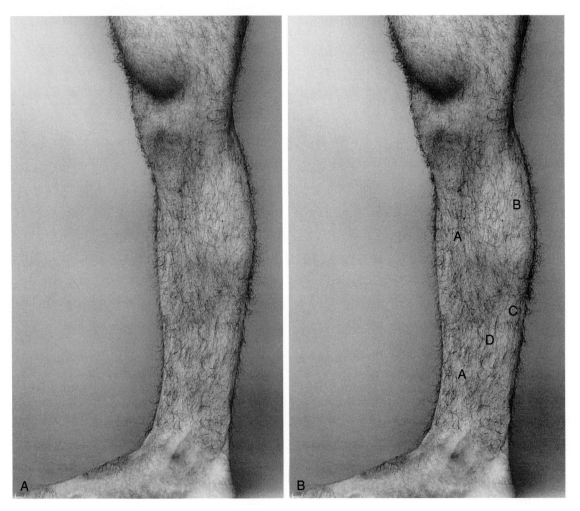

Figure 7–23. *A* and *B,* Medial aspect of the leg. A, tibia; B, gastrocnemius; C, soleus; D, most common site of tibial stress fracture.

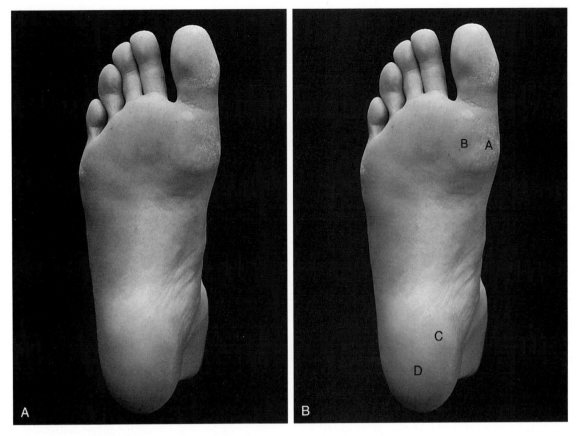

Figure 7–24. *A* and *B*, Plantar aspect of the foot. A, medial sesamoid; B, lateral sesamoid; C, typical site of plantar fasciitis; D, plantar fat pad of the heel.

posterior margin is defined by the contours of the **soleus** and the medial head of the **gastrocnemius.**

Plantar Aspect

Of course, the plantar aspect of the foot must be examined when the patient is not weightbearing (Fig. 7–24). However, careful inspection of the skin of the plantar surface allows the examiner to deduce information concerning the function of the foot during weightbearing. Areas of thickened or callused skin should be noted because they reflect the weightbearing pattern of the foot and can thus help identify areas of excessive weightbearing. Such areas of thickened skin commonly occur along the lateral foot and underneath the metatarsal heads. **Intractable plantar keratosis** is the term usually applied to the frequently painful accumulations of callused skin that can form beneath the metatarsal heads (Fig. 7–25). The formation of these keratoses is usually secondary to deformities of the toes. In *hammer toe* or *claw toe* deformities, the associated hyperextension of the metatarsophalangeal joint plantar

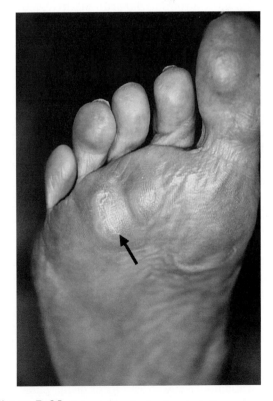

Figure 7–25. Intractable plantar keratosis *(arrow)*.

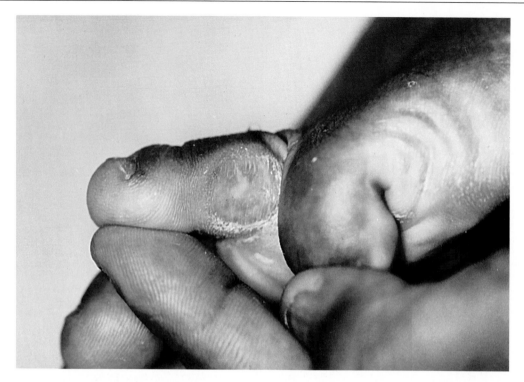

Figure 7–26. Heloma molle of fourth toe.

flexes the metatarsal head and pulls the metatarsal fad pad distally, leaving only skin and thin subcutaneous tissue between the metatarsal head and the ground. Subsequent heavy usage produces the protective callus known as an intractable plantar keratosis.

In general, thickening of the stratum corneum of the skin is referred to as a *hyperkeratosis* or *callus*. When hyperkeratoses are distinct and isolated, they are usually referred to as *corns* or *helomas*. Helomas may be further subdivided into heloma durum, or *hard corn*, and **heloma molle**, or *soft corn*. The heloma durum is a collection of dense compacted keratotic tissue usually found over pressure areas on the toes, especially the dorsolateral aspect of the fifth toe (see Fig. 7–2). Heloma molle is usually located deep in the web spaces between the toes, where it forms from pressure of an adjacent toe against an osteophyte or prominence of one of the phalanges (Fig. 7–26).

In the normal foot, the skin involved in weightbearing describes a specific pattern: the areas beneath the distal phalanges of the toes, the metatarsal heads, a thin strip along the lateral border of the foot, and an oval area beneath the plantar surface of the calcaneus. Not only is the skin thickened in these areas but also increased subcutaneous tissue in the form of fat pads further cushions the tips of the toes, the metatarsal heads, and the calcaneus.

The skin beneath the middle and proximal phalanges of the toes and the plantar surface of the arch is normally softer and less cushioned. As an individual's tendency toward pes planus increases, the weightbearing strip along the lateral border of the foot widens until, in more severe cases, it involves the entire width of the foot. In the presence of more severe deformities, such as the *rocker bottom* foot, the weightbearing pattern may be even more bizarre. The skin beneath abnormal prominences becomes thickly cornified or even ulcerated. **Ulcerations** are also associated with diabetic neuropathy (Fig. 7–27A).

The skin should also be inspected for cutaneous disorders such as warts or rashes. **Plantar warts** are cutaneous excrescences a few millimeters in diameter that can be the source of considerable pain if they form beneath the metatarsal head or the tuberosity of the calcaneus (see Fig. 7–27B). The most common rash seen on the foot is due to **tinea pedis**, or athlete's foot. This fungal infection produces characteristic peeling of the skin between the toes and a dry red scaly appearance on the sole of the foot that, in extreme cases, may involve the entire plantar surface or spread onto the dorsum (Fig. 7–27C).

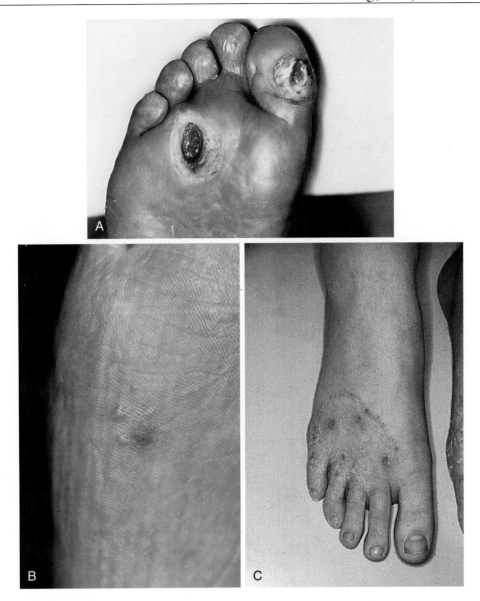

Figure 7–27. *A*, Ulcerations of the plantar aspect of the foot. *B*, Plantar wart. *C*, Tinea pedis.

ALIGNMENT

Inspection of the foot and the ankle for malalignment begins with the patient standing and facing the examiner. Any gross abnormalities or deformities such as bumps or swelling are usually be noted immediately from this perspective.

Anterior Aspect

GREAT TOE. Detailed examination begins with inspection of the hallux, or great toe. Normally, the great toe should point directly forward when the patient is standing with the feet together. **Hallux valgus** is by far the most common abnormality of the great toe. In this condition, a valgus deformity occurs at the first metatarsophalangeal joint, which causes the great toe, the hallux, to deviate away from the midline (Fig. 7–28*A*). In severe cases, the great toe may be *pronated* or even overlap the second toe. A pronated hallux is one that is rotated along its longitudinal axis, so that the toenail faces supramedially instead of directly superior.

Hallux valgus may be associated with a bunion deformity, although the two terms are not synonomous. The term *bunion* specifically refers to the accumulation of bone and thickened soft tis-

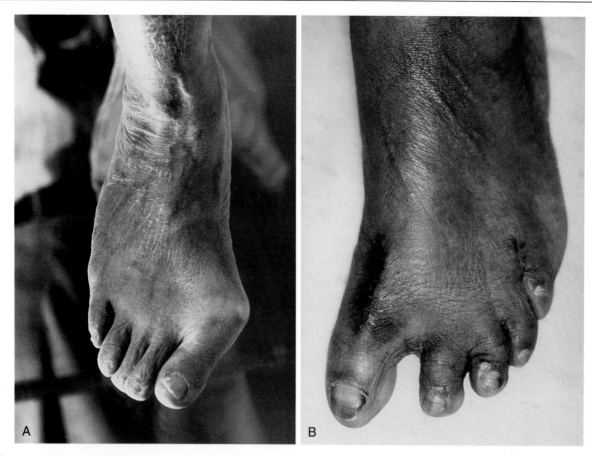

Figure 7–28. *A*, Hallux valgus. *B*, Hallux varus.

sue on the medial aspect of the first metatarsal head that results in a large prominent bump, whereas the term *hallux valgus* describes the deviation of the great toe away from the midline. Hallux valgus may also be associated with a **splayfoot** or **metatarsus primus varus.** *Splayfoot* is a condition in which the metatarsals tend to spread broadly during weightbearing, whereas the term *metatarsus primus varus* refers specifically to a first metatarsal that angles excessively toward the midline.

The opposite deformity, **hallux varus,** almost never occurs spontaneously, but it may be found as an unwanted complication of surgery to correct hallux valgus. In hallux varus, the great toe deviates away from the rest of the toes toward the midline (see Fig. 7–28*B*). This deformity can cause severe difficulties with shoe wear.

LESSER TOES. The remaining four toes are often collectively referred to as the *lesser toes*. Normally, the second through fourth toes should be straight and the fifth toe should be slightly supi-

nated and curved in toward the fourth. Common deformities of the lesser toes include hammer, claw, and mallet toe.

Hammer toe usually involves a single digit and consists of hyperextension of the metatarsophalangeal and distal interphalangeal joints combined with hyperflexion of the proximal interphalangeal joint (Fig. 7–29*A*). In hammer toe deformity, a callus often develops on the dorsal aspect of the proximal interphalangeal joint due to friction from the top of the shoe.

In **claw toe** deformity, both the proximal and the distal interphalangeal joints are held in flexion and multiple toes are usually involved (see Fig. 7–29*B*). In the presence of a claw toe deformity, a callus may develop both over the proximal interphalangeal joint and at the tip of the toe, which is pressed into the bottom of the shoe. At times, even the hallux may be clawed. Although clawing may be idiopathic, widespread clawing may signify a neurologic disorder, such as Charcot-Marie-Tooth disease, or an adaptive change from a longstanding rupture of the Achilles tendon.

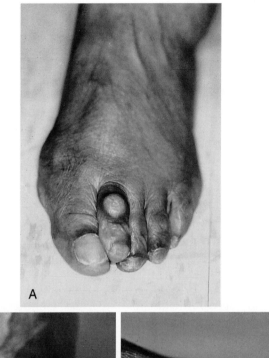

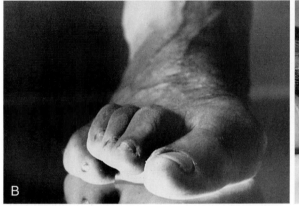

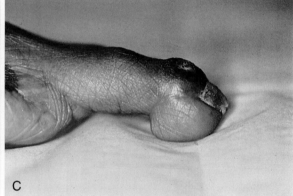

Figure 7–29. *A,* Hammer toe. *B,* Claw toes. *C,* Mallet toe.

The term **mallet toe** is usually applied to a digit with an isolated flexion deformity of the distal interphalangeal joint. This deformity results in excessive pressure on the tip of the involved toe, often producing a callus (see Fig. 7–29*C*).

A major factor in the production of all these deformities is thought to be the long term use of ill-fitting footwear because they occur more commonly in shoe wearing societies than in un-shod populations. Another important factor in the etiology of these deformities is thought to be the overpowering of weak or nonfunctional intrinsic muscles of the foot by the long flexors and extensors of the toes. A specific underlying cause is rarely identified, although occasionally a diagnosable neurologic disorder such as muscular dystrophy, polio, or Charcot-Marie-Tooth disease may be present. Rheumatoid arthritis can produce an amazing variety of abnormalities of toe alignment (Fig. 7–30).

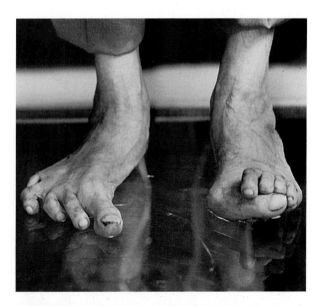

Figure 7–30. Multiple toe deformities associated with rheumatoid arthritis.

FOOT. The examiner's attention should now move proximally to the metatarsals. Normally, all the metatarsal heads should appear to bear weight evenly, and the alignment of the forefoot to the hindfoot should be neutral. If the forefoot appears deviated laterally in relation to the hindfoot, then **forefoot abduction** (forefoot abductus) is considered to be present. Forefoot abduction is usually associated with pronation of the forefoot. Forefoot abduction can occur as a consequence of flatfoot, either congenital or acquired, or following a midfoot fracture. If the forefoot seems deviated medially in relation to the hindfoot, **forefoot adduction** (forefoot adductus) is considered to be present (Fig. 7–31A). Forefoot adduction may be the residuum of a pediatric clubfoot or skewfoot deformity.

LOWER LEG. The anterior viewpoint is the best perspective for assessing tibial alignment. Normally, the tibia should appear straight. **Tibia vara,** or bowed tibia, may be due to a malunited fracture, metabolic disorders such as ricketts, or congenital or developmental anomalies, such as Blount's disease. Evaluation of **tibial torsion,** or rotational alignment, is described in the Alignment section of Chapter 5, Pelvis, Hip, and Thigh.

Medial Aspect

ARCH. Inspecting the foot from its medial aspect allows the examiner to assess the alignment and the integrity of the **medial longitudinal arch.** Although there are no universally accepted criteria for what constitutes a normal arch, the medial border of the foot from just behind the first metatarsal head to a point about 2 cm distal to the calcaneal tuberosity should be elevated from the floor when the subject is standing. The apex of this arch is usually about 1 cm. Jack described a general system for grading the morphology of the medial longitudinal arch. A **grade I** arch is subjectively normal or slightly depressed on weightbearing. In a **grade II** arch, the entire medial border of the foot touches the floor but its edge is straight. In a **grade III** arch, the entire medial border of the foot not only touches the floor but also bulges toward the examiner in a convex manner.

A foot with a high arch is called **pes cavus** (see Fig. 7–21A). When present, it is usually bilateral. Pes cavus may be idiopathic or associated with a congenital anomaly, muscle imbalance, or neurologic disorder such as Charcot-Marie-Tooth disease. Unilateral pes cavus may be secondary to tethering of the spinal cord.

When the medial arch is minimal or entirely absent, **pes planus** is said to be present (see Fig. 7–21B). Pes planus is more common in some ethnic groups and may be genetically determined. Pes planus can also be acquired in the adult in association with trauma, contracture of the Achilles tendon, degeneration and rupture of the posterior tibial tendon, or rheumatoid arthritis and other rheumatologic disorders. Although frank pes planus is readily observed, milder deformities are easy to overlook. In subtle cases, comparison with the other foot is important. Unilateral pes planus is usually associated with the *too-many-toes* deformity, which is described later as part of the posterior inspection.

Diabetic patients may present with an even more profound deformity, in which the bottom of the foot has a convex or **rocker bottom** appearance where the longitudinal arch should be (see

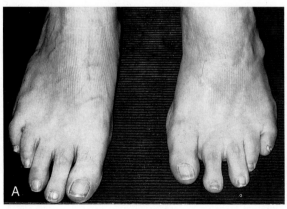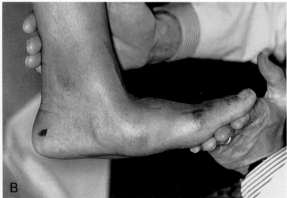

Figure 7–31. *A,* Residual forefoot adduction from a clubfoot deformity of the left foot. *B,* Rocker bottom deformity.

Fig. 7–31*B*). This deformity is due to the neuropathic *Charcot arthropathy* that is itself a consequence of the peripheral neuropathy common in diabetic patients. In Charcot's arthropathy, the loss of protective sensation leads to progressive deterioration of the articular structures of the foot. In the earlier stages of this disorder, the foot may have minimal deformity while showing swelling and erythema suggestive of an acute infection. In these cases, careful evaluation is needed to differentiate infected ulcerations or deep abscesses from early neuropathic arthropathy. In the advanced stages of Charcot's arthropathy, the foot is deformed but has normal skin color and minimal swelling. At times, the resultant deformity may include a bony prominence that leads to secondary ulceration of the overlying soft tissues. Rocker bottom deformity may sometimes be seen in a nondiabetic person in association with a congenital anomaly or malunited fracture.

Posterior Aspect

HINDFOOT. Assessment of standing foot and ankle alignment continues from the posterior aspect. The standing patient is asked to face away from the examiner.

The **alignment of the hindfoot** with the lower leg is then evaluated. This alignment is assessed by estimating or measuring the angle formed by a line bisecting the calf with another line bisecting the heel (Fig. 7–32*A*). Normally, the midline of the heel is at 5° to 10° of valgus in relation to the midline of the calf. Excessive **valgus** may occur following calcaneus fracture, in the presence of advanced degenerative or rheumatoid arthritis or Charcot's arthropathy, or in association with severe pes planus (Fig. 7–32*B*). A **varus** inclination of the heel can be seen following a malunited fracture of the calcaneus or ankle, or in the presence of neuropathic arthropathy or other neurologic disorders (Fig. 7–32*C*).

Figure 7–32. *A*, Normal heel alignment. *B*, Valgus heel alignment (right foot). *C*, Varus heel alignment (left foot).

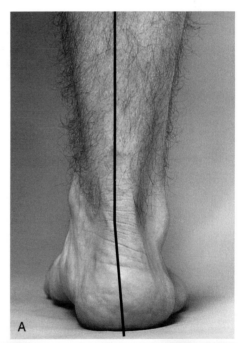

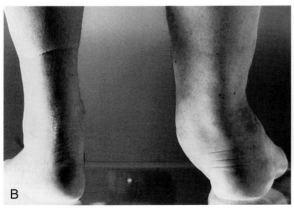

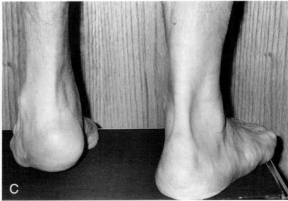

STIFF FIRST METATARSOPHALANGEAL JOINT.
A patient with a painful or **stiff first metatarsophalangeal joint** often compensates by supinating the entire foot and walking predominantly on its lateral border during stance phase (Fig. 7–35A). Such a situation would arise from osteoarthritis of the first metatarsophalangeal joint with secondary *hallux rigidus,* for example. This adaptation can be subtle and difficult to detect simply by observing the patient's gait. Supplementary examination of the patient's shoes may reveal evidence that reflects this gait adaptation. The dorsum of the shoe is asymmetrically creased compared with the other shoe, and inspection of the heel reveals increased wear on the lateral side.

EQUINUS CONTRACTURE. Patients who have an **equinus contracture**, with loss of normal ankle dorsiflexion, may exhibit a number of gait abnormalities. They may lift the affected limb higher during swing phase, as in the steppage gait, to facilitate ground clearance, or they may externally rotate the involved limb to decrease the amount of dorsiflexion necessary during stance phase (see Fig. 7–35B). The lack of dorsiflexion may force the ipsilateral knee into hyperextension during midstance, and heel rise on the affected side occurs earlier.

RANGE OF MOTION

The foot and ankle are a complex mechanism containing many individual joints. For a complete assessment, examination of each joint in a systematic manner with comparison to the opposite extremity is necessary. However, the patient's complaints and other physical signs often permit the clinician to focus the examination on the area of principal interest. It is usually most efficient to integrate the active and passive motion examinations by first asking the patient to move a joint actively and then manipulating it passively when indicated. The gross functional tests described under the Muscle Testing section—heel walking, toe walking, and walking on the medial and lateral borders of the feet—provide a useful quick assessment of the functioning capabilities of the ankle and the subtalar joints in particular. For more detailed information, each joint needs to be isolated individually.

Ankle

DORSIFLEXION. The principal motions of the ankle joint are **dorsiflexion** and **plantar flexion**. Both of these motions are usually assessed with the patient in the sitting position.

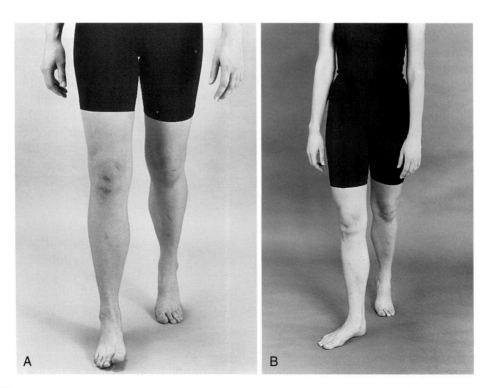

Figure 7–35. *A,* Walking on the lateral border of the right foot. *B,* Externally rotating the lower limb to accommodate an equinus contracture of the ankle.

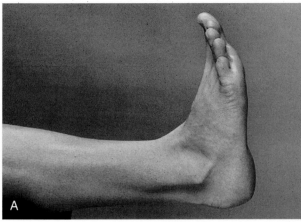
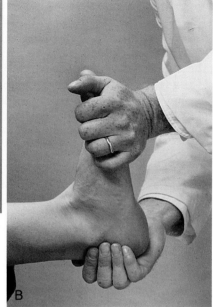

Figure 7–36. *A*, Active ankle dorsiflexion. *B*, Passive ankle dorsiflexion.

To examine **active dorsiflexion,** the patient is asked to pull the foot up toward the leg as far as possible (Fig. 7–36*A*). To compare **passive dorsiflexion,** the examiner grips the hindfoot in neutral, inverts the forefoot, and passively dorsiflexes the ankle to the maximal degree possible (Fig. 7–36*B*). Inversion of the forefoot minimizes the contribution of the forefoot joints to sagittal motion, so that a more accurate recording of pure ankle motion is achieved.

The magnitude of ankle dorsiflexion is assessed by measuring or estimating the angle between the plantar surface of the foot and a line perpendicular to the longitudinal axis of the lower leg. Normal ankle dorsiflexion averages about 20°.

CAUSES OF LOST DORSIFLEXION. Loss of dorsiflexion may be due to *contracture* of posterior structures, such as the Achilles tendon complex; *loss of flexibility* in the ankle syndesmosis; or *impingement* of anterior soft tissue or osteophytes. An ankle that cannot even dorsiflex to a neutral position is said to be in **equinus.**

If the Achilles tendon complex appears to be responsible for limiting dorsiflexion, further testing may allow the examiner to determine whether or not this is caused by an isolated contracture of the **gastrocnemius** portion of the Achilles complex. To make this determination, the examiner assesses the passive dorsiflexion of the ankle in two positions: with the knee fully extended and with the knee flexed 90°. Extending the knee tightens the gastrocnemius portion of

the Achilles complex because it originates above the knee. Flexing the knee allows the gastrocnemius to relax. Thus, when an isolated contracture of the gastrocnemius is present, less passive dorsiflexion is present with the knee fully extended than when it is flexed. If contracture of the **soleus** is the limiting factor, the position of the knee does not affect the amount of ankle dorsiflexion possible.

Because the dome of the talus is wider anteriorly, the distal fibula and tibia must slightly separate at the tibiofibular syndesmosis to allow full dorsiflexion to occur. Thus, any situation that causes the syndesmosis to scar or to ossify in a contracted configuration also limits dorsiflexion. This situation commonly arises following sprain or fracture, especially if the ankle has been immobilized in a plantar flexed position.

Finally, **impingement** of tissue anteriorly may also limit dorsiflexion. Following an ankle sprain, pinching of anterior soft tissues, such as fragments of damaged ligaments or tongues of inflamed synovium, may occasionally cause such a syndrome to develop. If anterior impingement is present, passively forcing the ankle into maximal dorsiflexion with a quick sharp movement may elicit pain localized at the site of the soft tissue impingement (see Fig. 7–36*B*). Anterior ankle impingement may also be due to the accretion of osteophytes on the anterior rim of the tibial plafond and the neck of the talus. Such osteophytes are common among athletes in jumping sports, such as volleyball and basketball, and in ballet dancers.

PLANTAR FLEXION. To assess **active plantar flexion,** the patient is asked to point the foot downward as far as possible (Fig. 7–37A). **Passive plantar flexion** may be assessed by again grasping the hindfoot, inverting the forefoot, then plantar flexing the ankle as far as possible (Fig. 7–37B). Normal plantar flexion is about 50°. An ankle that cannot even plantar flex to neutral is said to be in **calcaneus.**

CAUSES OF LOST PLANTAR FLEXION. Limited plantar flexion may be due to anterior capsular contracture following trauma or posterior joint impingement. *Capsular contracture* may be a nonspecific sequela of a major ankle injury such as a fracture. *Posterior impingement* may be associated with chronic ankle instability or trauma to a prominent processus trigonum or os trigonum. The *processus trigonum* is a normal bony prominence of the posterior talus, and the *os trigonum* is a small ossicle that occurs at the same location. If posterior impingement is suspected, the examiner may test for it by quickly and sharply plantar flexing the ankle passively (Fig. 7–37B). Posterior ankle pain in response to such a maneuver suggests the possibility of posterior impingement.

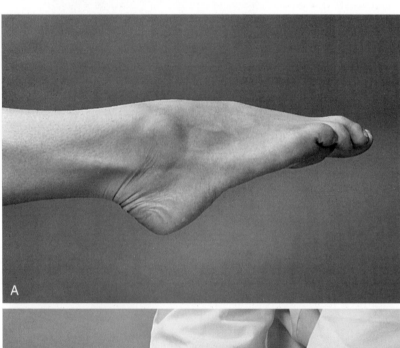

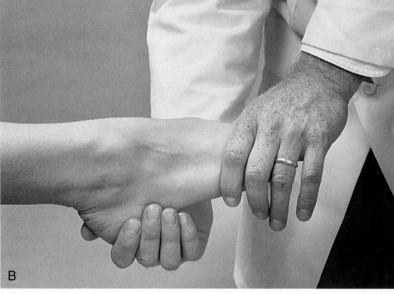

Figure 7–37. *A,* Active ankle plantar flexion. *B,* Passive ankle plantar flexion.

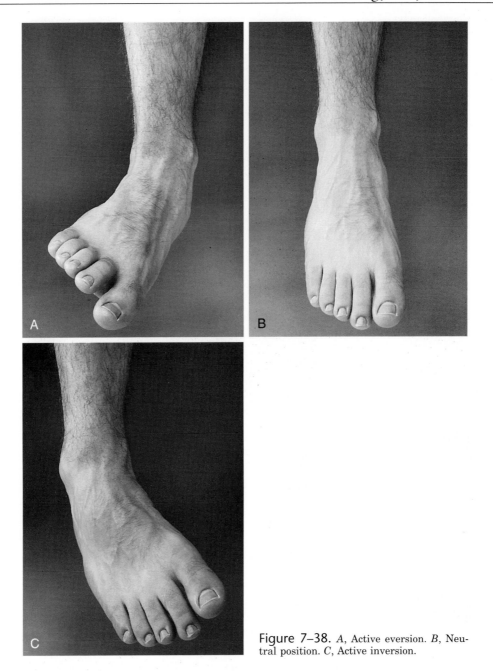

Figure 7–38. *A*, Active eversion. *B*, Neutral position. *C*, Active inversion.

Subtalar Joint

INVERSION AND EVERSION. The principal motions of the subtalar joint are inversion and eversion. Active inversion and eversion may be roughly assessed in the *seated* patient (Fig. 7–38), although the motion of the heel may be more precisely assessed with the patient lying *prone*. In this position, the examiner grasps the patient's heel and gently inverts it and everts it as far as possible. The amount of motion is assessed by estimating the angle between a line bisecting the heel and another line bisecting the posterior leg (Fig. 7–39). Average eversion is about 20° and inversion about 40°, although considerable variation exists in the normal population. Severe restriction or absence of subtalar motion in a child or adolescent suggests the possibility of *tarsal coalition;* in an older individual, it is the common sequela of hindfoot fractures, particularly those involving the calcaneus.

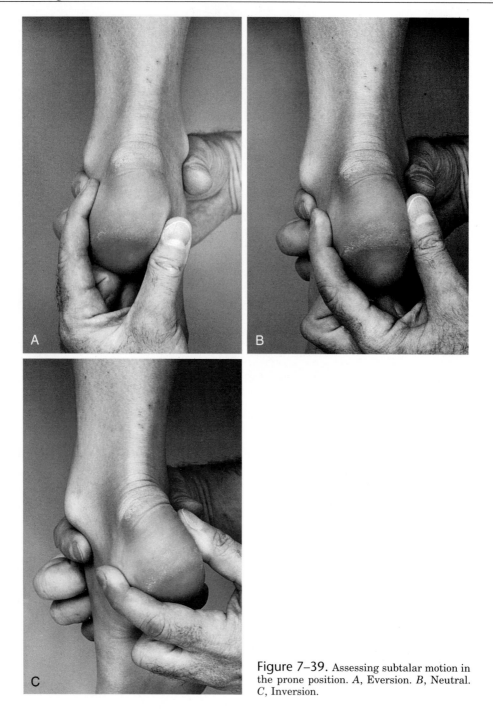

Figure 7–39. Assessing subtalar motion in the prone position. *A*, Eversion. *B*, Neutral. *C*, Inversion.

Forefoot

ABDUCTION AND ADDUCTION. Forefoot abduction and adduction are usually evaluated by passively stabilizing the calcaneus in neutral position with one hand and pushing the forefoot laterally and medially, respectively, with the other hand (Fig. 7–40). The transverse tarsal joints are responsible for the small amount of motion that exists. This motion totals about 5° in most individuals. Clinically, it is sufficient to document that motion is present because it is very difficult to measure accurately.

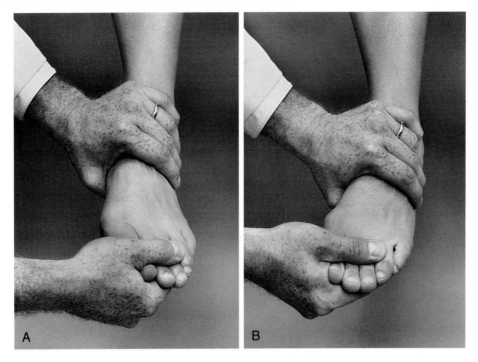

Figure 7–40. *A,* Forefoot abduction. *B,* Forefoot adduction (left foot).

Great Toe

Motion of the great toe occurs through both the **metatarsophalangeal joint** and the **interphalangeal joint.** Both joints are capable of **extension,** or dorsiflexion, and **flexion,** or plantar flexion. **Active range of motion** of these two joints is normally tested simultaneously by asking the patient to extend the great toe as far as possible (Fig. 7–41) and then to flex it (Fig. 7–42).

The individual movements of these two joints may be isolated during passive testing. To test the **passive extension and flexion** of the **first metatarsophalangeal joint,** the examiner stabilizes the foot in a neutral position by grasping the foot with one hand. The other hand then grasps the great toe and passively dorsiflexes, then plantar flexes it as far as possible. **Passive extension** of the normal first metatarsophalangeal joint averages 70° (Fig. 7–43A), and **pas-**

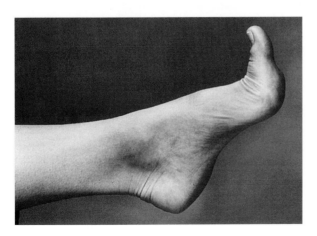

Figure 7–41. Active extension of the great toe.

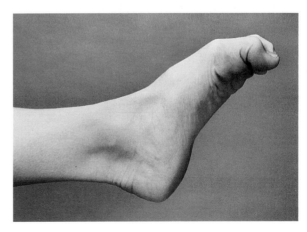

Figure 7–42. Active flexion of the great toe.

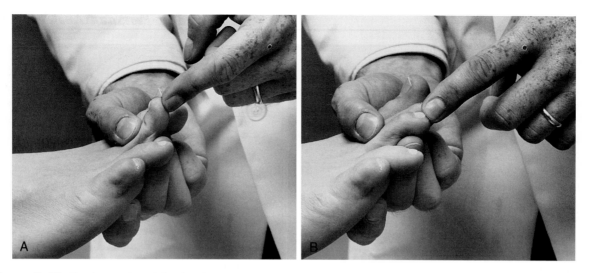

Figure 7–48. Passive motion of the distal interphalangeal joints of the lesser toes (third toe). *A*, Extension. *B*, Flexion.

joints, normal **passive extension** is 30° (Fig. 7–48*A*), and normal **passive flexion** is 60° (Fig. 7–48*B*). These motions vary considerably among individuals. In the smaller toes, the middle phalanx is quite short, making it difficult to distinguish distal interphalangeal joint motion from proximal interphalangeal joint motion. As in the great toe, loss of motion in the metatarsophalangeal joints has the greatest functional significance. Loss of motion in the interphalangeal joints is common following fracture or in the presence of hammer toe, claw toe, or mallet toe deformities. The primary significance of the associated contractures of these joints is their tendency to cause friction against the adjacent shoe surfaces and, ultimately, to cause callus or even ulcer formation.

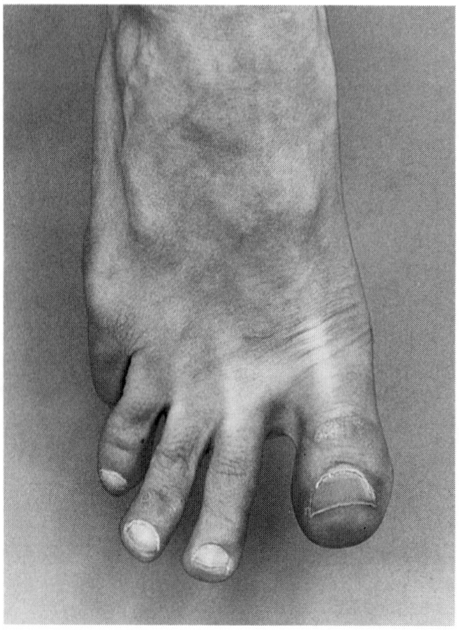

Abduction and **adduction** of the toes is possible to a limited degree, although it is not of great functional significance. As in the hand, *abduction* is considered motion away from the midline of the foot, rather than the midline of the body. In the foot, *abduction* is judged in relation to the second toe, which is considered the midline axis of the foot. Motion away from the second toe is considered abduction and motion toward the second toe, *adduction*. **Active abduction** may be roughly assessed by asking the patient to spread the toes (Fig. 7–49). This is not normally measured in degrees but merely by noting the patient's ability to separate the toes. Similarly, **active adduction** may be documented by asking the patient to squeeze the toes together.

Figure 7–49. Active abduction of the toes.

Palpation

Palpation is usually performed with the patient seated with the lower part of the leg dangling comfortably off the end or the side of the examination table. For comfort, the examiner is usually seated on a low stool. The examiner grasps the patient's foot with one hand to provide resistance and stability while palpating with the other hand. A common mistake is to use too little or too much force when palpating. Our rule of thumb is to use just enough force to blanch the examiner's nailbed.

Anterior Aspect

LOWER LEG AND ANKLE. Palpation can be helpful in diagnosing several unusual conditions of the anterior leg (see Fig. 7–10). Although stress fractures more commonly occur on the posteromedial aspect of the tibia, they occasionally arise on the **anterior tibial crest.** These lesions are usually associated with point tenderness at about the midpoint of the anterior tibial crest and sometimes a small visible bump at this location. These fractures are important to detect because they may progress to nonunion or even a completely displaced fracture.

Another cause of anterior leg pain in athletes is an *exercise-induced anterior compartment syndrome.* In such individuals, the **anterior compartment muscles** seem normal at rest but tender and abnormally firm if the examiner palpates them immediately after the patient has exercised. The physical findings of the exercise-induced anterior compartment syndrome are transient and subtle compared with those of the classic *acute compartment syndrome,* in which the anterior compartment muscles are extremely firm and tender.

The **anterior inferior tibiofibular ligament** connects the distal fibula and tibia just proximal to the ankle joint (see Fig. 7–8). It forms the anterior portion of the syndesmotic complex, which stabilizes the ankle mortise. Tenderness over the anterior-inferior tibiofibular ligament may be associated with a syndesmosis sprain or a Maisonneuve fracture. In the more severe injuries, the tenderness continues up the leg owing to injury of the interosseous membrane.

The **tibialis anterior** tendon may be easily identified by asking the patient to actively dorsiflex the ankle. At the level of the ankle joint, the tendon is closer to the medial malleolus than to the lateral malleolus, but the muscle itself lies lateral to the tibial crest in the anterior compartment. *Peritendinitis,* or inflammation of the tissue around the tibialis anterior tendon, occasionally occurs where the more proximal portion of the tendon courses over the anterior surface of the tibia (see Fig. 7–10). In the presence of this condition, the tibialis anterior is tender about a hand's breadth proximal to the ankle joint. If the examiner lightly palpates the tendon at this point while the patient alternately dorsiflexes and plantar flexes the ankle, soft tissue crepitus surrounding the tendon is often appreciated.

Acute or chronic degenerative ruptures of the tibialis anterior tendon occasionally occur. In complete ruptures, the retracted tendon stump is felt as a firm, palpable mass just proximal to the joint line of the ankle. In such cases, active dorsiflexion of the ankle is accompanied by involuntary eversion of the foot due to overpull of the extensor hallucis longus and the extensor digitorum communis. In longstanding undiagnosed tears, this overpull of the toe extensors may cause all the toes to become clawed, and the unbalanced activity of the muscles of plantar flexion may lead to contracture of the Achilles tendon and ankle equinus.

Rarely, the **superficial peroneal nerve** may be compressed at the point where it pierces to the deep fascia of the ankle to supply sensation to the dorsum of the foot. In such cases, percussing the nerve about 12 cm proximal to the lateral malleolus may reproduce the patient's pain or produce dysesthesias. Laceration of the superficial peroneal nerve is a more common occurrence that results in numbness of the majority of the dorsum of the foot.

FOOT. As the anterior tibial artery courses across the ankle into the foot, it becomes the **dorsalis pedis artery** (see Fig. 7–1). The extensor hallucis longus tendon crosses the artery at about the level of the ankle, so that in the ankle and the foot, the artery is located immediately lateral to the extensor hallucis longus tendon. The best place for palpating the dorsalis pedis pulse is on the dorsum of the foot at a point just lateral to the extensor hallucis longus tendon and just proximal to the prominence of the metatarsal-cuneiform joints (Fig. 7–50).

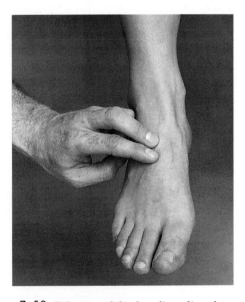

Figure 7–50. Palpation of the dorsalis pedis pulse.

The **deep peroneal nerve,** which travels with the dorsalis pedis artery, may become entrapped under the extensor retinaculum over the dorsum of the foot. Trauma, tight shoes, and space-occupying lesions are the most common causes of this condition, known as *anterior tarsal tunnel syndrome.* To check for anterior tarsal tunnel syndrome, the examiner should percuss the dorsum of the foot in the vicinity of the dorsalis pedis artery in the same manner used to perform **Tinel's test.** In the presence of an anterior tarsal tunnel syndrome, such percussion usually generates a burning pain that radiates to the web space between the first and the second metatarsals, the area of primary sensory distribution of the deep peroneal nerve.

The tendons of the **extensor digitorum longus** and the adjacent **peroneus tertius** lie just lateral to the dorsalis pedis artery. Just distal to the ankle joint, these tendons are restrained by the inferior extensor retinaculum. The extensor digitorum tendons then fan out to each of the lateral four toes. These tendons are usually readily visible and palpable, especially when the patient is actively dorsiflexing the toes (see Fig. 7–7). Although the tendons themselves are rarely involved in a pathologic process other than laceration, pressure from shoes laced excessively tight can cause a *tenosynovitis* on the dorsum of the foot surrounding the extensor digitorum longus tendons. This condition may cause diffuse tenderness and mild swelling around the extensor digitorum longus tendons in the vicinity of the tarsometatarsal joint.

Maximal passive plantar flexion of the ankle exposes the anterolateral aspect of the **talar dome** to palpation (Fig. 7–51A). With this maneuver, the anterolateral portion of the talar dome becomes palpable and often visible between the lateral malleolus and the extensor digitorum longus tendon (Fig. 7–51B). Oscillating the ankle while palpating can help orient the examiner. Tenderness of the talar dome may reflect *osteochondritis dissecans* or a transchondral fracture of the dome of the talus.

While maintaining maximal plantar flexion of the ankle, the examiner may palpate the **tarsal navicular** and intervening **talonavicular joint** just distal to the ankle. Identification of the **navicular tuberosity** helps with orientation. Prominent osteophytes are palpable when advanced degeneration of the talonavicular joint is present. Tenderness of the body of the navicular in an athlete should cause the examiner to suspect a navicular stress fracture. Such fractures are difficult to diagnose radiographically. In children, a tender navicular may signify *Kohler's disease,* or navicular osteochondrosis.

The medial, intermediate, and lateral **cuneiforms** articulate with the distal navicular. Tracing the **tibialis anterior** tendon distally to its insertion leads the examiner to the medial cuneiform. The other two cuneiform bones are lateral to it. Tenderness in these bones is usually attributable either to posttraumatic arthrosis or to inflammatory arthritis. Prominent osteophytes may be identified in these circumstances.

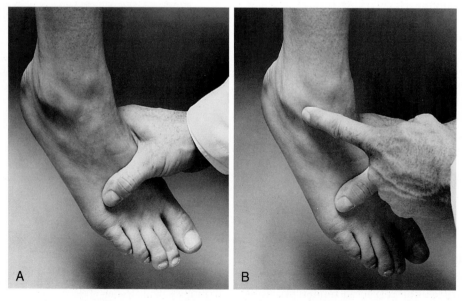

Figure 7–51. *A* and *B,* Palpation of the anterolateral aspect of the talar dome.

Further distally, the examiner palpates the articulations of the five **metatarsals** with the cuneiforms and the cuboid. These articulations are collectively called the **tarsometatarsal joint** or **Lisfranc's joint.** Tenderness and swelling in the vicinity of Lisfranc's joint suggests a sprain, or in its more severe forms, a subluxation or even dislocation. The subtler forms of these injuries are difficult to diagnose radiographically. In a chronic situation, tenderness of Lisfranc's joint usually signifies arthritis, whether posttraumatic, inflammatory, or idiopathic. Palpable tender osteophytes are a frequent finding. Arthritis of Lisfranc's joint can cause deformities including forefoot abduction and arch collapse.

The individual metatarsals should be identified and palpated for tenderness. Localized tenderness suggests the possibility of a *stress fracture.* These stress fractures occur most commonly in the shafts of the second and the third metatarsals about two fingerbreadths proximal to the metatarsophalangeal joints. Early in their course, these stress fractures may be associated with local edema or even ecchymosis. In more longstanding cases, a palpable lump of callus may be detectable. Stress fractures of the fifth metatarsal tend to occur in the proximal metaphysis about 2 cm distal to the palpable base of the metatarsal. Such stress fractures are often called *Jones fractures,* although Jones fractures may also occur owing to acute trauma as well as recurrent stress.

METATARSOPHALANGEAL JOINTS. The first metatarsophalangeal joint may be tender medially in the presence of a bunion or hallux valgus deformity, although in such cases the associated deformity should be obvious. Osteoarthritis of the first metatarsophalangeal joint may produce a subtler finding of palpable osteophytes on the dorsum of the joint without associated angular deformity. These osteophytes may be tender and may limit joint motion. Extreme tenderness, especially when associated with swelling, warmth, and erythema around the joint, is more suggestive of acute gout or septic arthritis.

The four **lesser metatarsophalangeal joints** should also be palpated for tenderness. These joints may be painful and swollen in the presence of active synovitis. Synovitis can occur owing to active rheumatoid arthritis, or it can be the result of pressure overload in a foot with a shortened, hypermobile first metatarsal that increases pressure distribution to the lesser metatarsophalangeal joints. Isolated tenderness of the **second metatarsophalangeal joint** may signify overuse synovitis or, less commonly, *Freiberg's infrac-*

tion, which is avascular necrosis of the second metatarsal head. Freiberg's infraction may occasionally involve multiple toes. Isolated tenderness of the **fifth metatarsophalangeal joint** may be associated with a *tailor's bunion,* or bunionette. Although this deformity is not always tender, active bursitis may occur over the prominence in extreme cases.

The spaces between the **metatarsal heads** should be firmly palpated for tenderness. The examiner may either compress the tissue between the thumb and the index finger of one hand or support the forefoot with one hand while compressing with the index finger of the other (Fig. 7–52). Tenderness between the metatarsal heads, which reproduces the patient's pain, is most commonly due to an *interdigital neuroma,* also known as *Morton's neuroma.* If the neuroma is very large, the examiner may actually be able to feel a firm nodule between the metatarsal heads. The interspace between the third and the fourth metatarsal heads is the most common location for such neuromata. In advanced cases, the patient also reports hypoesthesia or dysesthesia in response to light touch on the side of the toes adjacent to the interspace. For example, a neuroma in the interspace between the third and fourth metatarsal heads may be associated with sensory changes of the lateral side of the third toe and the medial side of the fourth toe. If an interdigital neuroma is suspected, the examiner should also perform Morton's test, described in the Manipulation section.

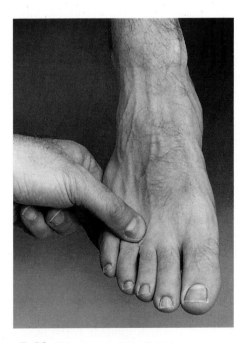

Figure 7–52. Palpation for interdigital neuroma.

TOES. In the toes, the deformities already described may be associated with tender **calluses**. The toes should be spread so that **heloma molle**, soft interdigital corns, may be identified and palpated for tenderness (see Fig. 7–26). Ingrown toenails should be palpated for tenderness and fluctuance that suggest an active infection. In the presence of such an infection, palpating the nail border may cause purulent material to be expressed.

Lateral Aspect

ANKLE AND FOOT. On the lateral aspect of the foot and the ankle, the **lateral malleolus** provides orientation. Tenderness of the lateral malleolus, especially when accompanied by localized edema or ecchymosis, suggests the possibility of a fracture (see Fig. 7–11). In the case of a displaced fracture seen acutely, the examiner may actually be able to palpate a step-off at the fracture site or feel crepitus when the bone is compressed. In the presence of an unstable fracture, the examiner may note crepitus when simply grasping the foot to examine it.

The lateral malleolus is also the principal landmark for palpating the lateral ankle ligaments. Connecting the anterior flare of the lateral malleolus with the talar neck, the **anterior talofibular ligament** is the most common ankle ligament to be injured (see Fig. 7–11). Although the ligament itself cannot be distinctly identified, the finding of tenderness in this region, in association with swelling and ecchymosis, is clinical evidence of a sprain of the ligament. The functional integrity of the anterior talofibular ligament is assessed with the anterior drawer test, described in the Manipulation section.

The **calcaneofibular ligament**, the second most commonly injured ankle ligament, runs from the tip of the lateral malleolus in a postero-inferior direction to insert on the calcaneus. Full delineation of the entire ligament is not possible because it runs deep to the peroneal tendons. However, tenderness over this ligament, in association with localized swelling and ecchymosis, is clinical evidence of a sprain. The functional integrity of the calcaneofibular ligament is evaluated with the inversion stress test, described in the Manipulation section.

The **peroneus longus** and **peroneus brevis** tendons can usually be identified and palpated posterior to the lateral malleolus. Asking the patient to evert the foot against resistance makes these tendons more palpable (see Fig. 7–12). The

peroneus brevis can usually be followed distally to its insertion at the base of the fifth metatarsal. Tenderness over these tendons suggests the possibility of tendinitis. In more severe cases, palpable or visible thickening of the tenosynovium posterior to the lateral malleolus is noted. Peroneal tendinitis may be associated with instability of the peroneal tendons. The clinical test for peroneal tendon instability is described in the Manipulation section.

Just distal to the lateral malleolus, the examiner may palpate a small bony prominence of the calcaneus known as the **peroneal tubercle**, which separates the peroneus brevis tendon from the peroneus longus tendon. This tubercle may occasionally become enlarged and tender. Below the peroneal tendons, the lateral aspect of the **calcaneus** is subcutaneous and easily palpated. Tenderness of the calcaneus in an athlete suggests the possibility of a calcaneal stress fracture. Tenderness of the posterior portion of the **calcaneal tuberosity** in a child or adolescent may indicate the presence of calcaneal apophysitis, also called *Sever's disease.*

The **sinus tarsi** is a space between the lateral talus and the calcaneus in which reside the muscle belly of the **extensor digitorum brevis** and an associated fat pad. The sinus tarsi may be palpated as a depression immediately beneath the anterior talofibular ligament. Slight inversion of the heel accentuates the space, allowing deeper palpation to the lateral talar neck. Tenderness in the sinus tarsi often indicates injury or arthritis involving the posterior facet of the subtalar joint.

Distal to the sinus tarsi, the examiner can palpate the bony prominence of the **anterior process of the calcaneus.** This process may fracture owing to a twisting injury. Detecting tenderness over the anterior process of the calcaneus is important because such fractures are often overlooked by routine radiographs.

Beyond the anterior process of the calcaneus lies the **calcaneocuboid joint.** Although the margins of the joint may be difficult to palpate, alternate abduction and adduction of the forefoot may allow the examiner to identify it. Tenderness of this articulation may be due to degenerative joint disease or increased stress secondary to disruption of the plantar fascia. The **cuboid** should also be palpated for tenderness because it is occasionally the site of stress fractures or avascular necrosis.

LOWER LEG. Palpation further proximally on the **fibula** can alert the clinician to the presence of fractures that may not be otherwise clinically obvious. *Stress fractures of the fibula* most commonly occur in the narrow portion of the diaphysis just proximal to the point where the fibula widens to become the lateral malleolus (see Fig. 7–11). Point tenderness on the fibula about 8 cm proximal to the tip in an athlete who runs suggests the possibility of such a fracture. The midshaft of the fibula is covered by the overlying musculature and therefore felt only as a firm resistance deep to the muscle. Traumatic fractures of this portion of the bone may occur owing to a direct blow. Such fractures often go undiagnosed because the patient is still able to bear weight on the intact tibia. Significant tenderness of the lateral leg in the vicinity of the midshaft fibula following trauma should raise the suspicion of such a fracture and not be passed off as a muscle bruise. Tenderness along any portion of the fibular shaft, in conjunction with tenderness of the deltoid and the syndesmotic ligaments of the ankle, suggests the possibility of a *Maisonneuve fracture*. This eponym refers to the combination of a spiral fracture of the fibula with a ligamentous disruption of the ankle mortise. It is important to search for tenderness of the fibular shaft when a syndesmosis sprain is diagnosed because the fracture portion of a Maisonneuve injury is usually missed by routine ankle radiographs.

Posterior Aspect

CALF. The posterior leg, ankle, and foot are best palpated with the patient lying prone with the feet dangling over the end of the examination table. The gastrocsoleus muscle complex and the associated Achilles tendon are common sites of injury. Muscle tears most commonly occur at the junction of the **medial gastrocnemius** muscle belly with the ensuing aponeurosis (see Fig. 7–17). This site is visible in many individuals as a distinct demarcation where the bulge of the medial calf terminates and the leg becomes thinner. Tenderness at this site suggests an acute tear. In severe injuries, the examiner is able to detect a small divot at this location. This injury is sometimes called *tennis leg*. Injuries may also occur at the lateral musculotendinous junction or further distally in the aponeurotic section of the gastrocsoleus. Such injuries should not be associated with an abnormal response to the Thompson test (see Manipulation section).

Injuries of the Achilles tendon itself usually occur a few centimeters proximal to the insertion of the tendon on the calcaneus. In the presence of an acute rupture, localized swelling usually obscures the outlines of the tendon, but careful palpation reveals a gap in the firm tendon about 2 cm or 3 cm proximal to the calcaneus. The response to the Thompson test is abnormal in the presence of a complete Achilles rupture.

In chronic *Achilles' tendinitis*, the tendon is most commonly tender at the same site, approximately 2 cm to 3 cm proximal to the calcaneus (see Fig. 7–15). In milder cases, the tendon appears normal, but in more severe cases, a palpable and even visible thickening is present.

HEEL. Tenderness at the insertion of the Achilles tendon into the posterior tuberosity of the calcaneus is most commonly caused by *retrocalcaneal bursitis*, inflammation of the **retrocalcaneal bursa.** Tenderness at this location may less commonly be caused by calcific tendinitis of the Achilles insertion itself. Although these two entities may be difficult to distinguish clinically, tenderness on both sides of the Achilles insertion as well as over the insertion itself supports a diagnosis of retrocalcaneal bursitis. Retrocalcaneal bursitis may be associated with *Haglund's deformity*, an increase in the normal prominence of the posterior calcaneal tuberosity. Haglund's deformity itself may encourage the development of subcutaneous bursitis owing to the extrinsic pressure of the adjacent shoe. Such bursitis involves inflammation of the **subcutaneous bursa** between the calcaneal tuberosity and the overlying skin (see Fig. 7–11).

SURAL NERVE. **Sural nerve** entrapment may occur owing to posttraumatic scarring, most commonly following surgery or ankle sprains. In the distal leg, the nerve runs along the lateral border of the Achilles tendon. About 2 cm above the ankle it branches. One branch supplies sensation to the lateral heel, and the other frequently anastomoses with the lateral branch of the superficial peroneal nerve. The nerve then runs inferior to the peroneal tendon sheath in a subcutaneous position (see Figs. 7–11 and 7–15). As it reaches the tuberosity of the fifth metatarsal, the nerve ramifies to provide sensation to the lateral aspect of the fifth toe and the fourth web space. Sural nerve entrapment may occur anywhere along this course. Patients may give the history of a previous twisting injury with the subsequent development of shooting pain and paresthesias. If such a history is elicited, the examiner should check for tenderness and a Tinel sign along the course of the nerve just described. Characteristically, the nerve is tender, and the Tinel sign is elicited at the site of nerve entrapment.

Medial Aspect

LOWER LEG AND ANKLE. The **medial malleolus** is normally the most prominent structure of the medial ankle and foot. As on the lateral side, traumatic fractures involving the medial malleolus are usually associated with considerable swelling, ecchymosis, tenderness, and sometimes crepitus. Stress fractures of the medial malleolus are unusual and thus easy to overlook. Tenderness in such stress fractures usually occurs about 2 cm to 3 cm proximal to the tip of the malleolus (see Fig. 7–20). Continuing to palpate further proximally, the examiner's hand may explore the entire posteromedial subcutaneous border of the **tibia.** The most common site for stress fractures of the tibia is on the posteromedial cortex at the junction of the middle and distal thirds of the bone (see Fig. 7–23). Localized bony tenderness at this site usually is highly suggestive of a stress fracture. If the stress fracture has been present for several weeks or more, the examiner may be able to detect a small, firm, tender lump on the posteromedial tibia that represents the periosteal new bone formation in response to the stress fracture. More diffuse tenderness along the posteromedial tibia is more likely to represent the overuse syndrome known as *shin splints* or *periostitis.*

The **deltoid ligament** connects the medial malleolus with the adjacent talus and medial calcaneus. The individual fascicles of this ligament cannot be distinguished by palpation; however, tenderness, swelling, and ecchymosis over the deltoid ligament suggest a sprain involving this structure. Such an injury may be difficult to differentiate from damage to the **posterior tibial tendon.**

Passive eversion of the hindfoot also exposes the medial **head of the talus,** located just distal and anterior to the medial malleolus. In a patient with severe flatfoot, the medial talar head is already prominent. In the most severe cases of flatfoot, a diffuse callus caused by friction or weightbearing can be found overlying the medial aspect of the talar head.

About 2 cm distal and anterior to the tip of the medial malleolus lies the **navicular tuberosity.** Eversion of the foot increases the prominence of the tuberosity. Tenderness of the tuberosity, especially when it is more prominent than usual, suggests a symptomatic *accessory navicular.* This developmental variant may become painful through chronic overuse or acute trauma.

The **posterior tibial tendon** courses from behind the medial malleolus to insert on the navicular tuberosity. The tendon can be rendered more easily palpable by asking the patient to invert the foot against resistance (see Fig. 7–22). Tenderness posterior to the medial malleolus or further distal along the course of the tendon suggests the possibility of *posterior tibial tendinitis.* The association of localized swelling suggests more severe tendinitis or even rupture. Chronic tendinitis or rupture of the posterior tibial tendon can result in secondary collapse of the arch of the foot.

Immediately posterior to the tibialis posterior tendon lies the tendon of the **flexor digitorum longus.** The flexor digitorum longus tendon may be appreciated by firm palpation posterior to the tibialis posterior tendon while the patient actively flexes the toes (Fig. 7–53).

The **posterior tibial artery** is located immediately posterior to the flexor digitorum longus tendon. The posterior tibial pulse is usually easily felt by moderately firm palpation behind the medial malleolus using the tips of one or two digits.

The **posterior tibial nerve** is located immediately posterior to the posterior tibial artery. The **tarsal tunnel** is the name given to the space bounded anteriorly by the medial malleolus, laterally by the talus and calcaneus, and medially by the overlying flexor retinaculum. Compression of the posterior tibial nerve as it traverses this space is called *tarsal tunnel syndrome.* Possible contributory causes of tarsal tunnel syndrome include posttraumatic swelling, space-occupying lesions such as varicosities, ankle deformities, and severe pes planus. If tarsal tunnel syndrome is suspected, the examiner should percuss the nerve with the tip of one finger in the manner used for **Tinel's test** of the median nerve at the

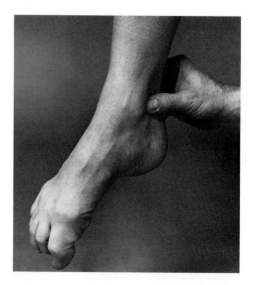

Figure 7–53. Palpation of the flexor digitorum longus.

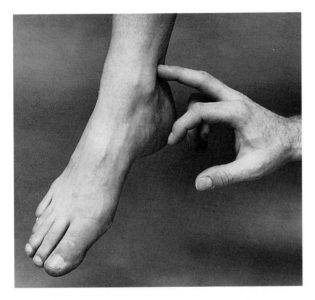

Figure 7–54. Tinel's test for tarsal tunnel syndrome.

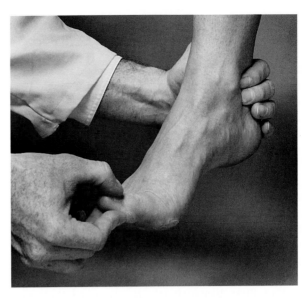

Figure 7–55. Palpation of the flexor hallucis longus tendon. Passive manipulation of the great toe makes the tendon easier to palpate.

wrist (Fig. 7–54). In a patient with tarsal tunnel syndrome, such percussion may reproduce or exacerbate the patient's pain or result in sharp or electric pains that radiate distally into the foot or proximally into the calf. Prolonged digital pressure over the nerve may also increase the symptoms or cause dysesthesias in the plantar portion of the foot, much in the same manner as Phalen's test exacerbates the symptoms of carpal tunnel syndrome in the hand.

The tendon of the **flexor hallucis longus** is located both posterior and lateral to the posterior tibial nerve. This deep position makes it relatively difficult to palpate. Excursion of the flexor hallucis longus can usually be appreciated by deep palpation posterior to the medial malleolus while passively extending the great toe or asking the patient to flex and extend it (Fig. 7–55). Tenderness of the flexor hallucis longus tendon suggests the possibility of flexor hallucis longus tendinitis, which characteristically occurs in ballet dancers. In the extreme case, enlargement of the tendon may cause palpable triggering of the tendon as it enters the fibrosseous sheath along the medial wall of the calcaneus, a condition analogous to trigger finger, which is sometimes called *hallux saltans*.

FOOT. It is important to continue percussion of the posterior tibial nerve distally to its bifurcation into the **medial and lateral plantar nerves** because these divisions may become individually entrapped. In the case of the medial plantar nerve, entrapment tends to occur at the *master knot of Henry*, the point in the medial plantar arch where the flexor hallucis longus and flexor digitorum longus tendons cross. In the presence of medial plantar nerve entrapment, the most characteristic place for tenderness is on the medial plantar aspect of the arch distal to the navicular tuberosity (Fig. 7–56). Palpating the nerve at this point may cause aching in the

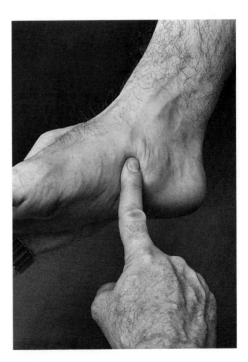

Figure 7–56. Typical site of tenderness in medial plantar nerve entrapment.

arch and dysesthesias in the medial plantar portion of the foot; **Tinel's sign** may also be present. Passively everting the patient's heel or asking the patient to stand on the toes may also reproduce the symptoms of medial plantar nerve entrapment. This syndrome may be associated with excessive adduction or abduction of the forefoot at the talonavicular joint, which may cause the medial plantar nerve to be compressed underneath the master knot of Henry. Other conditions that may be associated with medial plantar nerve entrapment include hallux valgus or hyperpronation of the foot. Medial plantar nerve entrapment is sometimes called *jogger's foot*. Decreased sensation may be found in such patients if the examination is conducted immediately after running.

The **first branch of the lateral plantar nerve** is more likely to become compressed than the entire lateral plantar nerve itself. This branch may become entrapped between the fascia of the abductor hallucis and the quadratus plantae muscles. Patients with this condition usually complain of chronic heel pain, often increased by running. This pain is often worse in the morning and may radiate to the inferomedial aspect of the heel and proximally into the medial ankle. In such patients, digital compression of the first branch of the lateral plantar nerve on the medial aspect of the heel should reproduce the patient's symptoms, including pain radiation (Fig. 7–57). No numbness should be associated with this syndrome.

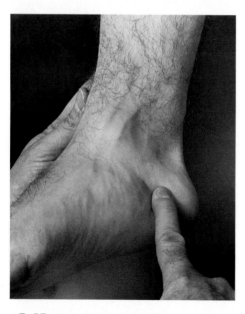

Figure 7–57. Digital compression of the first branch of the lateral plantar nerve.

Plantar Aspect

Examination of the plantar surface of the foot should include palpation of any abnormal **callosities** noted during inspection. Callosities reflect the weightbearing pattern of the foot, but they may not always be symptomatic. When a callosity is tender, particularly in areas such as beneath the metatarsal heads or abnormal bony prominences, it is likely that the tender area is a source of pain for the patient. Extreme tenderness suggests the possibility of an infection, particularly in the diabetic patient.

The plantar surface under the first metatarsal head should be palpated for tenderness of the **sesamoids** (see Fig. 7–24). These two small oval bones are embedded in the flexor hallucis brevis tendon beneath the first metatarsal head. The exact outlines of the sesamoids cannot be distinctly felt, but firm palpation should reveal the sensation of steady resistance provided by these bones. They are located about 15 mm apart underneath the medial and lateral borders of the first metatarsal head. Normally, the sesamoids should not be significantly tender to palpation. Tenderness localized to one of these sesamoids may be due to a variety of conditions including fracture, sesamoiditis, and avascular necrosis. The medial sesamoid is more commonly involved in such pathology.

Palpation of the middle portion of the plantar foot is directed primarily at detecting abnormal conditions of the **plantar fascia.** The plantar fascia is a sheath of tough tendon-like tissue that extends from the plantar surface of the calcaneal tuberosity anteriorly to the metatarsal heads and helps support the medial longitudinal arch. Passively hyperextending the toes tenses the fascia, making it more visible and facilitating palpation. In painful conditions of the plantar fascia, this maneuver may itself aggravate the pain. Palpable nodules of the fascia are usually evidence of *benign fibromatosis*. These nodules may or may not be tender. As previously noted, the medial plantar branch of the posterior tibial nerve may become entrapped within the medial longitudinal arch of the foot. This syndrome is usually associated with tenderness in the arch and sometimes dysesthesias in the medial plantar foot.

The proximal portion of the plantar fascia is the usual site of plantar fasciitis, a condition sometimes called *heel spur syndrome*. In its most common presentation, plantar fasciitis is an overuse injury to the proximal plantar fascia near its attachment to the plantar surface of the calcaneus. This condition is usually marked by tenderness, which may be extreme, at the anterior margin of the medial plantar surface of the calcaneal tuberosity.

Palpation of the rest of the plantar surface of the heel allows the examiner to assess the integrity of the **plantar fat pad** of the heel. Because this fat pad is normally thick and dense, the examiner is able to only vaguely delineate the outlines of the calcaneal tuberosity when palpating the normal heel. With atrophy of the plantar fat pad of the heel, which may be associated with aging or inflammatory arthritis, the contours of the plantar surface of the calcanel tuberosity are better delineated, and diffuse tenderness is usually elicited.

Manipulation

MUSCLE TESTING

Functional Tests

The general function of several major muscle groups may be rapidly assessed by asking the patient to perform various functional tests. The ability to walk on the toes is a good general indicator of the strength of the ankle **plantar flexors,** primarily the gastrocsoleus complex (Fig. 7–58A). Normally, the patient should be

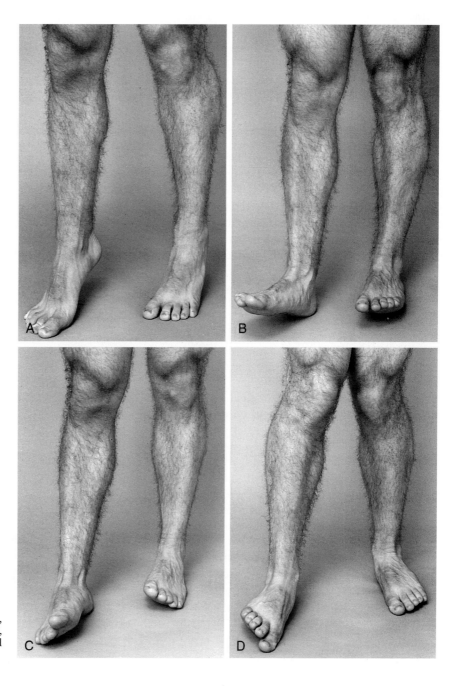

Figure 7–58. Functional tests. *A,* Toe walking. *B,* Heel walking. *C,* Lateral border walking. *D,* Medial border walking.

able to walk around the examination room with the heels several centimeters off the floor. Heel walking is a general test of the strength of the ankle **dorsiflexors,** particularly the tibialis anterior (Fig. 7–58*B*). Normally, the patient should be able to walk with the metatarsal heads several centimeters off the floor. Strength of **inversion** of the foot, primarily supplied by the tibialis posterior, may be grossly assessed by asking the patient to walk on the lateral borders of the feet (Fig. 7–58*C*). **Eversion** strength, supplied primarily by the peronei, may be grossly assessed by asking the patient to walk on the medial borders of the feet (Fig. 7–58*D*). These last two tests are somewhat awkward and may be difficult for the patient who is overweight or stiff. Individual manual resistance testing helps the examiner confirm suspicions raised by these functional tests. All these manual resistance tests are usually performed with the patient seated and the leg dangling off the side or the end of the examination table.

Ankle Dorsiflexors and Toe Extensors

The examiner tests the **tibialis anterior** by placing the patient's ankle in maximal dorsiflexion while supporting the patient's heel with one hand. The patient is then instructed to maintain the ankle position while the examiner attempts to passively plantar flex the ankle with the other hand (Fig. 7–59). This test should cause the tibialis anterior tendon to stand out prominently at the anterior ankle. In a normal patient, the examiner is unable to overcome the strength of the tibialis anterior. Although the tibialis anterior is the main ankle dorsiflexor, it is assisted by the **extensor hallucis longus,** the **extensor digitorum longus,** and the **peroneus tertius.** Therefore, if the tibialis anterior is lacerated, weak ankle dorsiflexion is still present. Because all four muscles are innervated by the *deep peroneal nerve,* a complete palsy of this nerve produces dramatic weakness of dorsiflexion, a condition known as **foot drop.** An injury to the *common peroneal nerve* weakens the peroneus longus and brevis as well.

To test the **extensor hallucis longus,** the examiner supports the patient's forefoot with one hand and instructs the patient to maximally extend the great toe. The patient is asked to maintain the extended position of the toe while the

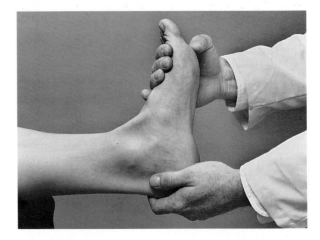

Figure 7–59. Assessing ankle dorsiflexion strength.

examiner attempts to passively plantar flex it by pressing downward on the dorsum of the distal phalanx (Fig. 7–60). In a normal individual, the examiner should have difficulty overcoming the strength of the extensor hallucis longus. The extensor hallucis longus tendon should be quite visible on the dorsum of the foot and the toe during such resistance testing. The more common causes of extensor hallucis longus weakness include lumbar radiculopathy and *peroneal nerve* palsy.

The **extensor digitorum longus** is tested in a manner similar to that used for the extensor hallucis longus. The four lesser toes are usually tested together with the resistance provided by the fingertips or the side of the examiner's hand. The examiner is able to overcome the strength of the extensor digitorum longus in most normal patients (Fig. 7–61). As with the extensor hal-

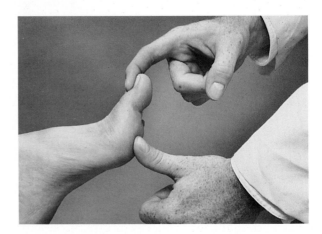

Figure 7–60. Assessing extensor hallucis longus strength.

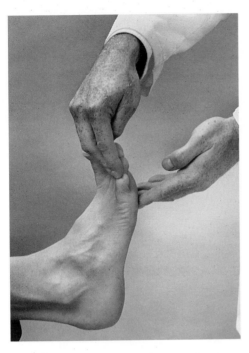

Figure 7–61. Assessing extensor digitorum longus strength.

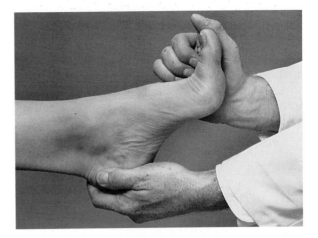

Figure 7–62. Assessing ankle plantar flexion strength.

lucis longus, the extensor digitorum longus tendons should be quite visible during this test. The more common causes of extensor digitorum weakness include lumbar radiculopathy and *peroneal nerve* palsy.

Ankle Plantar Flexors and Toe Flexors

To test the **gastrocsoleus complex,** the examiner asks the patient to maximally plantar flex the ankle. The patient is instructed to maintain the position of plantar flexion while the examiner attempts to force the ankle back into dorsiflexion. The examiner stabilizes the patient's leg with one hand while the palm of the other hand pushes upward against the plantar surface of the metatarsal heads (Fig. 7–62). In the normal patient, the examiner should be unable to overcome the strength of the patient's gastrocsoleus complex. The strength of this muscle group is so great that toe walking is usually a more sensitive test because the force generated by the patient's body weight is usually much greater than the resistance that the average examiner can supply. The more common causes of gastrocsoleus weakness include lumbar radiculopathy, prior Achilles' tendon rupture, and *sciatic or tibial nerve* injury.

The **flexor hallucis longus** and **flexor digitorum longus** are often tested together because they have tendinous cross-connections that make isolated testing difficult. The examiner stabilizes the patient's heel with one hand and instructs the patient to curl the toes downward. After instructing the patient to maintain this position against resistance, the examiner hooks his or her fingers beneath the patient's toes and attempts to passively dorsiflex them (Fig. 7–63). In a normal patient, the examiner should not be able to overcome the strength of the flexor hallucis longus and the flexor digitorum longus with this maneuver. The more common causes of weakness include lumbar radiculopathy, tendinitis, and *sciatic* or *tibial nerve* injury.

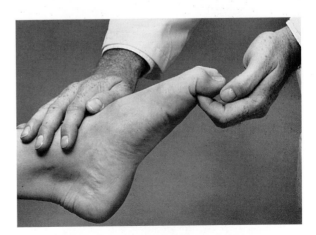

Figure 7–63. Assessing toe flexion strength.

Evertors of the Foot

Pure eversion strength is supplied primarily by the **peroneus brevis,** assisted by the **peroneus longus.** To test eversion strength, the examiner places the patient's foot in the everted position with the ankle plantar flexed. The patient is instructed to maintain the everted position while the examiner attempts to force the foot into inversion. The examiner stabilizes the limb with the palm of one hand against the medial aspect of the tibia just above the ankle. The examiner then pushes medially against the lateral border of the patient's foot in an attempt to invert the foot (Fig. 7–64). Normally, the examiner should be unable to overcome the patient's eversion strength. During this test, the peroneus brevis can normally be seen or palpated as it courses from the posterior aspect of the lateral malleolus to the fifth metatarsal.

Weakness of eversion may be due to tendinitis, instability of the peroneal tendons, or, if profound, Charcot-Marie-Tooth disease. Lumbar radiculopathy and *peroneal nerve* injury may also cause eversion weakness.

The **peroneus longus** is difficult to test in isolation. Because the peroneus longus passes beneath the plantar surface of the foot to insert on the plantar surface of the first metatarsal, it functions as a plantar flexor of the first metatarsal. The examiner may attempt to test this function by pushing upward with a thumb beneath the head of the first metatarsal. The patient is instructed to press the medial border of the foot downward to resist this force. Unfortunately,

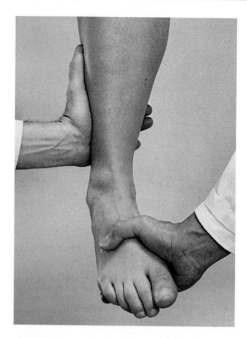

Figure 7–65. Assessing inversion strength.

most patients assist the peroneus longus with the toe flexors and gastrocsoleus complex. The examiner should attempt to verify that the peroneus longus is firing by palpating the tendon posterior to the lateral malleolus. Like the peroneus brevis, the peroneus longus is innervated by the *superficial peroneal nerve.*

Invertors of the Foot

Inversion of the foot is accomplished primarily by the **tibialis posterior,** with contributions from the **tibialis anterior, flexor digitorum longus,** and **flexor hallucis longus.** These are innervated by the *tibial nerve,* except for the tibialis anterior, which is innervated by the *deep peroneal nerve.*

To test inversion strength, the examiner places the patient's foot in an inverted position with the ankle plantar flexed. The patient is instructed to maintain this position while the examiner attempts to push the foot into eversion. The examiner supports the limb with one hand and pushes laterally against the medial border of the first metatarsal (Fig. 7–65). The tendon of the normal tibialis posterior sometimes can be seen and usually can be palpated between the medial malleolus and its insertion into the tuberosity of the navicular. Normally, the examiner should be unable to overcome the strength of the invertors. Tendinitis and rupture are common causes of tibialis posterior weakness.

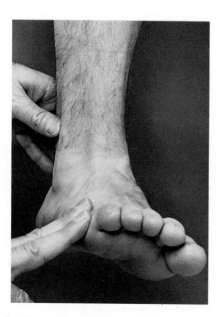

Figure 7–64. Assessing eversion strength.

Although completely isolated testing of the tibialis posterior is not possible, most of the effect of the tibialis anterior can be eliminated by modifying the test to have the patient begin the maneuver in the everted position.

Tibialis posterior function may also be assessed by asking the patient to rise up on the toes while the examiner observes from behind. If tibialis posterior function is normal, the heels should be observed to invert as they rise off the ground (see Fig. 7–34). The examiner should be aware, however, that stiffness in the subtalar joint may also prevent inversion of the heel, even in the presence of normal tibialis posterior strength.

SENSATION TESTING

The average distribution of the principal sensory nerves about the leg, ankle, and foot is delineated in Figure 7–66. The anatomy of the sensory nerves is quite variable; therefore, the exact pattern can vary considerably from one individual to another. Light touch or sharp-dull discrimination testing is generally used to screen for areas of altered sensation.

To detect a **sural nerve** deficit, the lateral border of the ankle and foot is usually tested. The **deep peroneal nerve** normally supplies the

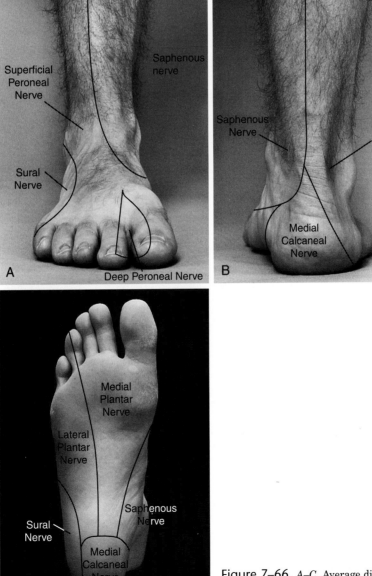

Figure 7–66. *A–C,* Average distribution of sensory nerves throughout the leg, the ankle, and the foot.

first web space between the great toe and the second toe, and the **superficial peroneal nerve** supplies most of the rest of the dorsum of the foot. The **saphenous nerve,** which is the most often injured or entrapped on the medial aspect of the knee, supplies most of the medial leg, usually extending down to the ankle or hindfoot.

Branches of the **posterior tibial nerve** supply most of the sensation to the plantar aspect of the heel and foot. These include the **medial calcaneal nerve,** which supplies the medial heel on both its medial and its plantar aspects, and the **medial and lateral plantar nerves,** which supply the medial and the lateral plantar surfaces of the foot, respectively.

Numbness in the distribution of the individual **digital nerve** branches can develop in the advanced stages of Morton's neuroma. Because these neuromata normally occur at an interspace, the adjacent sides of the digits that define the interspace can develop altered or decreased sensation. For example, the most common location of Morton's neuroma is at the interspace between the third and the fourth metatarsal heads. In the advanced stages of this condition, altered sensation is detectable along the lateral aspect of the third toe and the medial aspect of the fourth toe.

SPECIAL TESTS

Stability Testing

Two manipulative tests have been described for testing the passive laxity of the lateral ankle ligaments. The anterior talofibular ligament and the calcaneofibular ligament are the most common ankle ligaments to be injured and the most common to be associated with pathologic laxity. The test described may be performed after an acute injury or for evaluation of chronic instability, although examination in the face of an acute injury is more difficult owing to associated pain.

ANTERIOR DRAWER TEST. The *anterior talofibular ligament* is assessed with the **anterior drawer test.** This test is performed with the patient seated on the examination table and the lower limb relaxed and hanging loosely off the side of the table. With one hand, the examiner grasps the patient's leg just proximal to the ankle joint to stabilize it. The examiner should grasp the patient's foot and gently oscillate the ankle

to verify that the patient is relaxed. The examiner then grasps the patient's heel with the free hand and pulls forward while pushing posteriorly on the leg in a reciprocating manner (Fig. 7–67). The examiner focuses on the skin over the anterolateral dome of the talus to watch for anterior motion of the talus with this maneuver. The examiner assesses the amount of anterior translation by the feel as well as by the appearance of the talus. When greater degrees of displacement are present, the anterolateral dome of the talus is often seen tenting the skin. Because the deltoid ligament is usually intact, the talus tends to internally rotate in response to the anterior drawer stress. The examiner can maximize the excursion of the talus by internally rotating the foot as it is pulled forward.

In the normal patient, the talus is felt to move forward a few millimeters and then stop with a firm endpoint. Variation among individuals is great; comparison with the opposite side is extremely important.

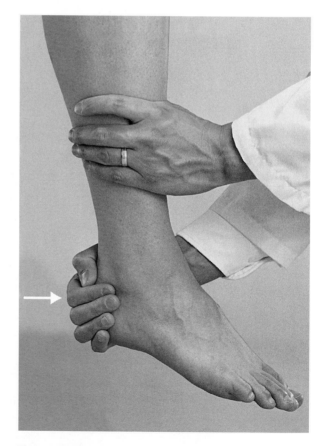

Figure 7–67. Anterior drawer test. The *arrow* indicates the direction of the force applied to the heel.

The key to diagnosing pathologic laxity of the anterior talofibular ligament is finding a difference of at least 3 mm to 5 mm in laxity between the two ankles. The *endpoint* may also be softer on the injured side. Unfortunately, it is not unusual for individuals to have sprained both ankles at some time in the past. In these cases, the examiner must use clinical judgment in assessing the result. If the anterolateral talus appears to sublux dramatically from the ankle mortise, the result is probably abnormal even if similar excursion is present on the other side.

INVERSION STRESS TEST. The integrity of the *calcaneofibular ligament* is evaluated with the **inversion stress test,** also called the **varus stress test.** The patient is seated in the same position used for the anterior drawer test. This time, the examiner grasps the patient's forefoot with one hand and maximally dorsiflexes the ankle to place the calcaneofibular ligament under tension and to lock the subtalar joint. While maintaining this position, the examiner grasps the patient's calcaneus with the opposite hand and attempts to invert the heel (Fig. 7–68). In the normal patient, very little movement is felt in response to this stress, and the resistance is firm. When the calcaneofibular ligament is compromised, the examiner feels the talus rock into inversion. Injury to the calcaneofibular ligament is diagnosed if an asymmetric increase in varus laxity is noted.

This test is more difficult to evaluate than the anterior drawer test because the motion of the talus is difficult to visualize and is usually assessed only by feel. If the examiner does not maximally dorsiflex the ankle when performing this examination, substantial inversion movement occurs at the subtalar joint, making it difficult to detect whether abnormal inversion is taking place at the ankle joint.

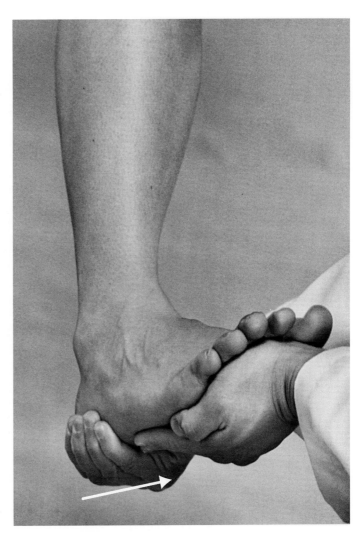

Figure 7–68. Inversion stress test. The *arrow* indicates the direction of the force applied to the heel.

Peroneal Tendon Instability Test

The **peroneal tendon instability test** is an active test that seeks to reproduce subluxation or dislocation of the peroneal tendons anterior to the lateral malleolus. To perform the instability test, the patient is seated on the table with the leg dangling. The patient is instructed to rotate the ankle and foot through maximal excursion, first in a clockwise manner, then in a counterclockwise manner. The motion begins with the ankle dorsiflexed and the foot in a neutral position. The ankle is actively rotated from a position of maximum dorsiflexion, to maximal eversion, to maximum plantar flexion, to maximum inversion, and back to dorsiflexion again. After several cycles, the direction of rotation is reversed. As the patient performs this maneuver, the examiner lightly palpates the posterior border of the lateral malleolus with two fingers (Fig. 7–69).

In the normal patient, the peroneal tendons are felt to move slightly anteriorly as they tense, but they remain behind the malleolus. When peroneal tendon instability is present, the tendons are felt to begin to sublux over the malleolus, or they may even dislocate. If the patient experiences pain when this occurs and identifies the sensation as duplicating his or her symptoms, the diagnosis is strengthened. In cases of longstanding instability, damage to the tendons may have occurred, resulting in signs of peroneal tendinitis.

Thompson's Test

The **Thompson test** is a manipulative test for confirming the diagnosis of *Achilles' tendon rupture*. Achilles' tendon rupture is sometimes overlooked because the patient is still able to plantar

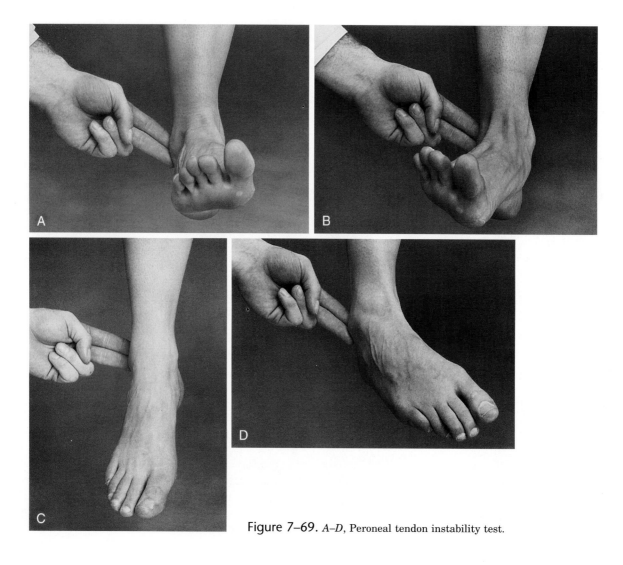

Figure 7–69. *A–D*, Peroneal tendon instability test.

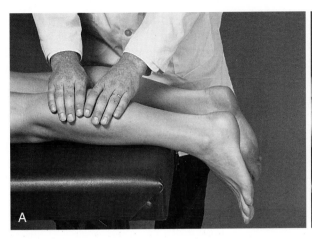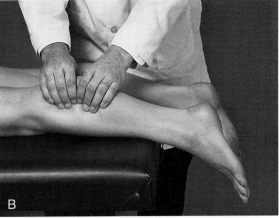

Figure 7–70. Thompson's test. *A,* Resting position. *B,* Normal plantar flexion response.

flex the ankle with the intact toe flexors. To perform the Thompson test, the patient is placed prone on the examination table with both feet dangling from the end. In this position, the examiner can see the swelling and ecchymosis usually associated with Achilles' tendon rupture and can palpate a gap in the tendon. The examiner should also observe the resting position of the foot when the patient is relaxed.

In the normal case, resting tension in the gastrocsoleus complex holds the foot in slight plantar flexion when the patient is lying prone (Fig. 7–70*A*). In the presence of Achilles' rupture, this resting tension is lost and the foot comes to rest in a more dorsiflexed position. The Thompson test itself is performed by grasping the patient's calf with one or both hands and gently squeezing the muscle. When the Achilles tendon is intact, the foot passively plantar flexes when the calf is squeezed (Fig. 7–70*B*). In the presence of Achilles' tendon rupture, virtually no motion of the foot is observed. In the presence of a partial tear of the Achilles or injuries to the gastrocsoleus aponeurosis, such as tennis leg, the normal plantar flexion response occurs.

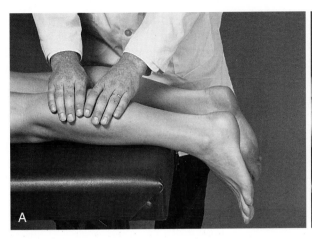

Figure 7–71. First metatarsal rise test. The *arrow* indicates the direction of the rise of the first metatarsal in response to external rotation of the lower leg.

First Metatarsal Rise Test

The **first metatarsal rise test** is a supplementary test for **posterior tibial tendon** dysfunction. The test is performed with the patient standing and facing away from the examiner. The examiner grasps the patient's lower leg and externally rotates it. This maneuver causes the heel to assume a varus position. In the presence of posterior tibial dysfunction, the patient's first metatarsal rises off the ground in response to the manipulation; in a normal patient, the first metatarsal remains in contact with the ground (Fig. 7–71). The test may also be done by grasping the heel directly and turning it into varus.

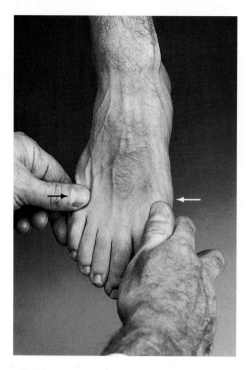

Figure 7–72. Morton's test. The *arrows* indicate the direction of the compressive forces applied to the first and fifth metatarsal heads.

Morton's Test

Morton's test is an adjunctive test for the detection of interdigital neuromas. The purpose of Morton's test is to reproduce the patient's symptoms by compressing the interdigital neuroma between the adjacent metatarsal heads. To perform Morton's test, the examiner grasps the heads of the first and fifth metatarsals and compresses them together (Fig. 7–72). Further irritation of the nerve may be produced by reciprocally moving the first and fifth metatarsals up and down in opposite directions. If this compression of the metatarsal heads reproduces the patient's characteristic pain, it is highly suggestive of the presence of an interdigital neuroma. Occasionally, the examiner may appreciate a palpable click while compressing the metatarsal heads. This is known as **Mulder's click**, and it is thought to be caused by a large neuroma being forced plantarly by the compressed metatarsal heads.

Homans' Test

Homans' test is a screening test for deep vein thrombosis of the calf; it is not a specifically orthopaedic test. Its sensitivity has been questioned because deep vein thrombosis may not always produce an abnormal Homans' test. Homans' test is usually performed with the patient supine or seated. The examiner then passively dorsiflexes the patient's foot. If this produces calf pain, then deep vein thrombosis of the calf may be present (Fig. 7–73). Obviously, injury to the gastrocsoleus complex may also be aggravated by this maneuver. Calf pain in response to Homans' test is called **Homans' sign.**

The physical findings in common conditions of the leg, ankle, and foot are summarized in Table 7–1.

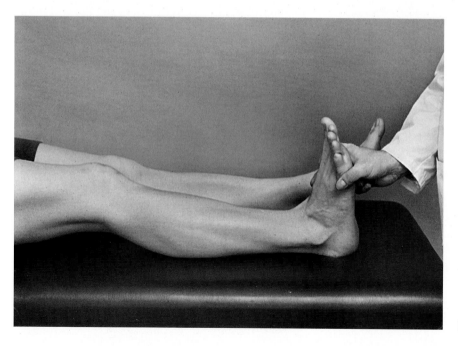

Figure 7–73. Homans' test.

TABLE 7–1.
PHYSICAL FINDINGS IN COMMON
CONDITIONS OF THE LEG, THE FOOT, AND THE ANKLE

Lateral Ankle Sprain

Swelling and ecchymosis over the lateral ankle ligaments
Tenderness over the anterior talofibular ligament
Tenderness over the calcaneofibular ligament (frequent)
Increased laxity to the anterior drawer test (frequent)
Increased laxity to the inversion stress test (more severe injuries)

Peroneal Tendinitis

Swelling posterior to the lateral malleolus
Tenderness over the peroneal tendons posterior to the lateral malleolus or over the peroneus brevis tendon between the lateral malleolus and the base of the fifth metatarsal
Pain reproduced or exacerbated by resisted eversion or walking on the medial borders of the feet
Subluxation of the tendons over the lateral malleolus noted during the peroneal instability test (if tendinitis is secondary to peroneal tendon instability)

Posterior Tibial Tendinitis or Tear

Swelling over the course of the posterior tibial tendon, posterior and distal to the medial malleolus
Tenderness over the posterior tibial tendon
Pain reproduced or exacerbated with resisted inversion or walking on the lateral borders of the feet
Asymmetric flattening of the longitudinal arch (frequent)
Abnormal first metatarsal rise test
Too-many-toes sign (more severe cases)
Absence of the normal windlass effect (more severe cases)

Achilles' Tendon Rupture

Swelling and ecchymosis over the distal Achilles tendon
Palpable defect in the Achilles tendon, usually 2 cm or 3 cm proximal to the calcaneal tuberosity
Weak and painful plantar flexion
Abnormal Thompson's test

Tibialis Anterior Tendon Rupture

Swelling and ecchymosis over the anterior ankle
Loss of the normal tibialis anterior prominence during active dorsiflexion
Tenderness and a palpable gap in the tibialis anterior tendon
Weakness to resisted ankle dorsiflexion and with heel walking
Achilles' tendon contracture and claw toes (chronic cases)

Hallux Rigidus

Prominent visible osteophytes on the dorsum of the first metatarsophalangeal joint
Swelling and erythema of the first metatarsophalangeal joint (variable)
Limited and crepitant arc of motion of the first metatarsophalangeal joint

Hallux Valgus

Great toe deviated laterally
Great toe rotated into pronation (more severe cases)
Bunion formation on the medial aspect of the first metatarsal head
Encroachment of the great toe on the lesser toes (more severe cases)

Morton's Neuroma

Tenderness of the involved web space (most commonly, between the third and the fourth toes)
Morton's test reproduces the patient's pain
Morton's test results in a palpable click (Mulder's click) (occasionally)
Numbness of the adjacent surfaces of the toes (advanced cases)

Metatarsal Stress Fracture

Tenderness of the distal shaft of the involved metatarsal (second and third metatarsals most common)
Edema and sometimes ecchymosis in the vicinity of the fracture (early stages)
Palpable callus on the metatarsal shaft (advanced stages)

Tibial or Fibular Stress Fracture

Point tenderness of the involved bone
Edema in the vicinity of the fracture (occasionally; early stages)
Palpable callus (advanced stages in more subcutaneous locations)

Compartment Syndrome of the Lower Leg

Muscles of the involved compartment feel extremely firm and tender (anterior compartment most common)
Pain exacerbated by active motion or passive stretching of the muscles in the involved compartment
Numbness in the distribution of nerves passing through the involved compartment (deep peroneal nerve for the anterior compartment) (more advanced stages)
Signs of compromised distal circulation (advanced stages)
N.B. In exercise-induced compartment syndrome, findings are transient and much more subtle

Bibliography

Anderson KJ, Lecocq JF, Lecocq EA: Recurrent anterior subluxation of the ankle. J Bone Joint Surg Am. 1952;34:853–860.

Arrowsmith SR, Fleming LL, Allman FL: Traumatic dislocations of the peroneal tendons. Am J Sports Med. 1983;11:142–146.

Brahms MA: Common foot problems. J Bone Joint Surg Am. 1967;49:1653–1664.

Buckley RE, Hunt DV: Reliability of clinical measurement of subtalar joint movement. Foot Ankle Int. 1997;18:229–232.

Cooper PS, Nowak MD, Shaer J: Calcaneocuboid joint pressures with lateral column lengthening (Evans) procedure. Foot Ankle Int. 1997;18:199–205.

Coughlin MJ: Second metatarsophalangeal joint instability in the athlete. Foot Ankle Int. 1993;14:309–319.

Dellon AL: Deep peroneal nerve entrapment on the dorsum of the foot. Foot Ankle Int. 1990;11:73–80.

DiStefano V, Sack JT, Whittaker R: Tarsal-tunnel syndrome. Clin Orthop. 1972;207:716–720.

Figura MA: Metatarsal fractures: an overview. Clin Podiatr Med Surg. 1985;2:247–257.

Frankel JP, Turf RM, King BA: Tailor's bunion: clinical evaluation and correction by distal metaphyseal osteotomy with cortical screw fixation. J Foot Ankle Surg. 1989;28:237–243.

Frey C, Rosenberg Z, Shereff MJ: The retrocalcaneal bursae: anatomy and bursography. Paper presented at: American Orthopaedic Foot and Ankle Society Meeting; 1986; Las Vegas.

Furey JG: Plantar fasciitis: the painful heel syndrome. J Bone Joint Surg Am. 1975;57:672–673.

Goldberg RS: Surgical treatment of the accessory navicular. Clin Orthop. 1983;177:61–66.

Hamilton WG: Stenosing tenosynovitis of the flexor hallucis longus tendon and posterior impingement upon the os trigonum in ballet dancers. Foot Ankle Int. 1982;3:74–80.

Hattrup SJ, Johnson KA: Subjective results of hallux rigidus following treatment with cheilectomy. Clin Orthop. 1988;226:182–191.

Holmes GB Jr, Mann RA: Possible epidemiological factors associated with rupture of the posterior tibial tendon. Foot Ankle Int. 1992;13:70–79.

Hunter LY: Stress fracture of the tarsal navicular. More frequent than we realize? Am J Sports Med. 1981;9:217-219.

Jack EA: The navicular-cuneiform fusion in the treatment of flat foot. J Bone Joint Surg Br. 1953;35:75–82.

Jahss MH: Evaluation of the cavus foot for orthopedic treatment. Clin Orthop. 1983;181:52–63.

Johnson ER, Kirby K, Lieberman JS: Lateral plantar nerve entrapment: foot pain in the power lifter. Am J Sports Med. 1992;20:619–620.

Johnson KA: Tibialis posterior tendon rupture. Clin Orthop. 1983;177:140–147.

Kavanaugh JH, Brower TD, Mann RV: The Jones fracture revisited. J Bone Joint Surg Am. 1978;60:776–782.

Kay DE: The sprained ankle: current therapy. Foot Ankle Int. 1985;6:22–28.

Krause JO, Brodsky JW: The natural history of type 1 midfoot neuropathic feet. Foot Ankle Clin. 1997;2:1–22.

Lidor C, Ferris L, Hall R, Alexander IJ, Nunley JA: Stress fracture of the tibia after arthrodesis of the ankle or the hindfoot. J Bone Joint Surg Am. 1997;79:558–564.

Mann RA, Thompson FM: Rupture of the posterior tibial tendon causing flat foot. Surgical treatment. J Bone Joint Surg Am. 1985;67:556–561.

Miller JW: Acquired hallux varus: a preventable and correctible disorder. J Bone Joint Surg Am. 1975;57:183–188.

Mulder JD: The causative mechanism in Morton's metatarsalgia. J Bone Joint Surg Br. 1951;33:94–95.

Myerson MS, Shereff MJ: The pathological anatomy of claw and hammer toes. J Bone Joint Surg Am. 1989;71:45–49.

Ouzounian TJ, Anderson R: Anterior tibial tendon rupture. Foot Ankle Int. 1995;16:406–410.

Rask MR: Medial plantar neuropraxis (jogger's foot): report of three cases. Clin Orthop. 1978;134:193–195.

Rogers BS, Leach RE: Achilles tendinitis. Foot Ankle Clin. 1996;1:249–259.

Saleh M, Murdoch G: Defence of gait analysis. J Bone Joint Surg Br. 1985;67:237–241.

Sangeorzan BJ, Veith R, Hansen ST: Fusion of Lisfranc's joint for salvage of tarsometatarsal injuries. Foot Ankle Int. 1989;10:193–200.

Slovenkai MP: Clinical and radiographic evaluation. Foot Ankle Clin. 1997;2:241–260.

Styf J: Entrapment of the superficial peroneal nerve. J Bone Joint Surg Br. 1989;71:131–135.

Thompson T, Doherty J: Spontaneous rupture of the tendo Achilles: a new clinical diagnostic test. J Trauma. 1962;2:126–129.

F. Todd Wetzel
Bruce Reider

8

Cervical and Thoracic Spine

*T*he spine performs two important functions in the human body. First, it provides stability and continuity, supporting the head on the thorax and the thorax on the pelvis. Second, it protects and transmits the neural elements of the central nervous system (CNS) from the brain to the periphery. The injuries and the disorders that affect the spine can interfere with one or both of these functions and may produce symptoms accordingly.

The structure of the spine reflects its function. The spine is composed of 24 distinct vertebrae—7 cervical, 12 thoracic, and 5 lumbar—perched on the solid base provided by the sacrum and the pelvis. The structure of each vertebra follows the same basic pattern, with modifications, as required, to fulfill its own particular function. The anterior portion of each vertebra (except C1) is a modified cylinder known as the *vertebral body*. The column formed by these bodies provides much of the stability of the spine. Linking each pair of vertebral bodies is an intervertebral disk that provides elements of stability, flexibility, and shock absorption. The portion of each vertebra posterior to the body is known as the *posterior elements*. These include the *pedicles*, which link the rest of the posterior elements to the vertebral body; the *laminae*; the *posterior facet joints*; and the *transverse* and *spinous processes*. The posterior elements create a protective canal for the spinal cord and its nerve roots, provide additional stability, and function as attachment sites for the intrinsic muscles of the spine. The intimate relationship of the structural elements to the neurologic elements of the spine means that structural abnormalities, such as herniated disks, fractures, or degenerative changes, can often produce neurologic symptoms.

The cervical spine serves as a pedestal for the head and is adapted to allow the mobility necessary to vary the position of the head in relationship to the surrounding environment. The increased exposure and mobility of the cervical spine place it at greater risk for trauma or chronic degenerative changes.

In contrast to the cervical spine, the thoracic spine is stiff and stable. Not only are the individual vertebrae designed to permit only limited movement but also the articulating ribs provide even greater stability and support. The thoracic spine's design provides much of the explanation for the low incidence of disk injuries and degenerative disorders in the thoracic spine compared with the cervical spine.

Inspection

SURFACE ANATOMY AND ALIGNMENT

When inspecting the cervical and the thoracic spine, the overriding goal should be to detect any departure from perfect symmetry. Possible causes of asymmetry include malunions or nonunions of fractures, developmental abnormalities such as scoliosis, muscular asymmetry such as that is seen in torticollis, or localized masses from tumors or glandular enlargement.

Posterior Aspect

To inspect the cervical and the thoracic spine from the posterior aspect, the patient is asked to stand facing directly away from the examiner (Fig. 8–1). Because the spine is located just deep to the dorsal surface of the body, posterior inspection reveals the most specific information regarding spinal pathology. From the top of the head to the natal cleft over the sacrum and the coccyx, all structures should appear perfectly symmetric. The head should be centered squarely on the neck. At the point where the cervical spine joins the occiput at the base of the skull, a definite bump, called the **inion**, should be either clearly visible or palpable, depending on the hairstyle and the build of the patient (Fig. 8–2). Beginning at the inion, the spine should be visible as a linear furrow running all the way to the sacrum, studded with small bumps that represent the **spinous processes** of the vertebrae. In the normal situation, the spine should be so straight that a plumb line dropped from the inion would pass perfectly over it and hang down in the natal cleft.

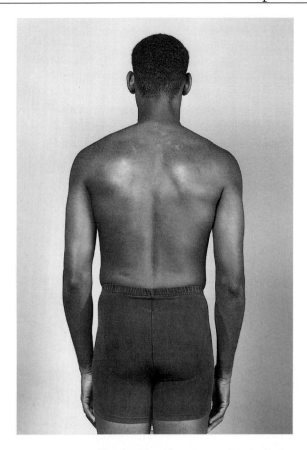

Figure 8–1. Posterior aspect of the spine.

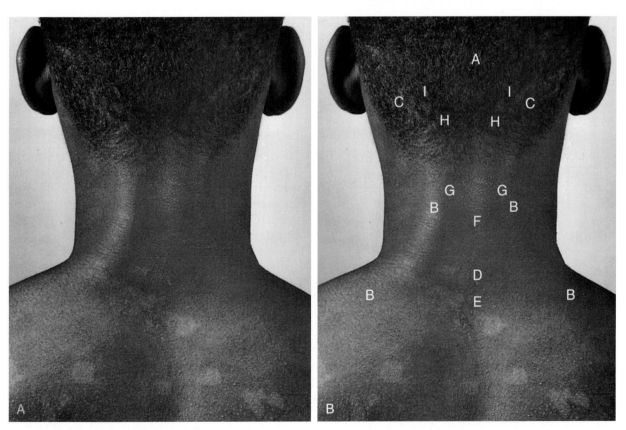

Figure 8–2. *A* and *B*, Posterior aspect of the neck. A, inion; B, trapezius; C, transversocostal muscle group; D, C7 spinous process; E, T1 spinous process; F, nuchal ligament; G, posterior facet joint; H, suboccipital muscles; I, greater occipital nerve.

VERTEBRA PROMINENS. At the cervicothoracic junction, one large spinous process is seen to stand out from those above and below it. This is often called the **vertebra prominens**, and it identifies the spinous process of C7. Above this, the spinous processes of the cervical vertebrae are bifid and less prominent. Forward flexion of the neck and back tends to make the C7 and T1 spinous processes more prominent in a thin individual (Fig. 8–3).

TRAPEZIUS. The **trapezius** is the most superficial and the most easily identifiable of the posterior neck muscles. Each trapezius is roughly triangular, originating from the occiput and the spinous processes of C7 through T12 and inserting laterally on the clavicle, the acromion, and the scapular spine. The upper border of the trapezius is quite prominent as it blends into the medial shoulder.

Deep to the trapezius lies the **transversocostal** group of muscles and the even deeper **transversospinal** group. The transversocostal group includes the *splenius capitis*, the *splenius cervicis*, the *iliocostalis cervicis*, and the *longissimus cervicis* and is visible in the proximal neck lateral to the superior trapezius.

LATERAL STRUCTURES. Lateral to the spine, the other structures visible from the posterior position should also appear symmetric. The shoulders should be level and the scapulae located equidistant from the spine. The rib promi-

nences on either side of the spine should be symmetric. When the patient is instructed to relax and to allow the upper extremities to hang limply at the sides, the size and the shape of the space between the arms and the sides of the body should be identical. At the base of the spine, the posterior landmarks of the pelvis should appear symmetric and level. A pelvis that does not appear to be level may be the result of either a leg length discrepancy in a patient with an otherwise normal spine or a fixed spinal deformity.

Departure from symmetry in any of these parameters may suggest a localized anomaly or a deformity of the spine in the coronal plane. An example of a localized anomaly is **Sprengel's deformity**, a congenital condition in which one of the scapulae remains fixed proximally in a tightly contracted position (see Fig. 2–21). Coronal deformities of the spine include a *list* and *scoliosis*.

LIST. A **list** is a pure planar shift to one side in the coronal plane (Fig. 8–4). It may be caused by pain, muscle spasm, or certain anomalies. When a list is present, the proximal part of the spine is shifted to one side, so that a plumb line dropped from the occiput or the vertebra prominens does not hang directly over the natal cleft and the spaces between the upper extremities and the trunk are asymmetric. Lists are more common in the lumbar spine than in the cervical or thoracic spine.

SCOLIOSIS. **Scoliosis** is a more complex, helical deformity in which a curve in the coronal plane is combined with abnormal rotation of the vertebrae in the transverse plane (Fig. 8–5). A well-compensated scoliosis, defined as one in which thoracic and lumbar curves are roughly equal in magnitude but opposite in direction, may be surprisingly difficult to detect during observation of the spine in the standing patient. In these cases, visually tracing the path of the spinous processes may help the examiner appreciate that they follow a subtle S curve, although the vertebra prominens is located directly above the natal cleft.

If a subtle scoliosis is suspected, looking for the **rib prominence** usually associated with thoracic scoliotic curves makes the deformity easier to detect. The rib prominence is a reflection of the rotational component of scoliosis. The ribs articulate with the transverse processes of the corresponding vertebrae. The vertebrae involved in the scoliotic curve are rotated around the lon-

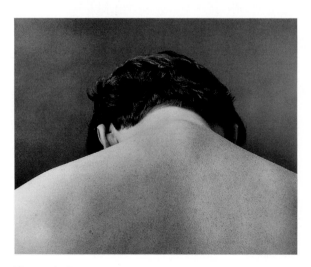

Figure 8–3. Posterior aspect of the neck in forward flexion.

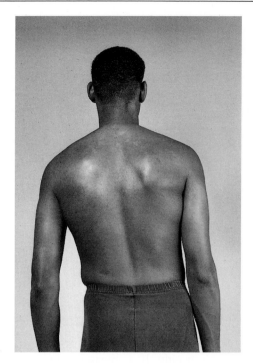

Figure 8–4. A list to the left side.

gitudinal axis of the spine, with the transverse processes on the convex side of the curve rotating posteriorly and those on the concave side rotating anteriorly. The ribs on the convex side, therefore, are more prominent, and those on the concave side are less prominent. The resulting rib prominence, therefore, appears on the convex side of the curve. In the most common type of scoliosis, *adolescent idiopathic scoliosis*, the thoracic convexity and, thus, the rib prominence are most

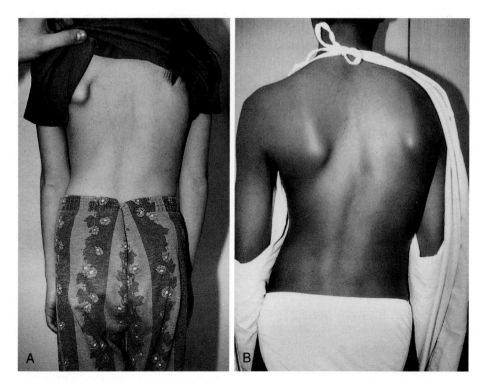

Figure 8–5. Scoliosis. *A*, Mild. *B*, More severe.

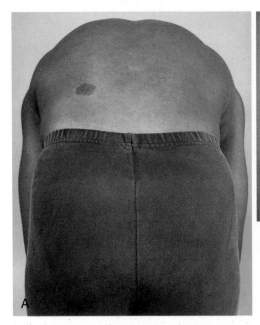

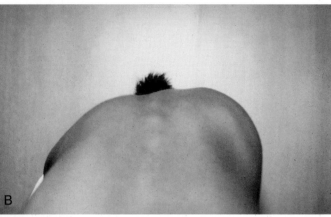

Figure 8–6. Examination for rib prominence. *A*, Normal. *B*, Abnormal.

often located on the right side. If scoliosis is suspected, asking the patient to bend forward as far as possible emphasizes the rib prominence (Fig. 8–6).

Idiopathic scoliosis is usually associated with a smooth, moderate curve, whereas scoliosis due to congenital or vertebral abnormalities more frequently produces short, sharp curves. If the scoliosis extends into the cervical spine, particularly in cases of congenital scoliosis, asymmetric twisting of the neck, known as **torticollis**, may be present. In very severe cases of scoliosis, the serpentine course of the spine may so shorten its effective length that the rib cage appears to rest on the iliac crests.

SKIN LESIONS. While examining the patient's back, the clinician should look for **skin lesions** that are known to be associated with conditions that may cause spinal deformity. Examples are a hairy nevus, which may be associated with spina bifida, and the café au lait spots or the cutaneous nodules of neurofibromatosis.

Lateral Aspect

CERVICAL LORDOSIS. From a lateral perspective, the cervical and the thoracic spine should be observed in both the sitting and the standing positions. When viewed from the side, the spine is not at all straight; it is a series of gentle, complementary curves (Fig. 8–7). A curve that is concave posteriorly is called a **lordosis**, and one

that is convex posteriorly is called a **kyphosis**. A **cervical lordosis**, with the head resting comfortably over the middle of the trunk, is present in normal individuals. A reduction in this normal lordosis, with straightening of the curve, is a common, nonspecific reaction to cervical spine pain. More dramatic reduction or even reversal of this lordosis may be seen in *ankylosing spondylitis*. In the most extreme examples of this condition, the patient's chin may come to rest against

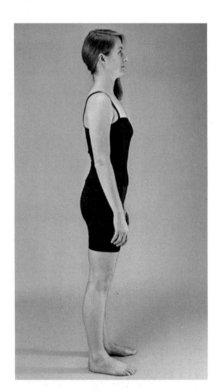

Figure 8–7. Lateral view of the spine.

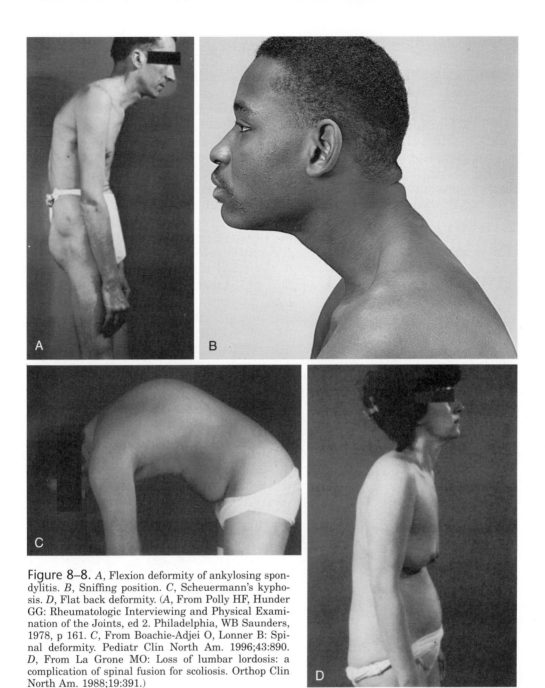

Figure 8–8. *A*, Flexion deformity of ankylosing spondylitis. *B*, Sniffing position. *C*, Scheuermann's kyphosis. *D*, Flat back deformity. (*A*, From Polly HF, Hunder GG: Rheumatologic Interviewing and Physical Examination of the Joints, ed 2. Philadelphia, WB Saunders, 1978, p 161. *C*, From Boachie-Adjei O, Lonner B: Spinal deformity. Pediatr Clin North Am. 1996;43:890. *D*, From La Grone MO: Loss of lumbar lordosis: a complication of spinal fusion for scoliosis. Orthop Clin North Am. 1988;19:391.)

the chest with the line of gaze fixed toward the ground (Fig. 8–8*A*). A milder deformity is the so-called **sniffing position**, in which the face of the patient appears to be thrust out anteriorly. Flexion at the cervicothoracic junction, with extension of the proximal segments, results in this position of cervical protrusion (Fig. 8–8*B*). The sniffing position is frequently associated with a cervicothoracic kyphosis.

THORACIC KYPHOSIS. The normal cervical lordosis is usually balanced by a smooth transition into a normal **thoracic kyphosis**. This kyphosis is particularly noticeable in the upper thoracic spine. Normal thoracic kyphosis is between 21° and 33° when measured radiographically by the Cobb method. Because the amount of thoracic kyphosis is difficult to quantitate by physical examination, departures from the normal degree of thoracic kyphosis are usually assessed by a general comparison with the examiner's prior experience of the normal range. Thoracic kyphosis that is increased above the normal range gives a distinct round-shouldered appearance (see Fig. 8–8*C*). Possible causes include *Scheuermann's disease*, which is an adolescent growth disturbance that produces wedge-shaped vertebral bodies; ankylosing spondylitis; congenital vertebral anomalies; and prior compression fracture.

In the presence of severely increased kyphosis, the head appears to be positioned far anteriorly of the thoracic spine and the trunk also appears to be shortened. A particularly sharp-angled kyphosis is called a **gibbus**. A gibbus usually reflects a sharp angulation of the spine at a single vertebral level. Possible causes include congenital anomalies, such as wedge-shaped vertebrae, or vertebral body collapse due to tumor, infection, or trauma.

A pathologic reduction in the normal thoracic kyphosis is unusual. Such a **flat back** appearance may be observed after surgery to correct thoracic scoliosis (see Fig. 8–8D).

Anterior Aspect

LANDMARKS. Anterior inspection of the spine is of limited usefulness owing to the dorsal location of the structure being examined. However, the examiner should again check carefully for the appearance of symmetry. The neck should appear straight, with the head sitting squarely on the shoulders and the chin positioned directly above the sternal notch (Fig. 8–9). Pain or fixed deformity may cause the head to be held at an angle. Prominent midline anterior landmarks include the hyoid bone, the thyroid cartilage, and the cricoid cartilage. Although evaluation of these structures does not fall within the domain of the orthopaedic physical examination, their identification allows the examiner to localize an abnormality at the corresponding level of the cervical spine. For this purpose, the examiner should keep in mind that the **hyoid** lies approximately at the level of **C3**, the **thyroid cartilage** at the level of **C4** and **C5**, and the **cricoid cartilage** at the level of **C6**.

Lateral to the midline, the two **sternocleidomastoid muscles** are prominent landmarks that are visible in most individuals. These muscles originate on the mastoid processes of the skull and insert on the sternum and the clavicle at the sternoclavicular joints, forming a prominent V configuration.

STERNUM. Proceeding distally, the examiner observes the **sternal notch** at the confluence of the two sternocleidomastoid muscles. The notch

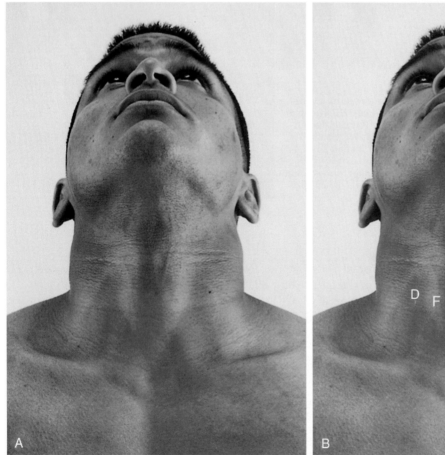
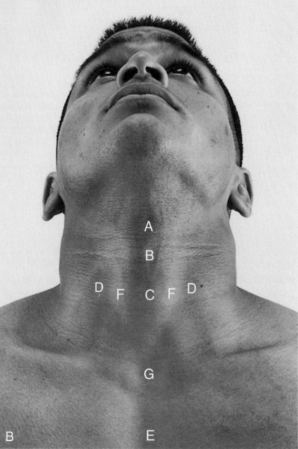

Figure 8–9. *A* and *B,* Anterior aspect of the neck. A, hyoid; B, thyroid cartilage; C, cricoid cartilage; D, sternocleidomastoid muscles; E, sternum; F, Chassaignac's tubercles; G, sternal notch.

is typically located at the level of the T3 and T4 vertebral bodies. Below this extends the **sternum**, a relatively narrow flat bone. Although it serves as the origin of the pectoralis major muscle, the sternum's central strip has little overlying soft tissue. It is, therefore, usually visible as a depression between the breasts in women or the pectoralis major muscles in men. Deformities of the sternum do occur. These include **pectus excavatum**, an abnormally concave sternum, and **pectus carinatum**, an abnormally convex sternum. The final significant anterior landmark (for orthopaedic purposes) is the **umbilicus**, which is contained in the T10 dermatome.

GAIT

An evaluation of gait is imperative for any thorough assessment of the spine. Some of the neurologic syndromes associated with disorders of the cervical or the thoracic spine produce characteristic gait disturbances. Observation of the spine during ambulation can also provide valuable information about the dynamic and the static behavior of the weightbearing cervical spine.

SHUFFLING AND SLAP FOOT GAITS. Injury to the posterior columns of the spinal cord produces a *posterior cord syndrome*, a condition characterized by the loss of proprioception in the extremities that are innervated below the lesion. When the individual with a posterior cord syndrome takes a step, he or she is unaware of the position of the swinging foot in space and thus is unable to predict the exact moment of heel strike. This uncertainty may be manifested by a **shuffling gait**, in which the feet are dragged on the ground during the swing phase, or a **slap foot gait**, in which the feet strike the ground in a violent, unpredictable manner. Although a shuffling gait is typical of posterior cord syndrome, it may also be seen in a variety of other neurologic disorders, such as Parkinson's disease.

BROAD-BASED GAIT. A **broad-based** or **halting gait** may be seen when stenosis of the cervical spine is complicated by compression of the spinal cord. In this gait pattern, which is caused by faulty programming of the sequence of muscle movements necessary for a normal gait, the patient's stance is widened owing to balancing difficulties during single leg stance. The rhythm of the gait is frequently jerky, again owing to central programming dysfunction. The pathogenesis of this pattern is unclear, but these patients frequently have difficulty walking over uneven ground and complain of loss of balance.

RANGE OF MOTION

Cervical Spine

To properly assess the range of motion of the cervical spine, it is important that the thoracic spine be supported. This is accomplished most easily by having the patient sit in a straight-backed chair. Ideally, the chair back should extend to the midscapular level but not above it (Fig. 8–10). In assessing each direction of movement, the examiner tries not only to measure the amount of motion possible but also to determine

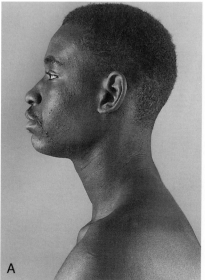 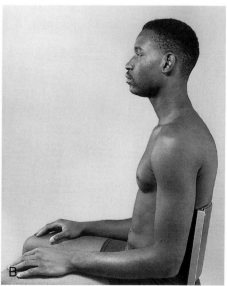

Figure 8–10. Neutral position for evaluation of flexion and extension. *A*, Cervical. *B*, Thoracic.

whether or not the various movements are painful. Any difficulties during the arc of motion, such as hesitation or midrange pain, should be noted. **Midrange pain** is typically due to instability of the structure being moved. When midrange pain is present, the total range of motion may be normal, but the movement is not conducted smoothly or with a constant velocity. This pain most commonly occurs in cases of subacute or chronic instability, such as would be produced by degenerative disk disease. For example, if the disk is painful when the neck is in a neutral position, the patient would be observed to hesitate in the neutral position when moving from full flexion to full extension.

FLEXION AND EXTENSION. To assess **flexion**, the examiner asks the patient to attempt to touch the chin to the chest. A patient with a normal cervical spine should be able to make firm contact between the chin and the chest or come very close to it (Fig. 8–11). Measuring the distance between the chin and the chest at the point of maximal flexion is the most useful way to quantify this movement for future comparison.

To assess **extension**, the patient is asked to tilt the head back and to look up toward the ceiling (Fig. 8–12). Maximum extension is a combination of cervical, thoracic, and occipitocervical motion. If normal extension is present, the patient should be able to tilt the head back until the face is parallel with the ceiling. Approximately 50% of flexion-extension motion occurs between the occiput and C1. The amount of extension may be reduced in the presence of degenerative arthritis or a fixed deformity such as scoliosis or kyphosis. In addition, acute cervical

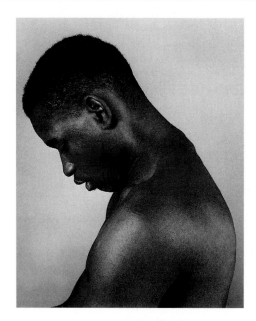

Figure 8–11. Active cervical flexion.

nerve root compression may also limit extension owing to pain.

LATERAL ROTATION. **Lateral rotation** to both the right and the left should be assessed. To measure lateral rotation, ask the patient to rotate the chin laterally toward each shoulder, in turn (Fig. 8–13). The spinous processes are seen to rotate away from the side to which the chin points. Normal lateral rotation is typically about 60° in each direction, but it may reach close to 90° in some individuals. This is best assessed by standing in front of or directly behind the patient and observing the arc of rotation as the head

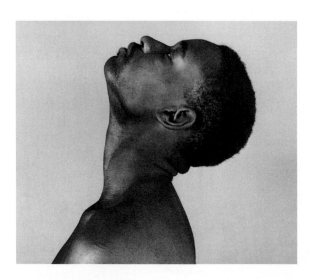

Figure 8–12. Active cervical extension.

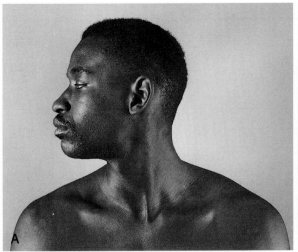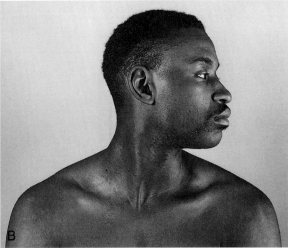

Figure 8–13. Active lateral rotation of the cervical spine. *A*, Right. *B*, Left.

moves. Approximately 50% of normal rotation occurs between C1 and C2, the atlas and the axis.

LATERAL BENDING. Lateral bending to both the right and the left sides is assessed by asking the patient to attempt to touch each ear to the ipsilateral shoulder (Fig. 8–14). When combined with a normal shoulder shrug, maximal lateral bending should permit the shoulder to nearly touch the ear. The amount of motion may be quantitated by measuring the distance between the shoulder and the ear at maximal effort or by estimating the angle that the midline of the face makes with the vertical.

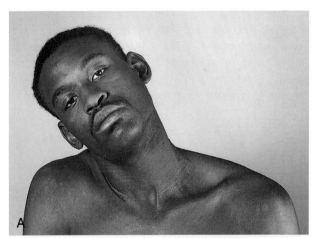

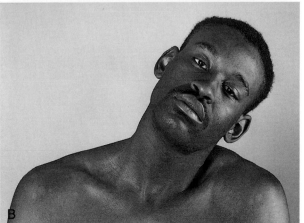

Figure 8–14. Active lateral bending of the cervical spine. *A*, Right. *B*, Left.

311

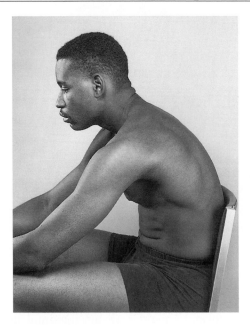

Figure 8–15. Active thoracic flexion.

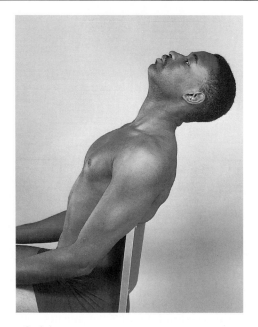

Figure 8–16. Active thoracic extension.

Thoracic Spine

FLEXION AND EXTENSION. In dramatic contrast with the cervical spine, the thoracic spine permits little motion. What is present consists of a small amount of flexion and extension. To assess flexion and extension of the thoracic spine, the patient is seated against a straight-backed chair in order to eliminate lumbopelvic motion. The patient is asked first to flex and then to extend the thoracic spine (Figs. 8–15 and 8–16). The small amount of motion present may be de-

tected by observing the change in relationship between the thoracic spine and the vertical chair back. In the presence of ankylosing spondylitis, the range of flexion and extension of the spine is limited.

A traditional way to detect this stiffness when ankylosing spondylitis is suspected is to use a tape measure to assess the **apparent change in length** of the spine between flexion and extension. This is done by measuring the distance between the vertebra prominens and the sacrum with a tape measure when the patient is standing

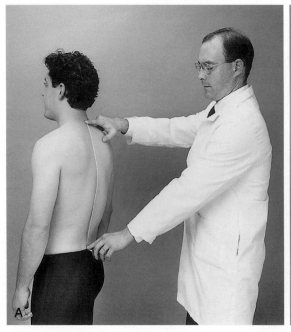

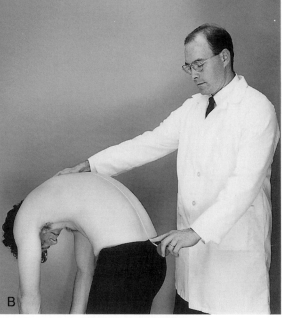

Figure 8–17. *A* and *B*, Measurement of apparent elongation of the spine with flexion.

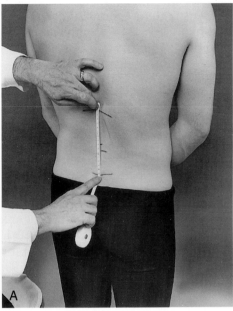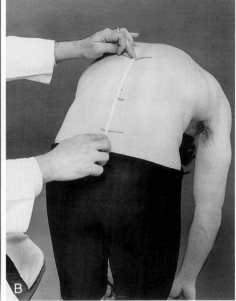

Figure 8–18. *A* and *B*, Modified Schober's test.

erect. The patient is then instructed to bend forward as far as possible and the same interval is measured (Fig. 8–17). A variant of this technique is the **modified Schober test**, which quantifies lumbosacral flexion. To perform this measurement, the examiner marks points 10 cm above and 5 cm below the lumbosacral junction in the extended spine. The patient is then asked to maximally flex, and the examiner measures the distance between the same two points (Fig. 8–18). Normally, the length of the dorsal aspect of the spine should appear to increase about 6 cm. Excursion of much less than this amount suggests the presence of ankylosing spondylitis, particularly if a kyphotic deformity is present.

Another screening test for ankylosing spondylitis is to measure the amount of **chest expansion** possible. This is normally done by encircling the patient's chest with a flexible tape measure at the nipple line. The patient is then asked to maximally exhale and the chest circumference is noted (Fig. 8–19*A*). Next, the patient is asked to maximally inhale and the circumference again is documented (Fig. 8–19*B*). The distance between these two measurements should be about 5 cm. If it is less than 2.5 cm, chest expansion is decreased. This may be a sign of ankylosing spondylitis. This measurement is more difficult to perform in females, in whom ankylosing spondylitis is fortunately less common.

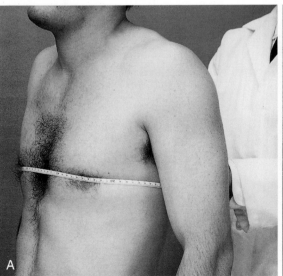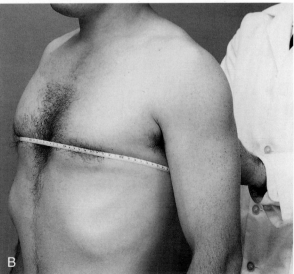

Figure 8–19. *A* and *B*, Measurement of chest expansion.

Palpation

Palpation has several uses in the evaluation of the cervical spine. First, it may reveal a subtle *deformity* or malalignment that was overlooked during inspection or hidden from visual examination because an acutely injured patient was encountered in a supine position. Second, palpation may detect paraspinous *muscle spasm*. Such spasm may reflect injury to the muscle itself or may merely be an involuntary response to a painful condition involving adjacent structures. Finally, careful palpation may identify an area of *point tenderness*. Point tenderness may allow the examiner to identify the level of a discrete lesion or even the exact site of injury, such as a posterior facet joint. In a patient with a history of recent trauma, point tenderness strongly suggests a fracture or a significant ligamentous disruption. Palpation of the spine is performed primarily from the posterior aspect.

Posterior Aspect

The cervical spine is most commonly palpated with the patient in either the supine or the seated position. The supine position allows the patient to relax more completely and may, thus, permit the identification of more anatomic detail (Fig. 8–20A). The disadvantage of the supine position is that the examiner cannot directly visualize the structures being palpated. The seated position (Fig. 8–20B) may compromise muscle relaxation, but it permits direct visualization of

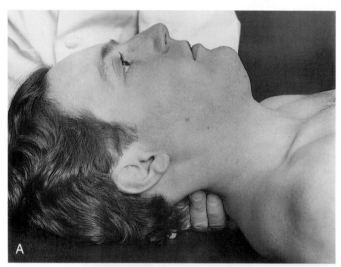

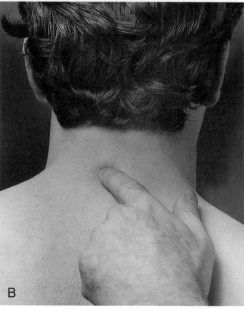

Figure 8–20. Palpation of the cervical spine. *A*, Supine position. *B*, Seated position.

the area being examined. The prone position, although not widely employed, permits a compromise between the two extremes. If the patient is initially seen in an emergency situation, such as on an athletic field or following a motor vehicle accident, the question of preferred position is moot. In the emergency situation, the patient should be examined in the position in which he or she is first encountered until the examiner is satisfied that the possibility of an unstable cervical spine has been ruled out. If the examiner is unable to make this decision with confidence, the patient should be transported to a hospital with the neck immobilized until a good radiographic evaluation can be conducted.

Cervical Spine

SPINOUS PROCESSES. Palpation of the cervical spine usually begins at the **inion**, located at the base of the skull (see Fig. 8–2). The examiner's palpating fingertips proceed distally in the midline, attempting to identify each **spinous process**. The first identifiable spinous process should be that of C2. Palpation proceeds distally toward the more prominent C7 and T1 spinous processes. The examiner should ask the patient whether gentle pressure on each of the spinous processes is painful. Such tenderness may signify an injury localized to that particular vertebra. In the emergency situation, documentation of localized tenderness is sufficient reason to consider the cervical spine potentially unstable and to immobilize and transport the patient accordingly.

In addition to palpating each of the spinous processes for *tenderness*, the examiner should also use palpation to evaluate their *alignment*. Normally, the spinous processes should be arranged in a perfectly linear fashion and regularly spaced. An acute lateral shift between two spinous processes may be due to a unilateral facet joint dislocation or fracture. An increase in the space between two otherwise normally aligned spinous processes raises the possibility of a posterior ligamentous disruption or fracture.

The **nuchal ligament** connects the cervical spinous processes, beginning at the base of the skull and extending to C7. Its prominence increases as the neck flexes. Conversely, the proximal spinous processes are easier to palpate when the cervical spine is extended.

POSTERIOR FACET JOINTS. After palpating in the midline, the examiner's fingers should move laterally about 2 cm to the region of the **posterior facet joints**. Owing to the overlying musculature, firmer palpation is needed to appreciate the resistance of the underlying bony structures. The examiner palpates from proximal to distal in a systematic manner. Although the specific outlines of the individual joints cannot usually be appreciated, the identification of localized tenderness over one of these joints may allow the examiner to identify the site of arthritic degeneration or ligamentous injury.

POSTERIOR CERVICAL MUSCULATURE. While palpating lateral to the midline, the examiner also is able to evaluate the posterior cervical musculature, consisting of the upper portion of the **trapezius** and the underlying intrinsic neck muscles. Occasionally, a localized mass owing to a hematoma or other lesion may be palpable. Muscle spasm may indicate injury to the muscle itself, or it may be an involuntary reaction to pain in an adjacent structure. Cervical spine pain may be referred to portions of the trapezius, either superior to the spine of the scapula or between the thoracic spinous processes and the medial border of the scapula. Palpation of these areas may reveal localized tender nodules, or *trigger points*.

The *splenius capitis* and other members of the **transversocostal** group are partly covered by the upper trapezius, but they may be palpated more distinctly in the proximal neck where they are exposed lateral to the trapezius. The deeper **transversospinal** group is not distinctly palpable but may contribute to the apparent tenderness of the overlying musculature.

Deep to the trapezius at the base of the skull lie the **suboccipital muscles**, the *rectus capitis (posterior) major*, the *rectus capitis minor*, and the *obliquus capitis superior* and *inferior*. The **greater occipital nerve**, also known as the **suboccipital nerve**, traverses the triangle formed by these muscles. Tenderness in this area may be due to occipital neuritis, muscle strain, or, in cases of rheumatoid arthritis, potential C1-C2 instability.

Thoracic Spine

The thoracic spine is stabilized by the associated ribs. Because of this, major injuries here require substantially more energy than in the cervical spine and, thus, are less common. However, palpation of the thoracic spine may be used to detect localized tenderness or discontinuity just as in the cervical spine.

Anterior Aspect

The principal landmarks of the anterior neck have already been described. When not readily visible, the hyoid bone, the thyroid cartilage, and the cricoid cartilage can be gently palpated. The primary purpose of identifying these structures is to orient the examiner to the corresponding vertebral level of spinal pathology.

The **hyoid** is a horseshoe-shaped bone that lies just caudal to the angle of the mandible at about the level of the **C3** vertebral body (see Fig. 8–9). The hyoid is rarely visible but usually easily palpable. The examiner may gently grasp this firm curved structure between the thumb and the index finger (Fig. 8–21).

Just inferior to the hyoid bone is the **thyroid cartilage**. The thyroid cartilage forms the Adam's apple, which is prominently visible in many men. This large superficial wing-like structure is freely mobile (Fig. 8–22). The thyroid cartilage is located at the level of the **C4** and **C5** vertebral bodies.

Inferior to the thyroid cartilage is a narrow groove followed by the prominent curved band that is the anterior portion of the **cricoid cartilage** ring (Fig. 8–23). This mobile ring is located approximately at the level of the **C6** vertebral body. The examiner's fingers may then be slid laterally to the right or the left of the cricoid in

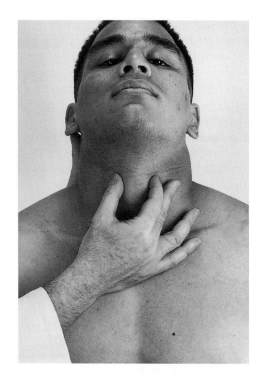

Figure 8–22. Palpation of the thyroid cartilage.

the small depression formed by the anterior strap muscles and the anterior borders of the sternocleidomastoid. Direct gentle posterior pressure should result in the detection of the **tubercles of Chassaignac**, or **carotid tubercles**, located

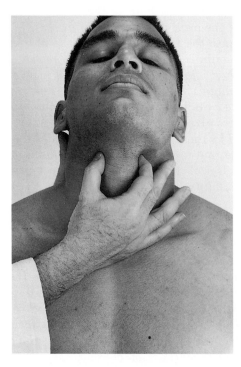

Figure 8–21. Palpation of the hyoid.

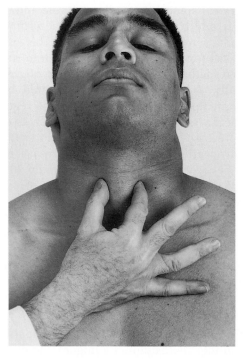

Figure 8–23. Palpation of the cricoid cartilage.

on C6. Typically, pulsations of the carotid artery are felt just medial to Chassaignac's tubercles. The examiner should take care not to compress both carotid arteries simultaneously.

Manipulation

MUSCLE TESTING

Strength testing of the muscles that move the cervical spine is not usually emphasized as much as the evaluation of the muscles that are innervated by the various cervical nerve roots. Nevertheless, it is important to establish that the protective function of the intrinsic cervical musculature is present. In addition, the identification of specific weak muscle groups, although not as significant as the identification of a specific central or peripheral neurologic deficit, may allow the clinician to formulate a treatment plan to restore normal function.

Muscle tests are normally conducted with the patient seated or standing. The patient's ability to support the neck in the erect position is an indication that the muscles are at least strong enough to overcome the force of gravity. All strength testing should be done gently, with the examiner providing firm, controlled resistance. This avoids sudden uncontrolled movements that could be painful or injurious.

Lateral Rotators

The **sternocleidomastoid** muscles function as both cervical rotators and flexors. Because they are innervated by the *spinal accessory nerves*, a complete injury to one of these nerves would paralyze the corresponding sternocleidomastoid muscle. Isolated contraction of one sternocleidomastoid rotates the cervical spine, so that the patient's chin points away from the contracting muscle: the *left* sternocleidomastoid produces **right lateral rotation** and the *right* sternocleidomastoid produces **left lateral rotation**.

To test a given sternocleidomastoid muscle, the examiner places the palm of one hand on the opposite side of the patient's head or face and instructs the patient to attempt to rotate the head to that side as strongly as possible. The tension in the sternocleidomastoid being tested should be quite visible (Fig. 8–24). Normally, the examiner should be unable to overcome the patient's strength of rotation.

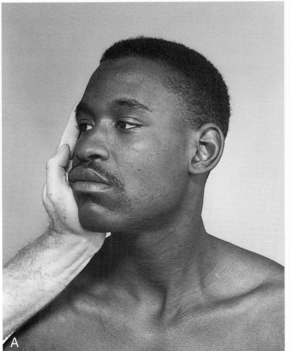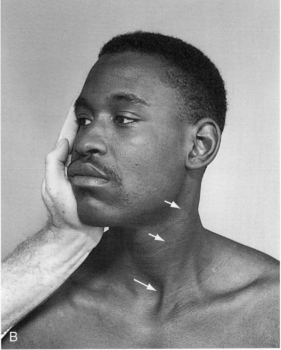

Figure 8–24. *A* and *B*, Assessing right lateral rotation strength. (*Arrows* in *B* indicate tensed left sternocleidomastoid muscle.)

Flexors

When fired together, the two **sternocleidomastoids** are the principal flexor muscles of the neck. To test **flexion** strength, the examiner places a resisting palm against the patient's forehead and stabilizes the thorax if necessary with the other hand. The patient is instructed to flex the neck against the examiner's resistance as forcefully as possible. Contraction of both sternocleidomastoid muscles should be quite visible, and the examiner should be unable to overcome the patient's inherent muscle strength (Fig. 8–25).

Extensors

Extension of the cervical spine is powered by the **posterior intrinsic neck muscles** and upper portion of the **trapezius**. Extension is tested in a manner analogous to the test of flexion strength. The examiner places the resisting hand on the patient's occiput and instructs the patient to extend the neck as forcefully as possible (Fig. 8–26). Again, the examiner should be unable to overcome the normal intrinsic muscle strength of the neck extensors.

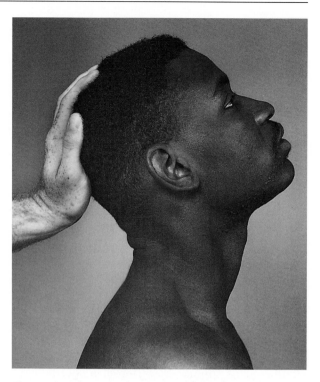

Figure 8–26. Assessing extension strength.

Lateral Benders

Lateral bending of the neck is powered primarily by the **scalene** muscles. To test the strength of these muscles, the examiner places the palm of one hand on the corresponding side of the patient's head and a stabilizing hand on the contralateral shoulder. The patient is then instructed to push against the examiner's palm as forcefully as possible (Fig. 8–27). In a normal case, the examiner is unable to overpower the patient's inherent lateral bending strength.

NEUROLOGIC EXAMINATION

A thorough neurologic examination is a basic part of cervical and thoracic spine evaluation. A neurologic examination should include a search for motor or sensory deficits, absent or abnormal reflexes, and root tension signs. Neurologic function is best evaluated in a systematic examination organized by dermatomes. The sensory, motor, and reflex tests for each dermatome are summarized in Table 8–1. Because the most common neurologic deficit associated with cervical spine disorders is a radiculopathy, such a systematic examination allows the clinician to identify the specific nerve root involved. In the case of

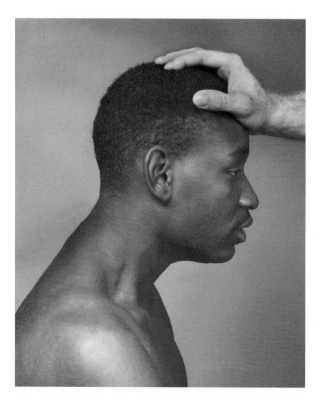

Figure 8–25. Assessing flexion strength.

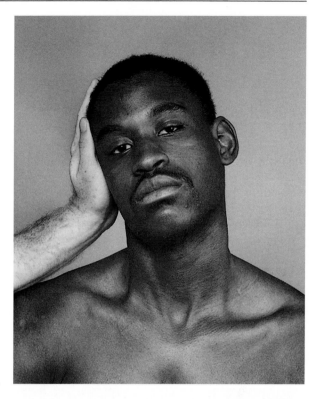

Figure 8–27. Assessing lateral bending strength.

more extensive deficits associated with spinal cord injuries, this same examination allows the clinician to determine the neurologic level of deficit.

Sensory Examination

PATTERNS OF SENSORY LOSS. Testing for light touch is a good screening tool for assessing the distribution of a sensory loss in order to characterize it as radicular, nonradicular, or global. **Radicular sensory loss** reflects the injury of a specific nerve root and should, therefore, correspond to the dermatome associated with that nerve root. A **nonradicular sensory loss** suggests a more peripheral nerve injury; the involved area is more diffuse and overlaps several dermatomes. A **glove** or **stocking distribution** of sensory dysfunction signifies a circumferential sensory deficit in the entire portion of the in-

TABLE 8–1.
PHYSICAL FINDINGS IN CERVICAL AND THORACIC RADICULOPATHIES

DERMATOME	SENSORY TESTING	MOTOR TESTING	REFLEX TESTING
C4	Lateral neck		
C5	Area over the middle deltoid	Deltoid Biceps brachii (secondary)	Biceps reflex
C6	Dorsum of the first web space and thumb	Biceps brachii Wrist extensors	Brachioradialis reflex Biceps reflex (secondary)
C7	Long finger	Wrist flexors Long finger extensors Triceps brachii	Triceps reflex
C8	Little finger and ulnar side of hand	Long digital flexors (grip)	
T1	Medial arm at the elbow	Finger abduction and adduction (interossei)	
T2	Medial upper arm and adjacent chest		
T4	Nipple line		
T10	Umbilicus	Trunk flexion (Beevor's sign)	Abdominal muscle reflex

volved limb distal to a certain point. Conditions that may be associated with a glove or stocking sensory deficit include diabetic peripheral neuropathy, reflex sympathetic dystrophy, and nonorganic disorders.

LIGHT TOUCH. All sensory testing is carried out with the patient's eyes closed. For screening purposes, **light touch** can be tested by lightly stroking the patient's skin with a soft object, such as a small paintbrush, a cotton wisp, or a tissue (Fig. 8–28*A*). The examiner strokes the area in question as well as adjacent areas and asks the patient to acknowledge each touch. In this manner, the examiner can gradually delineate an area that is anesthetic or hypoesthetic. The abnormal area can be marked on the patient and compared with diagrams of dermatomes and the sensory distribution of peripheral nerves. For more precise testing, special filaments made expressly for this purpose may be used.

SHARP-DULL DISCRIMINATION. Sharp-dull discrimination testing may be used to confirm the results of a light touch examination. In this case, the patient is asked to identify whether the area being examined is being touched with the sharp or dull end of a safety pin (Fig. 8–28*B* and *C*). This distinction should normally be an easy one for the patient to make; in an area of diminished sensation, the patient has difficulty distinguishing between sharp and dull.

VIBRATION SENSE. **Vibration sense** can be tested using a tuning fork of 256 Hz over bony prominences such as the humeral epicondyles or the radial styloid. The examiner rests the base of the vibrating fork on the bony prominence and

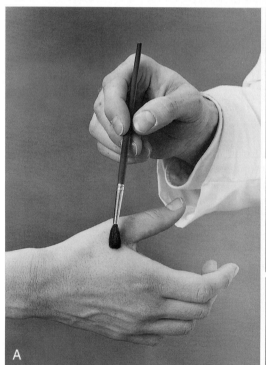
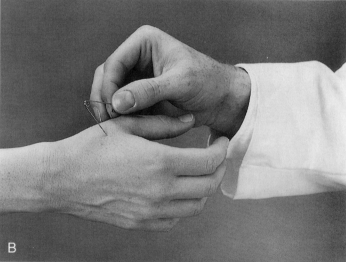
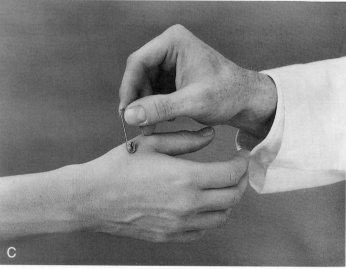

Figure 8–28. Sensory testing. *A*, Light touch. *B*, Sharp. *C*, Dull.

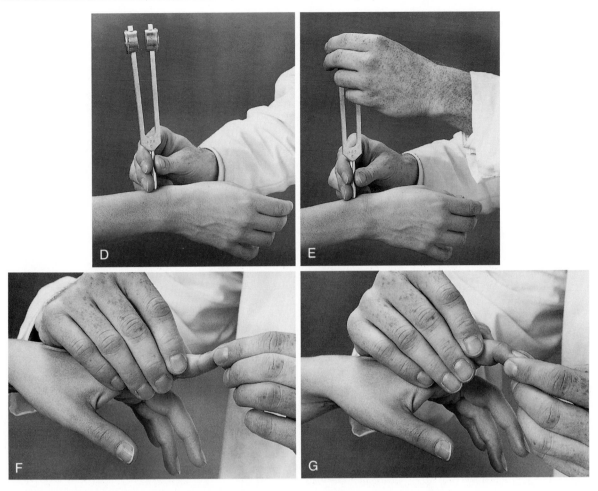

Figure 8–28 *Continued.* *D* and *E*, Vibration. *F* and *G*, Proprioception.

asks the patient to report when the vibration stops (see Fig. 8–28*D*). The examiner then stops the vibration suddenly with the free hand (see Fig. 8–28*E*). Normally, the patient identifies the cessation of vibration quite readily. Vibration sense should never be absent in the fingers or bony prominences. Some elderly individuals may, however, lose vibration sense distally. Otherwise, loss of vibration sense is associated with injury to the posterior columns of the spinal cord or peripheral nerves.

PROPRIOCEPTION. Loss of **proprioception**, also a sign of posterior column dysfunction, may be associated with aging, injury, or cerebellar dysfunction. To assess proprioception, the patient is instructed to close his or her eyes and the examiner grasps one of the patient's fingers or toes. The examiner then alternately flexes and extends the digit several times, randomly stopping in flexion or extension (see Fig. 8–28*F* and *G*). The patient should be able to identify whether the digit ends the maneuver in extension or flexion.

TWO-POINT DISCRIMINATION. The most sensitive means of assessing sensory loss in the upper extremities is two-point discrimination testing. This is most useful for deficits in the C6, the C7, or the C8 dermatomes. A subject with normal sensation should be able to distinguish points 5 mm apart on the fingertips. The technique for assessing two-point discrimination is described in Chapter 1, Terms and Techniques.

SENSORY DERMATOMES. The approximate areas of sensory innervation from the cervical and thoracic nerve roots are shown in Figure 8–29. There is considerable overlap in the sensory dermatomes, and the exact distribution of each dermatome varies somewhat from one individual to another. Sensory deficits are usually sought by evaluating sensation in relatively small areas that can reliably be expected to correspond to specific dermatomes in most individuals. The **C4** nerve root is most effectively assessed by testing the lateral neck (Fig. 8–30*A*). The **C5** nerve root can be evaluated by testing sensation

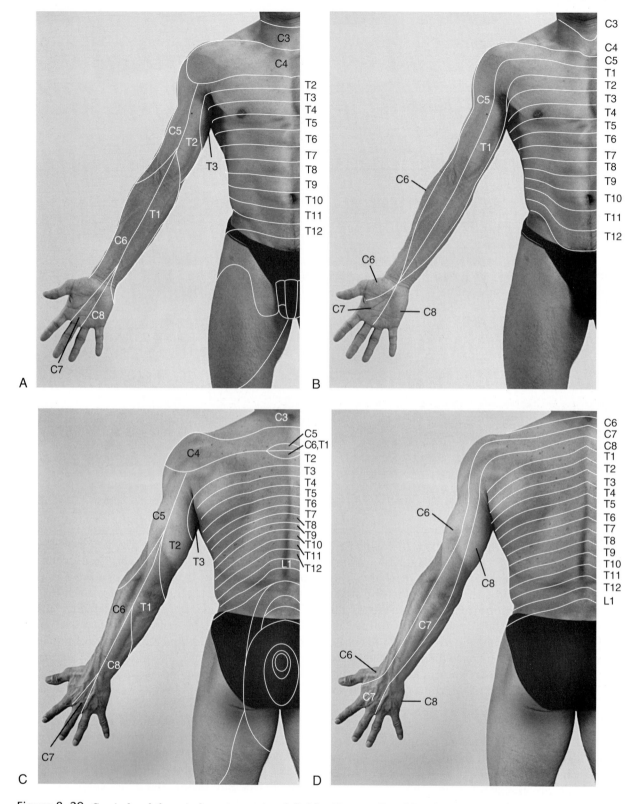

Figure 8–29. Cervical and thoracic dermatomes. *A* and *C*, After Foerster. *B* and *D*, After Reegan and Garrett.

over the middle deltoid (Fig. 8–30*B*). The **C6** nerve root supplies the dorsum of the first web space and the index finger (Fig. 8–30*C*), the **C7** nerve root supplies the long finger (Fig. 8–30*D*), and the **C8** nerve root supplies the little finger and the ulnar aspect of the hand (Fig. 8–30*E*). The **T1** nerve root can be evaluated by testing the medial arm about the elbow (Fig. 8–30*F*), and the **T2** nerve root supplies the upper medial arm adjacent to the axilla and a contiguous portion of

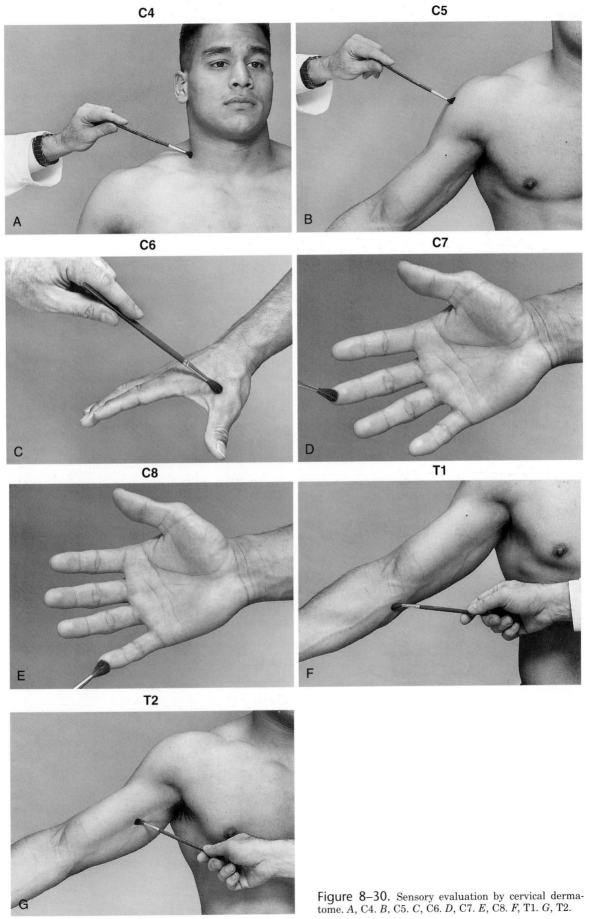

Figure 8–30. Sensory evaluation by cervical dermatome. *A*, C4. *B*, C5. *C*, C6. *D*, C7. *E*, C8. *F*, T1. *G*, T2.

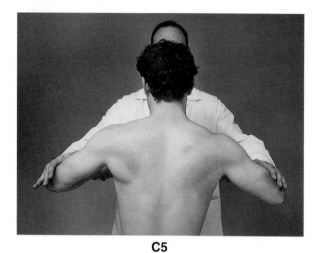

Figure 8–31. Assessing C5 motor function (deltoid strength).

C5 Nerve Root

The **C5 nerve root**, which exits the spine through the C4-C5 neuroforamen, is best assessed by testing **deltoid** strength. The patient is seated in a comfortable upright position and asked to abduct the arm with the elbow flexed. The examiner then exerts downward pressure on the elbow while the patient tries to resist with a pure abduction force (Fig. 8–31). In most normal patients, the examiner is not able to break the deltoid strength. The C5 nerve root also contributes to the **biceps brachii**. Because the innervation of the biceps is shared with C6, substantial neurologic dysfunction must be present before biceps weakness is perceived. Even in the face of a complete C5 motor deficit, moderate or normal biceps strength remains because of this dual innervation.

the chest (Fig. 8–30*G*). The other thoracic nerve roots supply sensation to successive strips of skin across the trunk. Remembering that the nipples identify the **T4** dermatome and the umbilicus, the **T10** dermatome helps the examiner identify the approximate level of sensory deficit in the distribution of the thoracic nerve roots.

Motor Examination

There is considerable overlap in the motor dermatomes of muscles supplied by the cervical nerve roots. In general, one or two muscles or muscle groups are selected to test each nerve root. These muscles or groups are usually chosen for their ease of examination or purity of innervation.

C6 Nerve Root

The **C6 nerve root**, which exits the spine through the C5-C6 neuroforamen, innervates the biceps brachii and the wrist extensors. To test the **biceps**, the examiner supports the patient's flexed elbow with one hand and grasps the patient's wrist with the other. The examiner then attempts to passively extend the elbow while the patient attempts to keep it flexed (Fig. 8–32*A*). In most normal patients, the examiner is unable to overcome the patient's biceps strength. Owing to the biradicular innervation of the biceps noted previously, even a complete C6 motor deficit may not lead to total biceps paralysis.

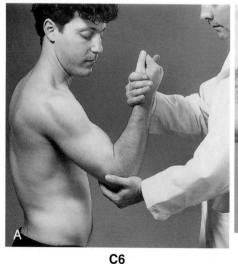

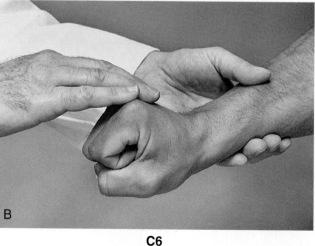

Figure 8–32. Assessing C6 motor function. *A*, Biceps. *B*, Wrist extensors.

To test the **wrist extensors**, the examiner asks the patient to flex the involved elbow and extend the wrist while the arm is held tightly at the side. The examiner stabilizes the patient's forearm with one hand while exerting downward pressure on the dorsiflexed wrist (see Fig. 8–32*B*). In most normal patients, the examiner is not able to overcome the patient's wrist extensor strength. Because the C5-C6 disk is the cervical disk most commonly involved in herniation or degeneration, a C6 radiculopathy is the most likely to be encountered.

C7 Nerve Root

The **C7 nerve root**, which exits the spine through the C6-C7 neuroforamen, is most easily assessed by testing the **wrist flexors**. The position is very close to that used for the assessment of wrist extensor strength. In this case, however, the patient is asked to make a fist and flex the wrist as strongly as possible while the examiner attempts to overcome the patient's strength and force the wrist into extension (Fig. 8–33*A*). Nor-

mally, the examiner can overcome the patient's flexion strength only with considerable difficulty.

The C7 nerve root may also be assessed by testing the strength of the **long finger extensors**. In this test, the examiner asks the patient to extend the fingers fully with the wrist in the neutral position. The examiner then stabilizes the patient's wrist with one hand and attempts to passively flex the patient's metacarpophalangeal joints while the patient resists maximally (see Fig. 8–33*B*). The examiner should be able to flex the fingers only with difficulty.

C7 also innervates the **triceps brachii**. To test triceps strength, the examiner grasps the patient's wrist and gently flexes the patient's elbow. The examiner's other hand stabilizes the patient's upper arm. The patient is then asked to extend the elbow as strongly as possible (see Fig. 8–33*C*). Normally, the examiner is unable to overcome the patient's triceps strength, and a strong patient may push the examiner away. Alternatively, the patient can be asked to hold the elbow in full extension while the examiner attempts to flex it. The examiner is not normally able to overcome the patient and flex the elbow.

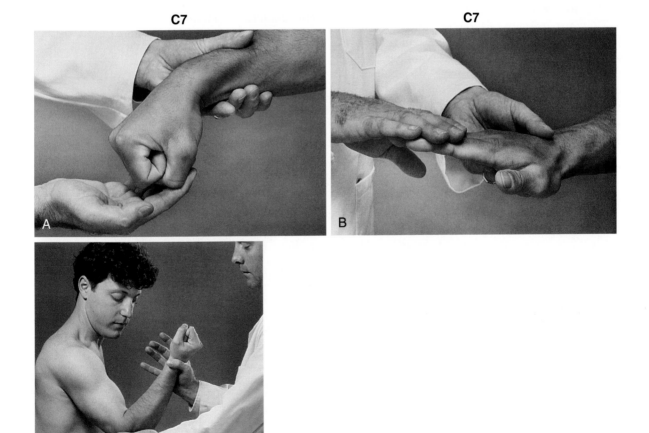

Figure 8–33. Assessing C7 motor function. *A*, Wrist flexors. *B*, Long finger extensors. *C*, Triceps brachii.

C8 Nerve Root

The **C8 nerve root**, which exits the spine through the C7-T1 neuroforamen, is best assessed by testing the **long digital flexors** and, thus, the patient's grip. One method of assessing the grip is to place the index and the long fingers in the patient's palm and ask him or her to squeeze these digits as tightly as possible (Fig. 8–34A). This method is sometimes difficult to quantitate and may be painful for the examiner if the patient is very strong.

An alternative method is for the examiner to place his or her flexed fingers against the patient's palm and ask the patient to make a tight fist. This causes the examiner's and the patient's fingers to be hooked together in a reciprocal manner. The examiner then instructs the patient not to allow the fist to be pulled open and then attempts to do so (see Fig. 8–34B). In most normal patients, the examiner is unable to overcome the patient's grip.

T1 Nerve Root

The **T1 nerve root** exits the spine through the T1-T2 neuroforamen. T1 motor function is usually assessed by testing the strength of the **interosseous** muscles, which govern abduction and adduction of the fingers. **Finger abduction** can be tested most easily by asking the patient to hold both hands out and spread the fingers as far apart as possible. The examiner then grasps the patient's spread fingers between the examiner's thumb and index finger and attempts to push them back together while the patient resists maximally (Fig. 8–35A). Normally, the examiner should be able to overcome the patient's efforts to maintain finger abduction with a moderate degree of difficulty. With this technique, both hands may be tested simultaneously and the strength of abduction compared.

An alternative technique is to test the **first dorsal interosseous** in isolation. To test the first dorsal interosseous, the examiner stabilizes the patient's hand with one of the examiner's own hands and places the index finger of the examiner's other hand against the radial aspect of the patient's index finger. The patient is then instructed to press the index finger being tested against the examiner's finger as hard as possible (see Fig. 8–35B). Not only can the strength be assessed by this method but also the contraction of the first dorsal interosseous can be confirmed visually or by palpation.

Finger adduction is also a motor function of the T1 nerve root. To test it, the examiner places an index card between the patient's extended long and index fingers and instructs the patient to squeeze the two fingers together as tightly as possible. The examiner then proceeds to withdraw the card from between the fingers, estimating the force required (see Fig. 8–35C). Normally, the examiner should be able to withdraw the card but with some difficulty.

Lower Thoracic Nerve Roots

Motor function of specific thoracic nerve roots is not normally assessed. **Beevor's sign**, however, may be used to screen for asymmetric loss of thoracic root motor function. Beevor's sign is a

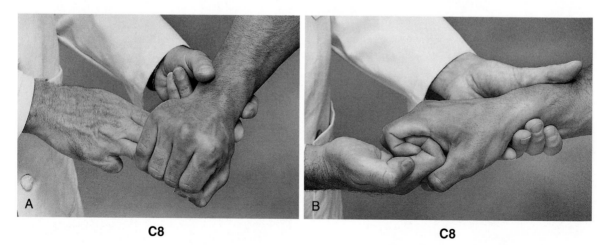

Figure 8–34. Assessing C8 motor function. *A,* Long finger flexors. *B,* Alternative technique.

T1

T1

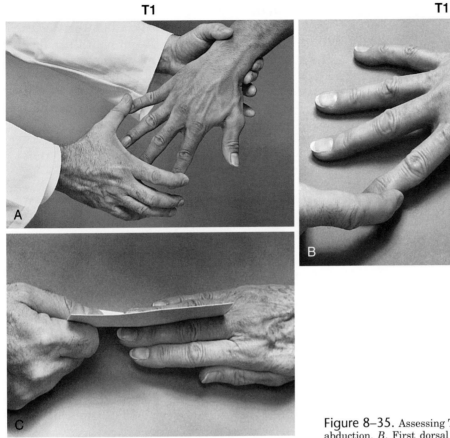

T1

Figure 8–35. Assessing T1 motor function. *A*, Finger abduction. *B*, First dorsal interosseous. *C*, Finger adduction.

gross test of muscular innervation from the thoracic spine. In this test, the patient is asked to do a half situp with the knees flexed and the arms behind the head (Fig. 8–36). In the normal patient, symmetric coordinated abdominal muscle contraction should keep the umbilicus in the midline during this maneuver. Compression or destruction of a thoracic nerve root, such as

might be caused by osteophyte or tumor, results in weakness of the musculature in the dermatome innervated by that root. This causes the umbilicus to deviate toward the stronger uninvolved side. This deviation is called Beevor's sign. Asymmetric weakness of the musculature innervated by the thoracic nerve roots may also be seen in cases of spinal dysraphism or poliomyelitis.

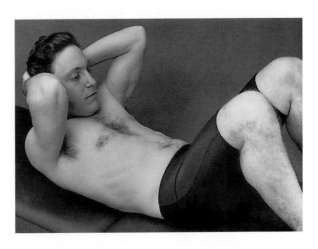

Figure 8–36. Test for Beevor's sign.

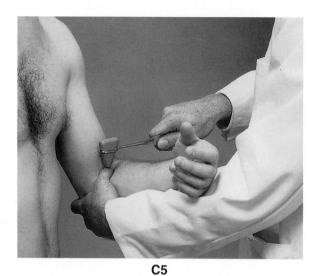

C5

Figure 8–37. Biceps reflex (C5).

Reflex Examination

Biceps Tendon Reflex (C5)

The biceps tendon reflex is usually used to assess the **C5 nerve root**. However, because the C6 nerve root also contributes to innervation of the biceps, the C5 radiculopathy may only result in diminution, not complete elimination, of the biceps reflex. To test the biceps reflex, the examiner grasps the patient's arm at the elbow, placing the examiner's own thumb on the patient's biceps tendon. The patient's forearm is allowed to rest on the examiner's forearm, in order to encourage complete relaxation. The examiner then lightly taps his or her own thumb with the reflex hammer (Fig. 8–37). In most normal patients, the examiner should feel a contraction of the biceps transmitted through the tendon in response to the tap. Usually, a contraction of the biceps is visible, as well.

Brachioradialis Reflex (C6)

The brachioradialis reflex is usually chosen to test the **C6 nerve root**. To test the brachioradialis reflex, the examiner supports the patient's forearm in a position of neutral rotation so that the radial aspect of the forearm is pointing upward. The wrist is allowed to fall into ulnar deviation. The examiner then taps the radial aspect of the forearm about 4 to 8 cm proximal to the radial styloid (Fig. 8–38). This should produce a visible contraction of the brachioradialis muscle and, in many cases, a quick upward motion of the forearm. Because the biceps brachii is innervated by C6 as well as C5, the biceps reflex can also be examined when a C6 radiculopathy is suspected.

Triceps Reflex (C7)

The triceps reflex is usually used to assess the **C7 nerve root**. The triceps reflex is best elicited with the patient in a position of 90° shoulder abduction and 90° elbow flexion. The examiner

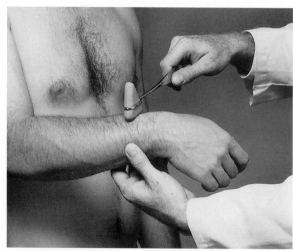

C6

Figure 8–38. Brachioradialis reflex (C6).

should support the arm completely, asking the patient to relax all musculature. The examiner should feel that the patient's limb would flop back to the side if the examiner released it. When adequate relaxation is sensed, the examiner strikes the triceps tendon just proximal to the olecranon (Fig. 8–39A). Normally, this should cause a visible contraction of the triceps and, sometimes, a slight extension of the elbow. The triceps reflex may also be elicited with the patient's arm at the side in a position similar to that used for the biceps reflex (Fig. 8–39B). This position is useful for patients who find the 90° of shoulder abduction uncomfortable.

Grading Reflexes

Because briskness of deep tendon reflexes varies considerably from one individual to another, the examiner should test several reflexes on both sides of the patient to verify that an apparently abnormal reflex is abnormal for that particular patient. Particularly significant is a reflex that is abnormal compared with the corresponding reflex on the opposite side of the body. Reflexes are typically graded as **hyporeactive, normal**, or **hyperreactive**. The examiner must make this subjective assessment through comparison with patients examined in the past. A normal reflex typically produces a palpable contraction, often associated with a slight movement of the limb. Strong or violent responses to reflex testing are suspicious for hyperreactivity. Hyporeactive reflexes are very difficult to elicit or are completely absent. Generalized areflexia may be present in metabolic states such as hypercalcemia. A *lower motor neuron lesion* is characterized by weakness and hyporeflexia, whereas an *upper motor neuron lesion* is typified by hyperreflexia and the presence of pathologic reflexes such as the Babinski reflex. A unilaterally diminished or absent reflex is the most common abnormal finding and suggests nerve injury at the root level or distal to it.

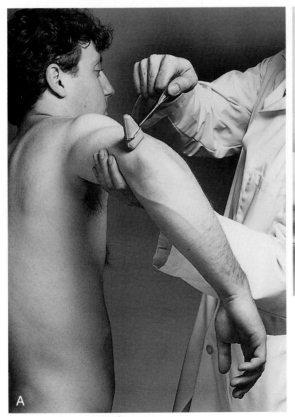

C7

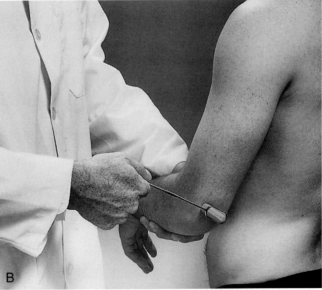

C7

Figure 8–39. *A*, Triceps reflex (C7). *B*, Alternative technique.

Plantar Reflex

The **Babinski sign** is a pathologic reflex that indicates upper motor neuron involvement. To test the **plantar reflex**, the examiner asks the patient to sit comfortably with the feet dangling from the examination table. The examiner grasps the patient's foot with one hand, then gently strokes the lateral border of the sole of the foot beginning about the level of the heel and moving distally (Fig. 8–40A). In a normal patient, the initial response is a downward reflection of the great toe (Fig. 8–40B), although the toes may subsequently dorsiflex. When the Babinski sign is present, the toes immediately dorsiflex when the plantar surface of the foot is stroked (Fig. 8–40C).

Clonus

Clonus is another sign of hyperreflexia that suggests an upper motor neuron lesion. It is usually assessed with the patient sitting on the examination table. While stabilizing the patient's leg with one hand, the examiner grasps the patient's forefoot with the other hand and quickly and forcefully pushes it into dorsiflexion (Fig. 8–41). When clonus is present, such a sudden dorsiflexion produces a rhythmic involuntary motion that alternates between plantar flexion and dorsiflexion. Each cycle of motion is called a *beat of clonus*. One or two beats of clonus may be present in otherwise normal individuals. When clonus is sustained beyond two beats, an upper motor neu-

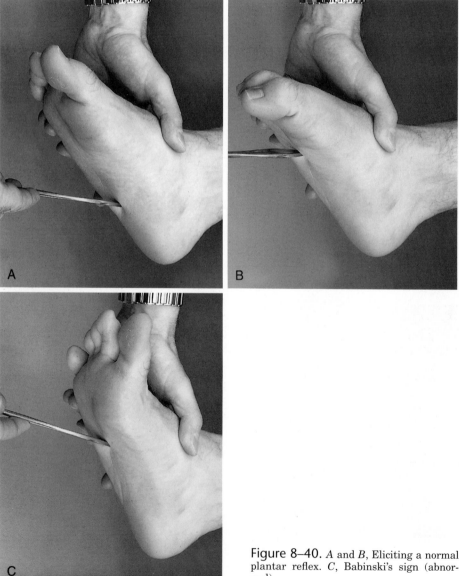

Figure 8–40. *A* and *B*, Eliciting a normal plantar reflex. *C*, Babinski's sign (abnormal).

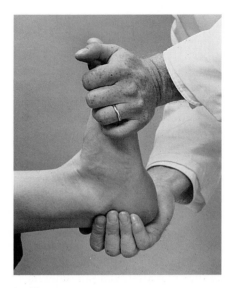

Figure 8–41. Eliciting ankle clonus.

ron lesion, such as proximal spinal cord compression, should be suspected.

Cervical Spinal Stenosis

Cervical spinal stenosis typically produces *lower motor neuron* findings at the level of the lesion and *upper motor neuron* deficits distal to the level of the lesion. For example, in the case of cervical stenosis at the C5-C6 level, one would normally find lower motor neuron signs of the C6 nerve root and upper motor neuron signs distal to that. Thus, in this particular example, the lower motor neuron deficit would be manifested by weakness in the biceps and the wrist extensors with diminution of the biceps and the brachioradialis reflexes. Upper motor neuron involvement distal to the level of the lesion would be reflected in hyperreflexia of the triceps, the quadriceps, and the gastrocnemius reflexes. Other upper motor neuron signs such as clonus and the Babinski reflexes might or might not be present.

Abdominal Muscle Reflexes

Abdominal muscle reflexes may be tested as a method of screening for thoracic spinal cord compression. To assess abdominal reflexes, the patient is positioned comfortably in a supine position with the abdomen exposed. The handle of the reflex hammer is then gently stroked across the abdomen in a radial manner beginning at the umbilicus and proceeding toward the 2-o'clock, the 4-o'clock, the 8-o'clock, and the 10-o'clock positions, in succession (Fig. 8–42). Normally, such stimulation should cause the abdominal musculature to involuntarily contract, resulting in movement of the umbilicus in the direction of the quadrant being stimulated. Absence of the normal response indicates thoracic spinal cord compression on the side of the diminished reflex. Remembering that the upper abdominal musculature is innervated by the T7 through T10 nerve roots and the lower abdominal musculature is innervated by the T10 through L1 nerve roots helps the examiner identify the approximate level of involvement.

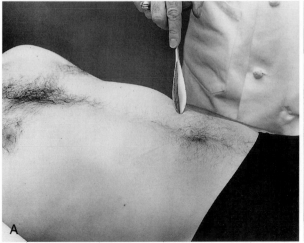
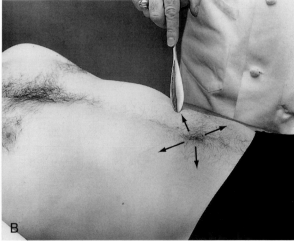

Figure 8–42. *A* and *B*, Eliciting abdominal reflexes. (*Arrows* in *B* indicate the direction of stroking.)

UPPER LIMB TENSION TESTS

A number of upper limb nerve tension tests have been described by authors including Elvey, Kennealy, and Butler. These are sometimes known as the straight-leg raising tests of the arm because they are analogous to the nerve root tension signs of the lower extremity, such as the Lasegue test, the slump test, and the femoral nerve stretch test. Like their lower extremity counterparts, these maneuvers aim to reproduce or exacerbate neurologically based symptoms by placing tension on the cervical nerve roots and the associated peripheral nerves. As in the lower extremity tension tests, these maneuvers often produce some degree of symptoms in normal individuals, such as aching or stretching sensations. The patient's response to the test is considered abnormal if the maneuver reproduces the patient's familiar pain, which usually radiates distal to the elbow.

Upper Limb Tension Test 1

The **upper limb tension test 1 (ULTT1)** is a series of maneuvers applied to the upper extremity to place tension on the **C5**, the **C6**, and the **C7 nerve roots**, and it is described as **median nerve dominant** because the median nerve is the peripheral nerve most stressed by these maneuvers. Thus, the test is not specific with regard to a given level, but indicates irritation or compression of any one, two, or three of the involved roots, all of which contribute to the median nerve. However, each portion of the maneuver should be done carefully and gently because considerable tension may be placed on sensitive nerve roots. Throughout the procedure, the examiner maintains communication with the patient to determine whether radicular symptoms are reproduced and, if so, at what point in the test.

To perform this test on the patient's right side, the patient is positioned in a relaxed supine position along the right edge of the examination table. The examiner stands next to the table at the patient's right side. The examiner's left hand then grasps the patient's right hand securely and gently abducts the patient's shoulder, allowing the patient's arm to rest along the examiner's right thigh. The examiner's right hand is placed in contact with the superior aspect of the patient's right shoulder and driven firmly against the examination table. This allows the examiner's right hand to serve as a post that prevents further elevation of the patient's shoulder girdle (Fig. 8–43A). The patient's shoulder is then abducted to about 110° (Fig. 8–43B). While maintaining this position, the examiner supinates the patient's forearm and extends the patient's wrist and fingers (Fig. 8–43C). The next step is to externally rotate the patient's shoulder to 90° (Fig. 8–43D). Next, the patient's elbow is slowly extended (Fig. 8–43E). Finally, the patient is asked to laterally bend the neck, first toward the shoulder being examined (Fig. 8–43F) and then away from it (Fig. 8–43G). If nerve root tension is present, laterally bending the neck toward the side being tested should relieve the symptoms, whereas bending it away from the side being tested should exacerbate them. Optionally, an assistant may perform a straight-leg raise to further increase nerve root tension (Fig. 8–43H).

The ULTT1 maneuver produces a sensation of stretching or aching in the antecubital fossa in almost all subjects. This is not considered an abnormal response. Pain suggestive of true radicular involvement would radiate to the lateral deltoid and the midarm (C5), down the dorsal radial aspect of the forearm to involve the index finger and the thumb (C6), or centrally down the forearm to involve the dorsum of the hand and the long finger (C7).

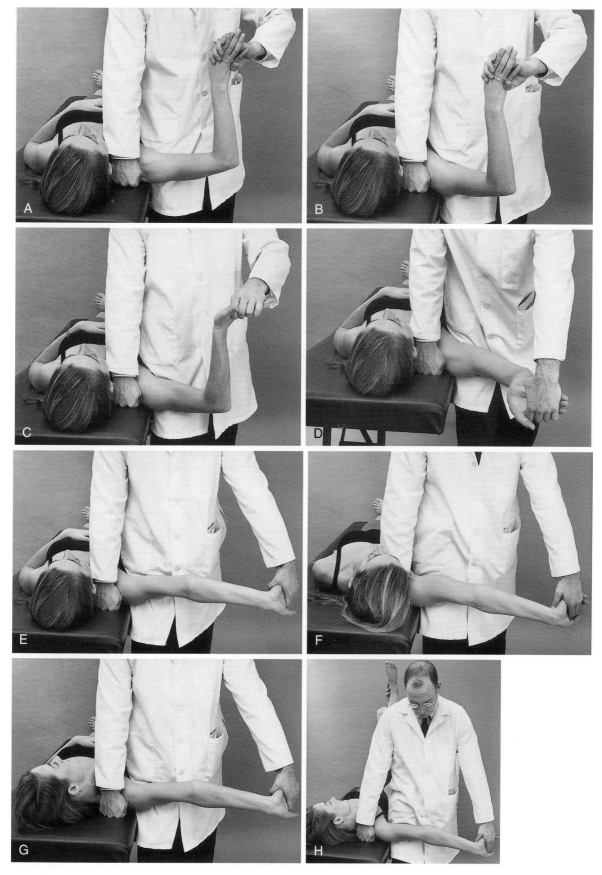

Figure 8–43. *A–H*, Upper limb tension test 1 (ULTT1).

Upper Limb Tension Test 2

The **upper limb tension test 2 (ULTT2)** also tests for irritation of the **C6** or **C7 nerve roots**. There are two variants of this test, one that is median nerve dominant and one that is radial nerve dominant. They are both performed with the patient lying supine on the examination table.

MEDIAN NERVE DOMINANT. To perform the median nerve dominant variation, the patient is positioned at an angle so that the scapula of the side being tested projects past the edge of the table. When the right side is being tested, the examiner stands at the head of the table with the examiner's left thigh resting against the superior aspect of the patient's right shoulder. The examiner's left hand holds the patient's right elbow

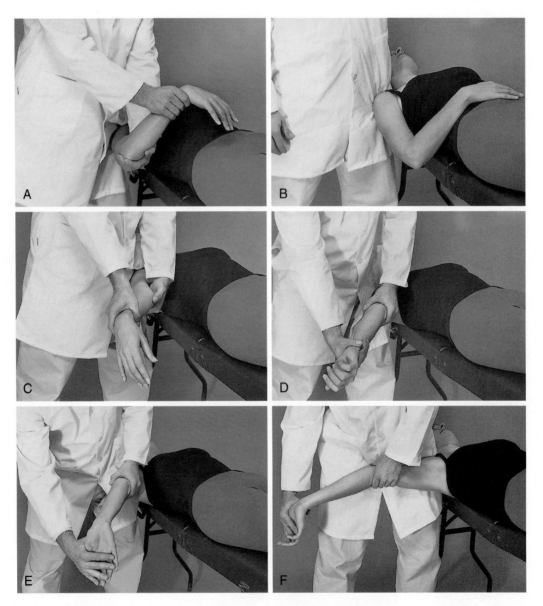

Figure 8–44. *A–F*, Upper limb tension test 2 (ULTT2), median nerve dominant variation. (In *B*, the examiner has temporarily released the patient's arm so that the shoulder depression can be seen by the reader.)

and the examiner's right hand holds the patient's right wrist (Fig. 8–44*A*). In a controlled manner, the examiner carefully depresses the patient's shoulder girdle with pressure from the examiner's thigh (Fig. 8–44*B*). The patient's shoulder is abducted about 10° so that the arm is clear of the table. While maintaining the shoulder depression, the examiner next extends the patient's elbow (Fig. 8–44*C*). Then, the examiner uses both hands to externally rotate the patient's upper limb at the shoulder (Fig. 8–44*D*). The examiner's right hand then grasps the patient's fingers securely and uses them to extend the metacarpophalangeal joints and dorsiflex the wrist (Fig. 8–44*E*). Abducting the patient's shoulder to 90° while maintaining the shoulder depression further increases nerve root tension (Fig. 8–44*F*). As in the ULTT1, the patient's response is considered abnormal only if radicular pain is elicited.

RADIAL NERVE DOMINANT. The radial nerve dominant variant of the ULTT2 begins in the same position. Again, the patient is positioned obliquely on the table so that the shoulder to be examined extends past the edge of the table. The examiner's left thigh is again used to depress the patient's right shoulder, and the patient's elbow is extended as it was for the ULTT1 (Fig. 8–45*A*). This time, the examiner's hands are used to internally rotate the entire upper extremity at the shoulder (Fig. 8–45*B*). While maintaining the shoulder depression, the elbow extension, and the internal rotation of the limb, the examiner's right hand is used to grasp the patient's right hand and flex the patient's wrist, thumb, and fingers (Fig. 8–45*C*). As with the previous test, the response is considered abnormal if this maneuver elicits radicular pain, particularly in the radial nerve distribution.

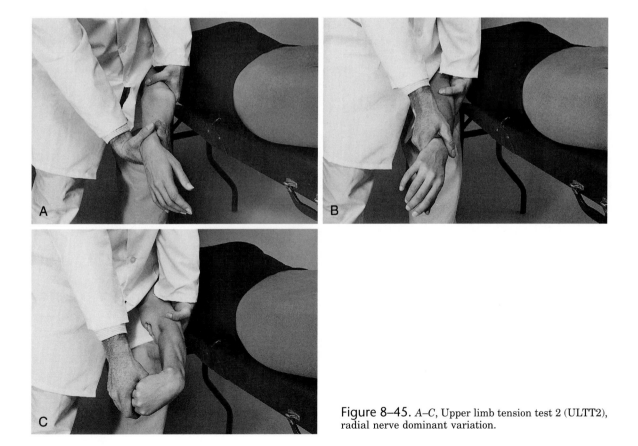

Figure 8–45. *A–C*, Upper limb tension test 2 (ULTT2), radial nerve dominant variation.

Upper Limb Tension Test 3

The **upper limb tension test 3 (ULTT3)** is performed to assess possible irritation of the **C8** and **T1 nerve roots**. It is designed to be **ulnar nerve dominant**. Owing to the relative hypomobility of the cervicothoracic junction, lesions of these lower nerve roots are more difficult to assess. For this test, the patient and the examiner are positioned as for the ULTT1. The examiner should assume a wide-based stance so that his or her weight can be shifted forward when required. To examine the right side, the patient's flexed right elbow is rested against the examiner's pelvis, just below the anterior superior iliac spine. The examiner's left hand grasps the patient's right hand by the fingers and the examiner's right hand is again pressed into the examination table against the superior aspect of the shoulder to prevent elevation (Fig. 8–46A). The patient's wrist is then dorsiflexed and the forearm supinated (Fig. 8–46B). While maintaining this position, the patient's elbow is maximally flexed (Fig. 8–46C). The examiner's right hand is then used to depress the patient's shoulder (Fig. 8–46D). The patient's shoulder is externally rotated and then abducted, approximating the patient's hand to his or her own ear (Fig. 8–46E). Asking the patient to laterally bend the neck away from the side being tested places additional tension on the nerve roots (Fig. 8–46F), whereas bending toward the side being tested relaxes the tension somewhat. In response to the ULTT3 maneuver, normal subjects feel a tugging sensation in the axilla. The response is considered abnormal if the patient feels pain radiating down the arm past the elbow to the ring and little fingers (C8) or into the axilla (T1).

Additional nerve root tension can be added by having an assistant perform a simultaneous straight-leg raise on the ipsilateral side or by performing the test in the slump position. If the slump variant is selected, the ULTTs are performed as described but with the patient seated. The patient is asked to maximally flex the trunk and hips while keeping the knees extended. This places the cauda equina under stretch and provides additional tension.

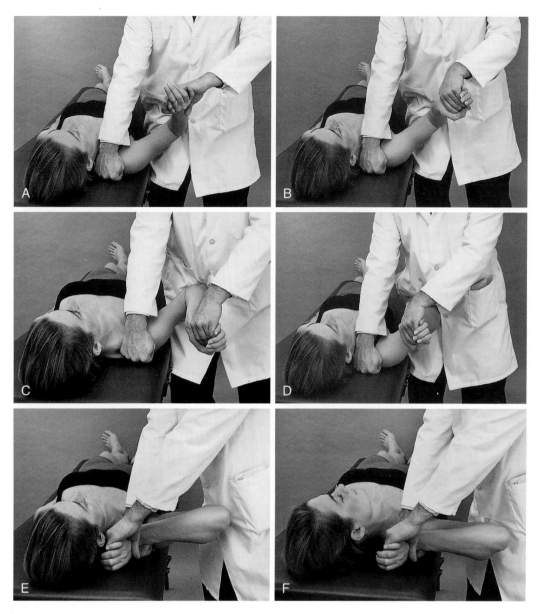

Figure 8–46. *A–F*, Upper limb tension test 3 (ULTT3).

MISCELLANEOUS SPECIAL TESTS

Axial Compression Test

The axial compression test and Spurling's test are designed to determine whether axial compression elicits or aggravates the patient's painful symptoms. They should not be performed when nerve root compression with a motor deficit is suspected or detected. To perform the **axial compression test**, the examiner stands behind the patient who is seated with the cervical spine in a neutral position. The examiner then places both hands at the crown of the patient's head and compresses, thus supplying an axial load (Fig. 8–47A). The application of the force should be gentle and gradual because it may elicit a very painful response. The patient is asked to report whether the maneuver produces pain or other unpleasant sensations, as well as the quality and distribution of the symptoms created. A **distraction test** of the neck may relieve the symptoms (Fig. 8–47B).

Spurling's Test

If the examiner is suspicious of lateralizing pathology, such as a disk prolapse, the compression maneuver may be repeated with various amounts of cervical flexion, extension, lateral bending, or rotation in an attempt to find the position that elicits the maximal response (Fig. 8–48). In

Spurling's test, the neck is extended and rotated toward the involved side prior to axial compression. This maneuver is designed to exacerbate encroachment on a cervical nerve root by decreasing the dimensions of the foramen through which the nerve root exits the spine. In response to the axial compression test or Spurling's test, a patient may feel no discomfort, a sensation of heaviness, nonradicular or pseudoradicular pain, or radicular pain. Pain related to muscular strains or mild ligamentous sprains is not normally aggravated by these tests. *Nonradicular* or *pseudoradicular* pain includes pain that radiates to the occiput, the scapula, or the shoulders, or occasionally down the arm but not distal to the elbow. Such pseudoradicular pain may be the result of a mechanical or degenerative process in the cervical spine such as spondylolisthesis or degenerative disk disease without nerve root compression. *Radicular* pain radiates into the upper extremity, usually below the elbow, along the distribution of a specific dermatome. In the younger individual, this is most commonly the result of nerve root compression owing to intervertebral disk prolapse. In the older patient, radicular pain is usually produced by foraminal stenosis owing to the combination of disk degeneration and secondary facet hypertrophy.

Lhermitte's Maneuver

Lhermitte's maneuver is performed by asking the seated patient to maximally flex the cervical

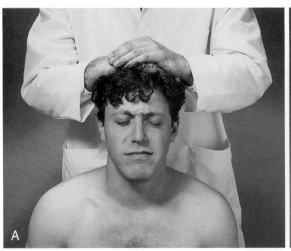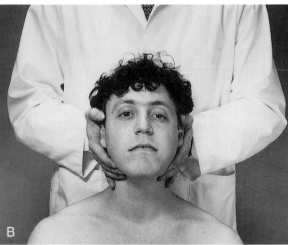

Figure 8–47. *A*, Axial compression test. *B*, Distraction test.

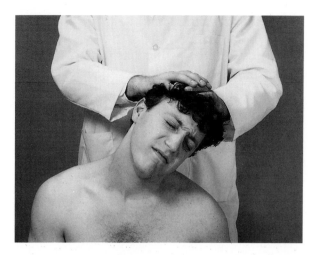

Figure 8–48. Spurling's test.

and the thoracic spine (Fig. 8–49). **Lhermitte's sign** is considered present when this maneuver produces distal paresthesias in multiple extremities or the trunk. Lhermitte's sign is thought to be indicative of spinal stenosis and resulting spinal cord compression. In the patient with a narrowed cervical spinal canal, flexion can further reduce the dimensions of the canal, causing cord compression and the paresthesias described. In the patient without cervical spinal stenosis, maximal flexion simply results in a pulling sensation at the cervicothoracic junction without any radiating symptoms at all.

NONORGANIC SIGNS OF WADDELL

Waddell described five signs that the examiner may note during the initial evaluation that suggest the possibility of nonorganic pathology. These are physical findings that cannot be explained by current knowledge of anatomy and physiology. They are thought to represent functional or behavioral maladaptations to the disease process or reaction to real or perceived pain. It should be borne firmly in mind that they are not pathognomonic of functional or nonorganic pathology, but rather they are just a component of the overall assessment. These signs were originally described in conjunction with the lumbar spine.

Nonanatomic Tenderness

The first of Waddell's signs is superficial **nonanatomic tenderness**. This sign is considered present when the patient reports disproportionate pain in response to extremely light touch or tenderness whose distribution does not correspond to the configuration of known anatomic structures (Fig. 8–50). The examiner must make this somewhat subjective judgment based on previous experience with the response of other patients to similar levels of pressure. If the examiner senses that the patient's pain response is out of proportion to the pressure applied during a normal examination, the examiner may wish to further test by palpating the involved area with extremely light pressure or by palpating structures that are seldom tender. It should be kept in mind that reflex sympathetic dystrophy and its variants may cause hypersensitivity in an extremity.

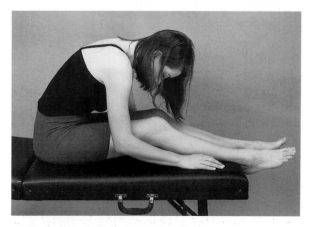

Figure 8–49. Lhermitte's maneuver.

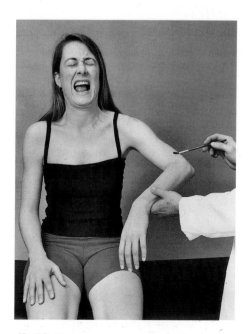

Figure 8–50. Nonanatomic tenderness.

Simulation Sign

Waddell's second sign is called the **simulation sign**. It is considered present if there is an exaggerated response to the axial compression test or a painful response to the rotation simulation maneuver. In the case of the **axial compression test,** organic pain should be experienced only in the neck, the shoulders, or the upper extremities. Patients who report pain in the low back or radiating down the entire spine in response to the axial compression test are judged as having a positive simulation sign.

The alternative way to test for simulation is by the **rotation simulation maneuver.** In this maneuver, the shoulders are rotated in a manner coplanar with the pelvis while the patient is standing (Fig. 8–51). This is essentially a logroll and puts no torsional force on the thoracic or lumbar spines. It should, therefore, not provoke pain from those regions. A report of pain in response to the rotation simulation maneuver is, therefore, considered a positive simulation sign and suggests nonorganic pathology.

Distraction Sign

The third sign of Waddell is called the **distraction sign**. When a positive distraction sign is

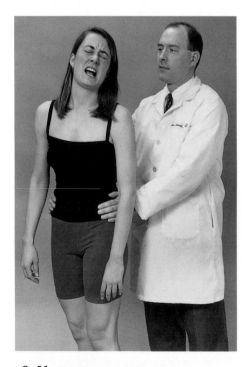

Figure 8–51. Rotation simulation maneuver.

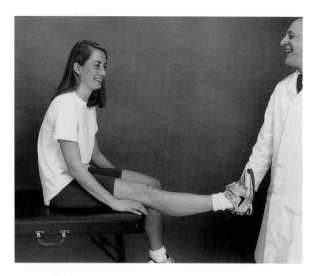

Figure 8–52. Distraction sign. Supine straight-leg raising reproduces symptoms, but seated-leg raising does not.

present, the response of the patient to the straight-leg raising test varies depending on whether it is performed with the patient in the supine or the seated position. In the presence of true nerve root tension, the patient should experience radiating pain in whichever position the straight-leg raising test is performed. Patients with nonorganic pain often know by experience that straight-leg raising in the supine position should be painful but may not realize that passive extension of their knee while seated produces the same position of tension on the sciatic nerve roots (Fig. 8–52). They may, thus, inconsistently fail to report pain in response to the seated-leg raising maneuver. Such an inconsistent response is said to represent a positive distraction sign because the patient is distracted from the nature of the test by the unfamiliar position.

Regional Sensory or Motor Disturbance

The fourth nonorganic sign of Waddell is called regional sensory or motor disturbance. A **regional sensory disturbance** is considered present when abnormal sensation is noted in a nonanatomic distribution such as a stocking or glove distribution in the leg or the arm, respectively. A **regional motor disturbance** is suspected if the examiner discovers diffuse motor weakness of multiple muscle groups, such as weakness of every muscle group tested in the upper extremity, or if the examiner senses, during strength testing, that the patient's muscles suddenly give way in a nonphysiologic manner.

Overreaction

The fifth nonorganic sign of Waddell is called **overreaction**. This sign is considered present when the patient reacts physically or verbally in an inappropriately theatrical manner to light forms of palpation or gentle examination techniques. Again, the evaluation of this sign depends on the examiner's previous experience with a broad range of normal patient behavior.

Waddell's original description of the five signs was in connection with a study of patients' responses to spine surgery. Waddell noted that three or more signs were present in patients who had had unsuccessful back surgery. Waddell also found that the most sensitive sign was overreaction. Because the assessment of these signs is subjective, their significance increases when several are present. It should be remembered that in certain organic disease states, individual Waddell signs may be present. This is clearly the case in the stocking distribution of numbness that can occur in the presence of diabetic neuropathy.

The physical findings in common conditions of the cervical and the thoracic spine are summarized in Table 8–2.

TABLE 8–2.
PHYSICAL FINDINGS IN COMMON CONDITIONS OF THE CERVICAL AND THE THORACIC SPINE

Cervical Radiculopathy

Restricted range of motion
Radiating pain exacerbated by the axial compression test and/or the Spurling test (frequent)
Upper limb tension test reproduces or exacerbates the patient's familiar radicular pain
Motor, sensory, and/or reflex deficit in the distribution of the involved nerve root (variable)

**Cervical Spondylitic Myelopathy
(Cervical Spinal Stenosis)**

Restricted range of motion
Lhermitte's maneuver produces distal paresthesias
Broad-based gait (variable)
Lower motor neuron findings of the nerve roots at the level of the lesion (motor, sensory, and/or reflex deficit in distribution of the involved nerve root) (variable)
Upper motor neuron deficit below the level of the lesion (hyperreflexia, ankle clonus, Babinski's sign)

Cervical Fracture

Point tenderness at the level of the injury
Palpable deformity, such as step-off or break in the normal alignment or spacing of the spinous processes
Neurologic deficit (may vary from none or partial spinal cord injury syndrome to complete spinal cord injury)
Partial spinal cord injury syndromes include anterior cord syndrome, central cord syndrome, Brown-Sequard syndrome, and posterior cord syndrome

**Cervical Strain
(Whiplash Injury, Mechanical Cervical Pain)**

Diffuse tenderness of the posterior neck muscles
Reduced range of motion
Normal neurologic examination

Bibliography

Apley AG: A System of Orthopaedics and Fractures, 4th ed. London, Butterworths, 1973.

Appleton AB, Hamilton WJ, Simon J: Surface and Radiological Anatomy, 2nd ed. London, Heffer and Sons, 1938.

Bickerstaff EF, Spillane JA: Neurological Examination in Clinical Practice, 5th ed. Oxford, Blackwell, 1989.

Bohannon RW, Gajodsik RL: Spinal nerve root compression: some clinical implications. Phys Ther. 1987;67:376–382.

Bradish CF, Lloyd GJ, Aldam CH, et al: Do nonorganic signs help to predict the return to activity of patients with low-back pain? Spine. 1988;13:557–560.

Breig A: Adverse Mechanical Tension in the Central Nervous System: An Analysis of Cause and Effect: Relief by Functional Neurosurgery. New York, Almqvist & Wiksell, 1978.

Butler DS: Mobilization of the Nervous System. Melbourne, Churchill Livingstone, 1991, pp 107–123, 127–139, 147–160.

Daniels L, Williams M, Worthingham C: Muscle Testing: Techniques of Manual Examination, 2nd ed. Philadelphia, WB Saunders, 1956.

Daniels L, Worthingham C: Muscle Testing: Techniques of Manual Examination, 3rd ed. Philadelphia, WB Saunders, 1972.

Elvey RL: Treatment of arm pain associated with abnormal brachial plexus tension. Aust J Physiother. 1986;32:224–229.

Fields H: Pain. New York, McGraw-Hill, 1987.

Foerster O: The dermatomes in man. Brain. 1933;56:1–39.

Grieve GP: Common Vertebral Joint Problems. Edinburgh, Churchill Livingstone, 1981.

Hadler NM: Regional back pain. N Engl J Med. 1986;315:1090–1092.

Haldeman S: The electrodiagnostic evaluation of nerve root function. Spine. 1983;9:42–48.

Hoppenfeld S: Scoliosis. Philadelphia, JB Lippincott, 1967.

Keegan JJ, Garrett FD: The segmental distribution of the cutaneous nerves of the limbs of man. Anat Record. 1948;102:409–437.

Khuffash B, Porter RW: Cross leg pain and trunk list. Spine. 1989;602–603.

MacNab I: Backache. Baltimore, Williams & Wilkins, 1977.

Macrae IF, Wright V: Measurement of back movement. Ann Rheum Dis. 1967;28:584–589.

Mathers LH: The peripheral nerve system. In Mayo Clinic: Clinical Examinations in Neurology, 5th ed. Philadelphia, WB Saunders, 1985.

McLeod JC, Lance JW: Introductory Neurology, 2nd ed. Melbourne, Blackwell, 1989.

O'Connell JEA: The clinical signs of meningeal irritation. Brain. 1946;69:9–21.

Peterson GW, Will AD: Newer electrodiagnostic techniques in peripheral nerve injuries. Orthop Clin North Am. 1988;19:13–25.

Propst-Proctor SL, Bleck EE: Radiographic determination of lordosis and kyphosis in normal and scoliotic children. J Pediatr Orthop. 1983;3:344–346.

Pullos J: The upper limb tension test. Aust J Physiother. 1986;32:258–259.

Richards JS, Nepomuceno C, Riles M, Suer Z: Assessing pain behavior: the UAB Pain Behavior Scale. Pain. 1982;14:393–398.

Schofferman JA: Physical examination. In White AH, Schofferman JA, eds. Spine Care. St. Louis, CV Mosby, 1995, pp 71–83.

Schofferman J, Zucherman J: History and physical examination. Spine State Art Rev. 1986;1:13–20.

Steindler A: Kinesiology of the Human Body. Springfield, Ill, Charles C Thomas, 1955.

Sunderland S: Nerves and Nerve Injuries, 2nd ed. Edinburgh, Churchill Livingstone, 1978.

Van Allen MW, Rodnitzky RL: Pictorial Manual of Neurologic Tests: A Guide to the Performance and Interpretation of the Neurologic Examination, 2nd ed. Chicago, Year Book Medical, 1981.

Waddell G, McCulloch JA, Kummel E, Venner RM: Nonorganic physical signs in low-back pain. Spine. 1980;5:117–125.

Waddell G, Somerville D, Henderson I, Newton M: Objective clinical evaluation of physical impairment in chronic low back pain. Spine. 1992;17:617–628.

Wohlfart G: Clinical considerations on innervation of skeletal muscle. Am J Phys Med Rehabil. 1959;38:223–230.

Frank M. Phillips
Bruce Reider

9

Lumbar Spine

*T*he examination of the lumbar spine may be seen as a continuation of the procedure already described for the cervical and the thoracic spine; the lumbar spine cannot be evaluated in isolation. Abnormalities of the lumbar spine may lead to compensatory or secondary abnormalities in other portions of the spine or pelvis. Symptoms that appear to emanate from the lumbar region may actually be due to abnormalities of adjacent structures. The principles already enumerated for evaluation of the cervical and thoracic spine continue to be of value in the assessment of lumbar disorders.

Because disorders of the lumbar spine often produce pain in the pelvis, the hip, or the thigh, a thorough evaluation of the lumbar spine usually includes examination of these regions. The details of this portion of the examination are outlined in Chapter 5, Pelvis, Hip, and Thigh, and are only alluded to here.

Inspection

SURFACE ANATOMY AND ALIGNMENT

Posterior Aspect

As with the rest of the spine, the dorsal location of the lumbar spine within the body makes the posterior viewpoint the most fruitful one for inspection (Fig. 9–1). When viewed from the posterior aspect, a longitudinal furrow is seen in most patients running down the midline from the thoracic spine to the sacrum. The **spinous processes** of the lumbar vertebrae run down the center of this furrow, and they are visible as a series of evenly placed bumps in thin individuals. Forward flexion at the waist usually makes the tips of the spinous processes more distinct and visible (Fig. 9–1C).

PARASPINOUS MUSCLES. On each side of the spinous processes runs a convex column of muscle. This contour is formed by the bulk of the paraspinous muscle mass. The more superficial column of paraspinous muscles is collectively known as the **erector spinae**, or **sacrospinalis**. The erector spinae is split longitudinally into three components. From medial to lateral on each side, they are the *multifidus*, the *longissimus*, and the *iliocostalis muscles*. The individual contours of these muscles cannot be discerned because they lie deep to the lumbodorsal fascia, and they are visualized as a group. The prominence due to the paraspinous muscles should be equal on both sides of the spine. In the presence of *paraspinous muscle spasm*, the contour of the muscles on one side of the spine may stand out in visibly greater prominence than those on the opposite side. Although almost any painful lesion of the lumbar spine may cause paraspinous spasm, the most common cause of asymmetric spasm is paraspinous muscle strain.

SYMMETRY. As in the rest of the spine, the verification of symmetry is an important part of inspection of the lumbar spine. It should appear that a plumb line suspended from the vertebra prominens at the base of the neck would bisect the lumbar spine and continue on through the center of the natal cleft between the buttocks. In addition to looking for straightness of the lumbar spine itself, the examiner should carefully inspect and compare the space created between the upper limbs and the trunk as the hands hang loosely at the patient's sides. Noting asymmetry of these spaces may allow the examiner to detect a subtle coronal deformity of the spine that would otherwise go undetected.

PELVIC OBLIQUITY. The examiner should also verify that the patient's pelvis is level. An imaginary line drawn between the posterior superior iliac spines or the iliac crests should be parallel to the floor. If these landmarks are not clearly visible, the examiner may have to palpate the

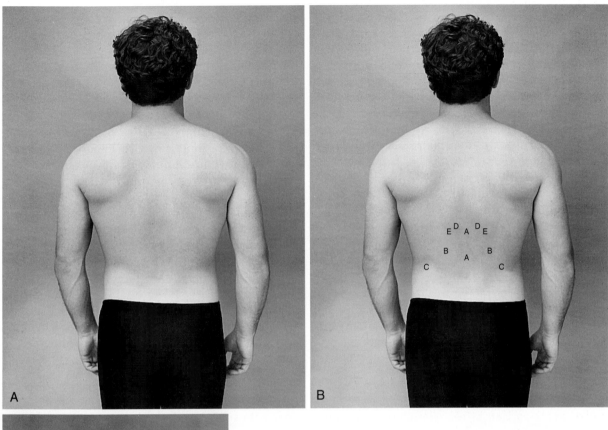

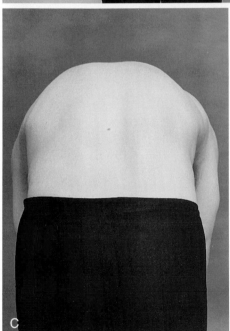

Figure 9–1. *A* and *B*, Posterior aspect of the lumbar spine. A, spinous processes; B, erector spinae; C, iliac crests; D, posterior facet joints; E, transverse processes. *C*, Posterior aspect of the lumbar spine in flexion.

iliac crests to verify that they are equidistant from the floor. If a **pelvic obliquity** is found, it may be the result of a deformity within the spine, such as scoliosis or an anomalous vertebra, or it may be secondary to a leg length discrepancy.

The possible causes of a leg length discrepancy are discussed in Chapter 5, Pelvis, Hip, and Thigh. In the case of a leg length discrepancy, a secondary compensatory deformity of the spine is usually present.

LIST. Any departure from symmetry in the lumbar spine is usually caused by a coronal plane deformity. A **list** is an abrupt planar shift of the spine, above a certain point, to one side (Fig. 9–2). This phenomenon typically occurs primarily in the lumbar spine. It is usually a reversible deformity related to pain and associated muscle spasm. A list may be caused by a herniated lumbar disk. In this case, the spine shifts away from the side of the nerve root that is being pinched by the herniated lumbar disk in an attempt to relieve pressure from the affected nerve root. Sometimes, local muscle strain can also result in a list.

SCOLIOSIS. Scoliosis is another major cause of coronal asymmetry (Fig. 9–3A). Although scoliosis is usually considered a coronal deformity of the spine, it is really a helical abnormality involving abnormal vertebral rotation along the axis of the spine. Lumbar scoliosis may be primary or secondary. In **primary scoliosis**, an actual structural abnormality of the spine is present. In **secondary scoliosis**, the curvature represents a compensatory adaptation of an otherwise normal spine to an extrinsic factor, such as muscle spasm or pelvic obliquity related to a leg length discrepancy. If the condition is secondary to a pelvic obliquity, leveling the patient's pelvis by placing blocks or books beneath the shorter limb should cause the deformity to disappear. If a pelvic obliquity has been present for a long time, however, permanent soft tissue contractures may develop; consequently, the deformity ceases to be reversible by leveling the pelvis.

As in the cervical and the thoracic spine, lumbar scoliosis may be idiopathic or due to neurologic disorders or vertebral anomalies. In general, lumbar scoliosis is less common than thoracic scoliosis and more difficult to detect by physical examination. The bulkier lumbar musculature may disguise the spinal curve, and the rib hump that often alerts the examiner to the presence of thoracic scoliosis may be mild or ab-

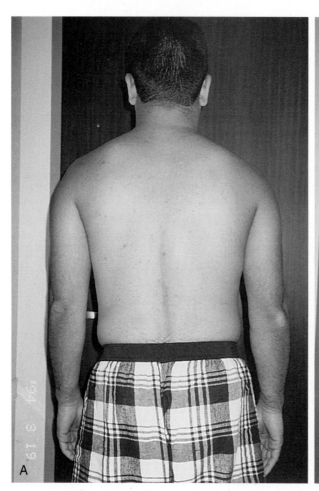 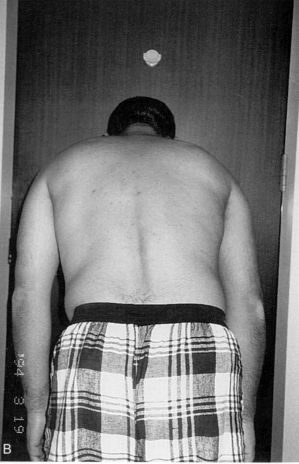

Figure 9–2. *A* and *B*, A list to the left. Note the asymmetry of the spaces between the arms and the trunk in *A* and the increase in the list with flexion in *B*.

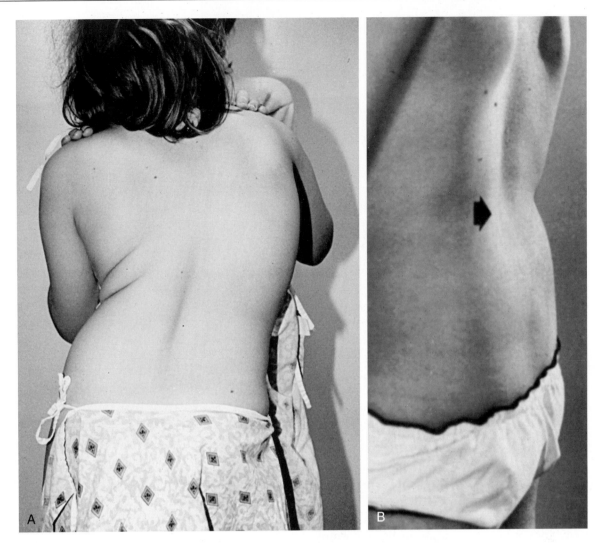

Figure 9–3. *A,* Thoracolumbar scoliosis. *B,* Spondylolisthesis (*arrow* indicates step-off). (*B,* From Rothman RH, Simeone FA. The Spine, 3rd ed. Philadelphia, WB Saunders, 1992, p 925.)

sent. Clues such as pelvic obliquity or asymmetry of the spaces between the upper limbs and the trunk are, therefore, extremely important in detecting lumbar scoliosis.

SKIN AND SUBCUTANEOUS TISSUE ABNORMALITIES. The examiner should also note any abnormalities of the skin or subcutaneous tissue of the lumbar region that may indicate underlying spinal abnormalities. A lumbar *lipoma,* an abnormal *hair patch,* or a *port wine stain* may be associated with spina bifida or even myelomeningocele. Large tan patches known as *café au lait spots* and nodular skin swellings may indicate neurofibromatosis, a condition that may cause secondary deformity of the spine.

STEP-OFF DEFORMITY. Severe degrees of spondylolisthesis may produce a visible **step-off deformity** of the lumbar spine. Normally, the tips of the lumbar spinous processes should protrude posteriorly about the same amount, producing a smooth hollow in the lumbar spine. When spondylolysis occurs, the spinous process and associated posterior elements of the involved vertebra are detached from the rest of the vertebra. In this setting, the body of the involved vertebra and the rest of the spine above it may slide forward, producing a spondylolisthesis. Spondylolisthesis is most likely to occur between L5 and S1. When the amount of spondylolisthesis is severe, an abrupt displacement or step-off is visible (see Fig. 9–3*B*). Less severe step-offs may only be palpable.

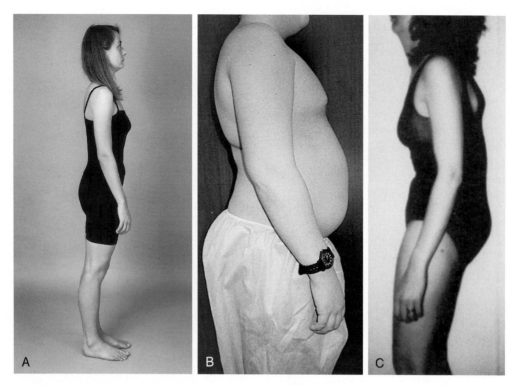

Figure 9–4. Lateral aspect of the lumbar spine. *A*, Normal alignment. *B*, Hyperlordosis. *C*, Flat back deformity. (*C*, From Rothman RH, Simeone FA. The Spine, 3rd ed. Philadelphia, WB Saunders, 1992, p 905.)

Lateral Aspect

Viewing the patient from the lateral aspect allows the examiner to judge the sagittal alignment of the spine. The lumbar spine is normally lordotic, that is, concave posteriorly. A normal **lumbar lordosis** should exactly complement the thoracic kyphosis and cervical lordosis, so that the base of the occiput rests directly above the sacrum (Fig. 9–4A).

The normal lumbar lordosis, which averages about 60°, is important in order to maintain healthy low back biomechanics. Several possible departures from normal lordosis may be seen, including hyperlordosis, decreased lordosis, lumbar flatback deformity, and gibbus deformity.

HYPERLORDOSIS. Hyperlordosis is usually a flexible postural deformity (see Fig. 9–4B). This deformity, also known as **swayback,** results in increased prominence of the buttocks. It is usually associated with flexion contracture of the hips, as described in Chapter 5, Pelvis, Hip, and Thigh.

DECREASED LUMBAR LORDOSIS. Decreased lumbar lordosis is often a temporary, reversible deformity related to pain and associated muscle spasm. Conditions in which pain is exacerbated by extension of the lumbar spine, such as *spondylolysis*, may be associated with a reflexive decrease in lumbar lordosis. *Ankylosing spondylitis* may produce a more rigid decrease in lumbar lordosis.

Lumbar flatback syndrome describes a rigid lumbar spine in which the normal lordosis has been completely lost (see Fig. 9–4C). Compression fractures that result in anterior wedging of the lumbar vertebral bodies can produce lumbar flatback syndrome. Advanced degeneration of the lumbar intervertebral disks may also result in this same deformity. Lumbar flatback syndrome may also occur following a long thoracolumbar spinal fusion for correction of scoliosis. This phenomenon occurs when the thoracic kyphosis has been abnormally reduced as part of a surgical procedure. In this case, the flatback deformity occurs in an effort to compensate for the decreased thoracic kyphosis and re-establish the sagittal balance of the spine.

GIBBUS. A **gibbus** is a sharp, angular kyphotic deformity. Gibbus is classically associated with tuberculosis of the spine. In this case, the infection destroys the anterior aspect of a vertebral body and the adjacent disk space, resulting in a localized collapse of the anterior portion of the vertebral column. Vertebral body collapse due to tumors, other infections, or fractures may also produce a gibbus.

348

GAIT

Although gait evaluation is not always considered an integral part of a lumbar spine examination, pain or deformity associated with certain conditions of the lumbar spine may produce characteristic gait abnormalities. A classic example is the gait abnormality that may be associated with sciatica. **Sciatica** is most commonly caused by a herniated disk at the L5-S1 or the L4-L5 interspace compressing a nerve root that feeds into the sciatic nerve. Because knee extension and hip flexion place further tension on the painful sciatic nerve, the patient with sciatica may attempt to walk with the hip more extended and the knee more flexed than normal. In addition, the patient may display an **antalgic gait**, putting as little weight as possible on the affected side and then quickly transferring the weight to the unaffected side.

The ability to toe walk and heel walk may also be used to screen for lumbar radiculopathy. These tests allow the examiner to quickly screen for radiculopathy related to the most common lumbar disk herniations. This method also allows the involved muscles to be tested with considerably higher loads than are exerted during manual testing of the same muscle groups.

HEEL WALKING. Heel walking tests the strength of the **ankle dorsiflexors**. The patient is asked to walk on his or her heels with the toes held high off the floor (Fig. 9–5). Because this is an unusual activity, the examiner may have to demonstrate the maneuver for the patient. The patient should be asked to take about 10 steps with each foot. This maneuver tests for weakness of the L4 innervated **tibialis anterior**, which would most commonly be weakened by a herniation of the L3-L4 disk. In the presence of severe weakness, the patient is unable to lift the front part of the foot off the floor at all. In milder degrees of weakness, the patient is not able to lift the forefoot as high off the floor as on the other side, or the muscles are noted to fatigue after a few steps have been taken.

TOE WALKING. Toe walking requires the S1 innervated **gastrocsoleus** muscle group that would most commonly be weakened by a herniation of the L5-S1 disk. The patient is asked to walk on the toes with the heels held high off the floor, again taking about 10 steps on each foot (Fig. 9–6). Again, severe weakness is manifested by the patient's complete inability to clear the

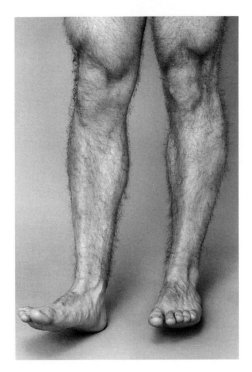

Figure 9–5. Heel walking.

heel of the involved side off the floor. When more subtle degrees of weakness are present, the heel of the involved side is not held as far off the floor as the heel of the opposite side or the muscles are noted to fatigue after a few steps.

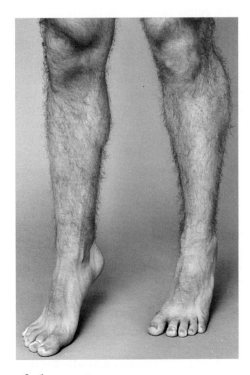

Figure 9–6. Toe walking.

RANGE OF MOTION

Motion of the lumbar spine is the result of a complex interaction among bony structures, articulations, and soft tissues. Abnormalities of any of these structures may limit the range of motion of the lumbar spine. The loss of motion may be due to pain, muscle spasm, mechanical block, or neurologic deficit. Range of motion of the lumbar spine is traditionally evaluated with the examiner standing or seated behind the patient. However, the examiner may also need to look from the side to more easily quantify the amount of flexion and extension present.

Flexion

To assess the **flexion** of the lumbar spine, the patient is asked to bend straight forward at the waist as far as possible (Fig. 9–7). Depending on the amount of flexibility present, the patient may be instructed to attempt to touch the fingertips or the palms to the floor. The amount of flexion present is estimated as the angle between the final position of the trunk and a vertical plane. Thus, 90° of flexion is present when the patient's trunk is parallel to the floor. When measured in this fashion, flexion averages about 80° to 90°.

Another way of quantifying lumbar flexion is to measure the distance from the patient's fingertips to the floor. In the average patient, the fingertips come to rest about 10 cm from the floor. The range of variation in lumbar flexion, however, is quite large. Flexion tends to decrease with age. Because lumbar flexion increases pressure on the intervertebral disks and places tension on sciatic nerve roots, herniation of L4-L5 and L5-S1 disks is frequently associated with painful, limited flexion of the lumbar spine. While assessing lumbar flexion, the examiner should also note whether the spine remains straight during flexion. The deformities associated with scoliosis and a lumbar list may both be accentuated by flexion of the spine (see Fig. 9–2).

It must be recognized that much, if not most, of the motion observed during forward bending is due to flexion at the hips, rather than true flexion of the lumbar spine. It is difficult to eliminate hip flexion and measure pure spine flexion. However, two methods are available to ensure that at least some of the flexion is taking place in the spine. The first is to observe the behavior of the normal lumbar lordosis as the patient bends forward. If flexion is actually taking place within the lumbar spine, the normal lordotic con-

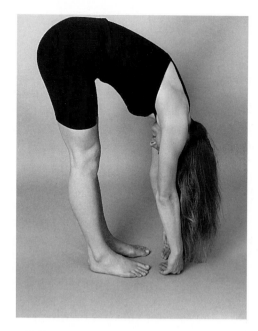

Figure 9–7. Lumbar flexion.

tour should flatten out and even mildly reverse itself into a slight kyphosis. If the contour of the lordosis remains unchanged during forward bending, the examiner may conclude that little flexion of the lumbar spine is actually occurring. The second technique for verifying that flexion is occurring within the spine is the tape measurement of the apparent increase in the length of the spine during flexion. This is done with the modified **Schober test** as described in Chapter 8, Cervical and Thoracic Spine. This method is really just a way of quantifying the change in spinal contour noted by observing the reversal of the lumbar lordosis.

Extension

To test for **extension** of the lumbar spine, the examiner asks the patient to lean backward as far as possible (Fig. 9–8). The amount of extension is quantified by estimating the angle between the trunk and a vertical line. In a normal patient, about 20° to 30° of extension is possible. As with the assessment of flexion, the examiner should not only observe the amount of motion possible but also determine whether the maneuver causes the patient pain. A number of different conditions may limit lumbar spine extension or cause it to be painful. Because extension tends to narrow the diameter of the spinal canal, patients with abnormal narrowing of the spinal canal tend to avoid further extension. The most

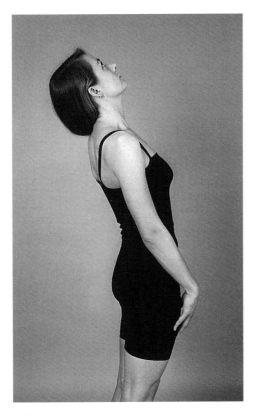

Figure 9–8. Lumbar extension.

common example of this is degenerative spinal stenosis, but posttraumatic deformities and space-occupying lesions, such as tumors, may produce the same picture. Lumbar spine extension may also be limited or painful in the presence of disorders of the posterior elements of the vertebrae. Examples include spondylolysis, tumors of the posterior elements, and degenerative arthritis of the posterior facet joints.

Lateral Bending

Lateral bending is tested by asking the standing patient to lean as far as possible to each side. The examiner should stabilize the patient's pelvis with a hand on each iliac crest (Fig. 9–9). This motion actually involves a combination of lateral bending and rotation of the vertebral column. The amount of lateral bending present is difficult to quantitate. It may be estimated by drawing an imaginary line between the vertebra prominens and the sacrum and estimating the angle between this line and the vertical. The average amount of lateral bending present in a normal patient is 20° to 30°.

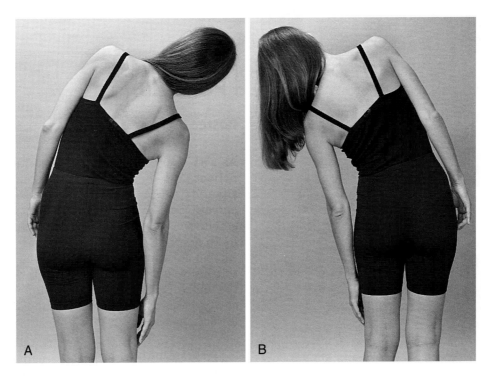

Figure 9–9. Lateral bending. *A*, Right. *B*, Left. Examiner has been omitted for clarity. Examiner should normally sit behind the patient with a hand on each iliac crest to stabilize the pelvis.

Manipulation

MUSCLE TESTING

Strength testing of the muscles that move the lumbar spine is not usually emphasized. Nevertheless, the abdominal and the lumbar musculature fulfills an important role by reducing the load on the static elements of the spine. A general assessment of the function of these muscle groups is, therefore, helpful in evaluating the common strain and overuse disorders that are frequent causes of low back pain.

Flexion of the lumbar spine is powered by the abdominal muscles, particularly the **rectus abdominis**. The function of these muscles may be assessed by having the patient perform a crunch, or modified sit-up. In this exercise, the patient lies supine on the examination table with the hip and the knees flexed, hands behind the head. The patient is then instructed to raise his or her shoulders off the table (Fig. 9–13). The height to which the shoulders can be raised and the number of repetitions possible vary tremendously among individuals according to flexibility, fitness level, and prior training. A patient who cannot raise the shoulders even once has significantly weak abdominal muscles.

Extension of the lumbar spine is powered by the **erector spinae** muscle groups. To assess the function of these muscles, the patient is placed in the prone position on the examination table with the hands behind the head. The patient is then asked to lift the chest off the table (Fig. 9–14). Again, the height that the shoulders rise off the table and the number of repetitions possible vary widely among patients according to flex-

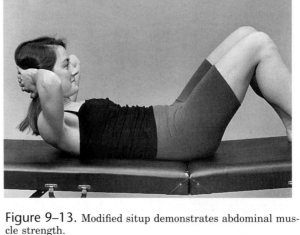

Figure 9–13. Modified situp demonstrates abdominal muscle strength.

ibility, fitness level, and training. The pain associated with disorders of the posterior elements of the lumbar spine, such as spondylolysis or facet joint arthritis, or of spinal stenosis may be exacerbated by this test.

NEUROLOGIC EXAMINATION

Sensory Examination

The approximate areas of sensory innervation from the lumbar and the sacral nerve roots are shown in Figure 9–15. As with the cervical and the thoracic nerve roots, there is considerable overlap in the sensory dermatomes, and the exact distribution of each dermatome varies somewhat from one individual to another. The initial screening for sensory deficits is usually done with light touch and sharp-dull discrimination testing, as described in Chapter 8, Cervical and Thoracic

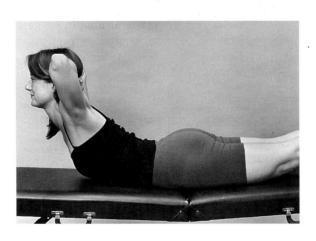

Figure 9–14. Active extension demonstrates erector spinae strength.

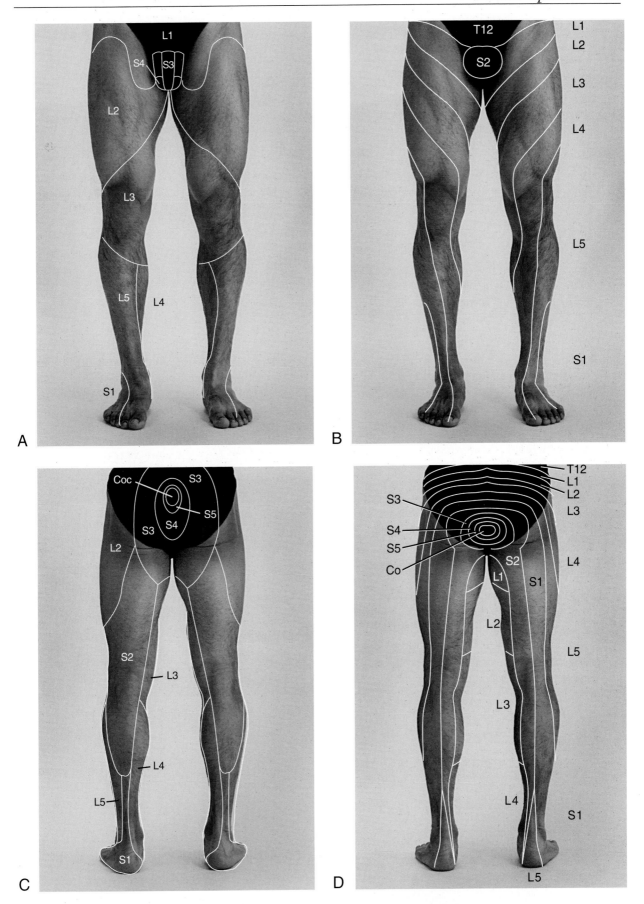

Figure 9–15. *A–D*, Lumbar and sacral dermatomes. (*A* and *C*, After Foerster. *B* and *D*, After Keegan and Garrett.)

TABLE 9–1.
PHYSICAL FINDINGS IN LUMBOSACRAL RADICULOPATHIES

DERMATOME	SENSORY TESTING	MOTOR TESTING	REFLEX TESTING
L1	Anterior proximal thigh near inguinal ligament	Iliopsoas (seated hip flexion)	
L2	Mid anteromedial thigh	Iliopsoas (seated hip flexion)	
L3	Just proximal or medial to patella	Quadriceps	Patellar tendon reflex (secondary)
L4	Medial lower leg and ankle	Tibialis anterior	Patellar tendon reflex
L5	Lateral and anterolateral leg and dorsal foot	Extensor hallucis longus Extensor digitorum brevis Gluteus medius	Tibialis posterior reflex Medial hamstring reflex
S1	Posterior calf, plantar foot, and lateral toes	Gastrocsoleus Peronei Gluteus maximus	Achilles' reflex
S2	Posterior thigh and proximal calf	Rectal examination	
S3, S4, S5	Perianal area	Rectal examination	

Spine. The sensory, motor, and reflex tests for each dermatome are summarized in Table 9–1.

The L1, L2, and L3 dermatomes run in broad bands obliquely across the anterior thigh. **L1** sensation is tested in the anterior proximal thigh near the inguinal ligament (Fig. 9–16A). Sensation supplied by the **L2** nerve root is tested over the anteromedial thigh, midway between the inguinal ligament and the patella (Fig. 9–16B). **L3** sensation may be evaluated by testing the skin

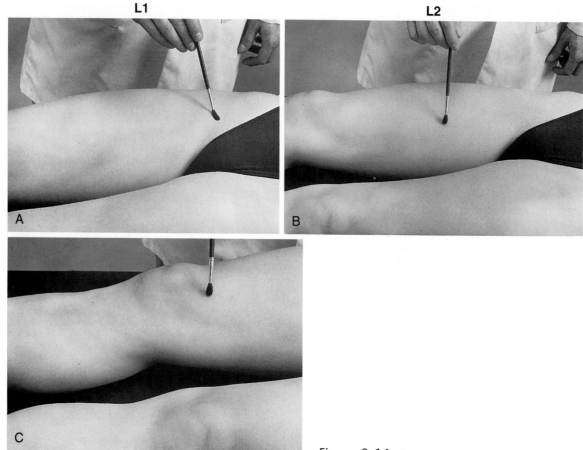

L1   **L2**

L3

Figure 9–16. Sensory evaluation by lumbar and sacral dermatome. *A*, L1. *B*, L2. *C*, L3.

L4　　　　**L5**

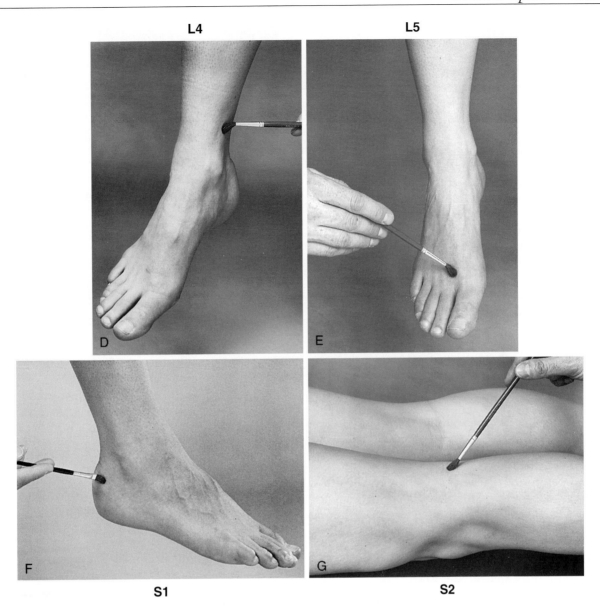

S1　　　　**S2**

Figure 9–16 *Continued. D,* L4. *E,* L5. *F,* S1. *G,* S2.

just proximal or medial to the patella (Fig. 9–16C). The **L4** nerve root supplies sensation to the medial leg and the ankle. It is best tested by examining the sensation in the area just proximal to the medial malleolus (Fig. 9–16D). The **L5** dermatome includes the lateral and the anterolateral leg and the dorsum of the foot. L5 sensation is usually tested by examining the area just proximal to the first web space (Fig. 9–16E).

The sensory distribution of the **S1** nerve root includes the posterior calf, the plantar surface of the foot, and the lateral toes. S1 sensation may be reliably tested over the posterolateral aspect of the heel (see Fig. 9–16F). The **S2** nerve root supplies the posterior thigh and the proximal calf. S2 sensory function may be tested by evaluating sensation in the center of the popliteal fossa (see Fig. 9–16G). The lower sacral nerve roots **(S3, S4, S5)** supply the sensation in the perianal area. The dermatomes are arranged in concentric rings around the anus, with the S3 dermatome being the most peripheral and the S5 being the most central.

Motor Examination

The spinal cord terminates at about the L1-L2 level, but its lower nerve roots continue distally as the cauda equina. Each pair of nerve roots exits the spine at the neural foramen formed by the vertebra of the same number and the one below. Thus, the L4 nerve root exits at the L4-L5 neuroforamen, the L5 nerve root exits at the L5-S1 neuroforamen, and so forth. However, when a lumbar disk herniation occurs, the disk tends to compress the next lower nerve root. Thus, the L5-S1 disk, the most common to herniate, usually compresses the S1 nerve root. Similarly, the L4-L5 disk usually compresses the L5 nerve root, and the L3-L4 disk, the least common of the three to herniate, usually compresses the L4 nerve root. Higher nerve roots are unlikely to be compressed by disk herniations. However, these higher nerve roots may be affected by other types of pathology, such as spinal fractures or dislocations; congenital malformations, such as spina bifida; tumors; and infections.

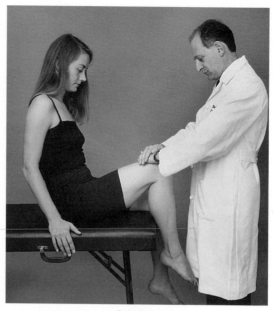

L1–L2

Figure 9–17. Assessing L1 and L2 motor function (iliopsoas strength).

L1 and L2 Nerve Roots

The **L1 and L2 nerve roots** supply the **iliopsoas** muscle, the primary hip flexor. To test the iliopsoas, the patient is seated with the knees flexed to 90° over the end or the side of the examination table. The patient is instructed to raise the thigh off the examination table while maintaining flexion of the knee. The examiner then presses downward on the patient's knee with both hands, asking the patient to resist as strongly as possible (Fig. 9–17). In a normal patient, the examiner should be able to overcome the iliopsoas with moderate difficulty.

L3 Nerve Root

The **L3 nerve root** is usually assessed by evaluating **quadriceps** strength, although the quadriceps is also innervated by L2 and L4. The quadriceps is also tested with the patient sitting on the end or the side of the examination table. The patient is asked to extend the knee fully and then to maintain the knee in full extension while the examiner pushes downward on the lower leg just above the ankle (Fig. 9–18). In a normal patient, the examiner should be unable to overcome the quadriceps and initiate knee flexion. In fact, in a strong patient, the examiner may begin

to lift the patient's pelvis off the examination table as the lower leg is pushed downward with the patient's knee locked in full extension.

L4 Nerve Root

The **L4 nerve root** is usually evaluated by testing the strength of the **tibialis anterior** muscle. As previously noted, the examiner may screen for

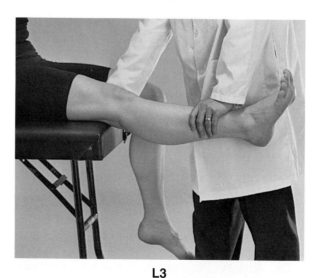

L3

Figure 9–18. Assessing L3 motor function (quadriceps).

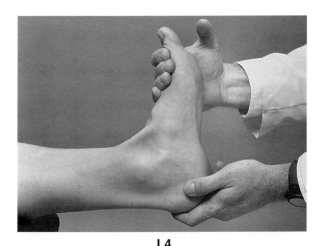

L4

Figure 9–19. Assessing L4 motor function (tibialis anterior strength).

tibialis anterior weakness by asking the patient to **heel walk**. Specific manual resistive testing of the tibialis anterior is accomplished with the patient seated on the end or the side of the examination table. The patient is asked to maximally

dorsiflex the ankle on the side being tested. The patient is then instructed to maintain this position while the examiner presses downward on the foot and attempts to passively plantar flex the ankle (Fig. 9–19). In a normal patient, the examiner should be unable to overcome the strength of the tibialis anterior.

L5 Nerve Root

The **L5 nerve root** provides the motor supply of the long toe extensors. It is most commonly tested by evaluating the strength of the **extensor hallucis longus**. To test the extensor hallucis longus, the examiner asks the seated patient to pull up or extend the great toe. The examiner then stabilizes the medial aspect of the patient's foot with one hand while pressing downward on the distal phalanx of the great toe with the fingers or the thumb of the other hand. The patient is instructed to resist the examiner's attempt to flex the interphalangeal joint of the toe (Fig. 9–20A).

When normal strength is present, it should be difficult for the examiner to overcome the

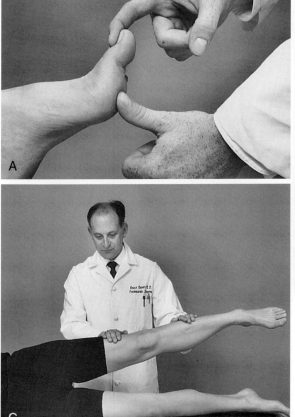

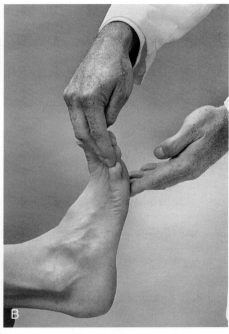

L5

Figure 9–20. Assessing L5 motor function. *A,* Extensor hallucis longus. *B,* Extensor digitorum longus. *C,* Gluteus medius.

strength of the extensor hallucis longus. In some patients, the patient's ability to demonstrate strength of the extensor hallucis longus may be limited by nonneurologic factors, such as the presence of severe bunions or the anatomic changes due to prior bunion surgery. In these patients, the examiner may assess the motor supply of the L5 nerve root by testing the other digital extensors or the gluteus medius.

The **extensor digitorum longus** is assessed in a manner analogous to that used for the extensor hallucis longus. In this case, the examiner stabilizes the forefoot with one hand and asks the patient to extend the toes as far as possible. The examiner then instructs the patient to maintain the extended position of the toes while the examiner attempts to passively flex the toes with his or her fingers (see Fig. 9–20B). In a normal patient, the examiner is able to overcome the strength of the toe extensors with moderate difficulty.

The **gluteus medius** is evaluated by assessing the strength of hip abduction. For this test, the patient is in the lateral position on the examination table and is asked to abduct the lower limb away from the table while maintaining knee extension. The examiner then instructs the patient to maintain the position of abduction while the examiner presses downward on the distal thigh, attempting to push the thigh back toward the table (see Fig. 9–20C). In a normal patient, the examiner has considerable difficulty overcoming the strength of the gluteus medius. In stronger patients, the examiner may be unable to do so.

S1 Nerve Root

The **S1 nerve root** provides motor supply to the plantar flexors, the evertors of the ankle, and the extensors of the hip. As previously described, the examiner may screen for weakness of the plantar flexors of the ankle by asking the patient to **toe walk**. Primary plantar flexion strength is provided by the gastrocsoleus complex, with assistance from the toe flexors. Manual resistance testing of the **gastrocsoleus** is usually carried out in the seated patient. The examiner stabilizes the patient's ankle with one hand and instructs the patient to passively plantar flex the ankle. The patient is told to maintain this position while the examiner attempts to force the ankle back into dorsiflexion by pressing upward on the patient's forefoot with the examiner's other hand

(Fig. 9–21A). In a normal patient, the examiner is unable to overcome the powerful plantar flexor muscles and initiate dorsiflexion.

The **peroneus longus** and **brevis** muscles, the principal evertors of the foot, are tested in the same basic position as the gastrocsoleus complex. The examiner stabilizes the patient's leg with one hand and asks the patient to rotate the foot outward. The examiner may have to passively place the patient's foot in eversion to communicate the desired position. The patient is then instructed to maintain the foot in the everted position while the examiner attempts to invert the foot by pressing inward on the lateral aspect of the foot (see Fig. 9–21B). In the normal patient, the examiner is able to overcome the strength of the evertors only with difficulty.

The **gluteus maximus** is also supplied by the S1 nerve root. To test it, the patient is asked to lie prone on the examination table and to flex the knee on the side being tested. The patient is then instructed to raise the thigh off the table. Finally, the examiner presses downward on the thigh with both hands while asking the patient to maintain the position of hip extension (see Fig. 9–21C). In a normal patient, the examiner experiences considerable difficulty pushing the thigh back to the table.

S2, S3, and S4 Nerve Roots

The **S2, S3, and S4 nerve roots** may be compressed or injured by tumors or fractures of the sacrum, or, more commonly, affected by spinal cord injury at a higher level. In the presence of spinal cord injury, the finding of sacral sparing, the preservation of some function of the sacral nerve roots, is a positive factor in predicting the potential for recovery of function.

The S2, S3, and S4 nerve roots are the principal nerve supply for the bladder, and they also supply the intrinsic muscles of the feet. Motor testing for these functions is difficult. The motor function of the sacral nerve roots is, therefore, usually tested by performing a **rectal examination**. When normal function is present, the examiner should note fairly firm resistance as the examining finger enters the rectum. The patient is then instructed to try to squeeze the examiner's finger, thus contracting the external anal sphincter. This should produce a strong, readily palpable feeling of constriction around the examiner's finger.

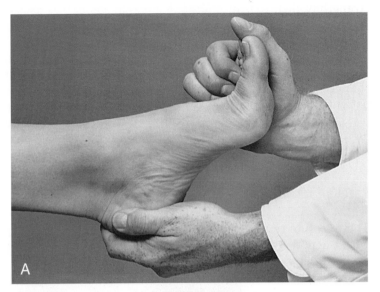

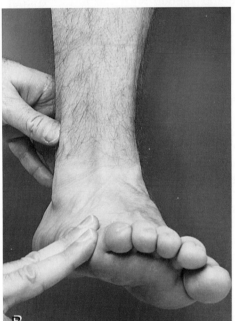

S1

Figure 9–21. Assessing S1 motor function.
A, Gastrocsoleus. *B*, Peroneus longus and brevis.
C, Gluteus maximus.

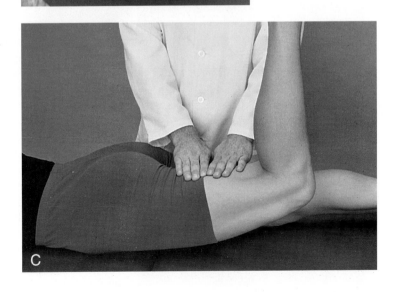

Reflex Examination

Deep tendon reflexes are not easily assessed for all the lumbar and sacral nerve roots. Two principal deep tendon reflexes are normally tested: the patellar tendon reflex, which primarily involves the L4 nerve root, and the Achilles tendon reflex, which primarily involves the S1 nerve root.

Patellar Tendon Reflex (L4)

The **patellar tendon reflex** is usually assessed with the patient seated on the side of the examination table with the knees flexed and the feet dangling. The examiner then sharply strikes the midportion of the patellar tendon with the flat side of a rubber reflex hammer. The examiner's other hand may rest lightly on the patient's quadriceps to feel for a muscle contraction (Fig. 9–22A).

In most patients, a contraction of the muscle is felt in response to the strike of the hammer, and in some patients the knee is seen to extend slightly. If no reflex is observed, the examiner may try to **reinforce** the reflex. To do this, the patient is instructed to hook the fingers of both hands together and pull against each other isometrically. While the patient is pulling, the examiner again strikes the patellar tendon (Fig. 9–22B). This technique may produce a patellar tendon reflex in patients in whom the reaction is otherwise unobtainable.

The patellar tendon reflex is more difficult to elicit than the Achilles tendon reflex. In some normal patients, the patellar tendon reflex is symmetrically absent. As in many other aspects of the physical examination, lack of symmetry is the key to evaluating this test. The patellar tendon reflex is primarily used to evaluate the **L4 nerve root**. Some contribution from L3 is also present.

Tibialis Posterior Reflex (L5)

The available reflexes for the **L5 nerve root** are difficult to elicit. They include the tibialis posterior reflex and the medial hamstring reflex. The **tibialis posterior reflex** is evaluated in the seated patient. The examiner holds the patient's foot in a small amount of eversion and dorsiflexion and strikes the posterior tibial tendon just below the medial malleolus. The examiner may also place a finger on the posterior tibial tendon and strike the finger instead of striking the tendon directly (Fig. 9–23A). When the reflex is elicited, a slight plantar flexion inversion response is noted.

Medial Hamstring Reflex (L5)

To elicit the **medial hamstring reflex**, the patient is placed in the prone position. The examiner passes one hand underneath the patient's

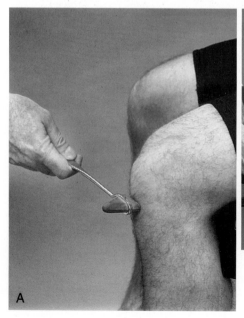
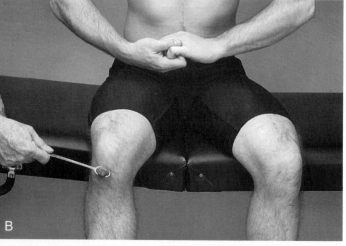

L4

Figure 9–22. *A*, Patellar tendon reflex (L4 nerve root). *B*, Reinforcement technique.

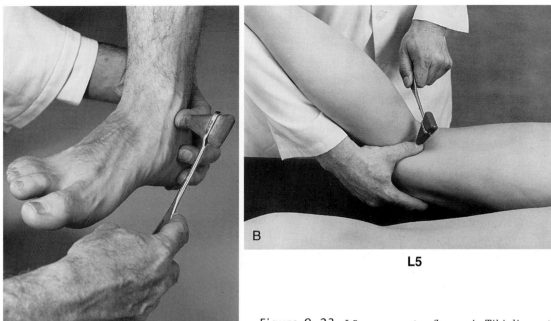

L5

Figure 9–23. L5 nerve root reflexes. *A*, Tibialis posterior. *B*, Medial hamstring.

leg and places the thumb of that hand on the semitendinosus tendon in the popliteal fossa. The patient's leg is allowed to rest on the examiner's forearm so that the patient's knee is somewhat flexed. The examiner then strikes the thumb, which is pressing on the semitendinosus tendon, with the pointed end of the hammer (see Fig. 9–23*B*). When the reflex is elicited, the examiner feels a contraction transmitted through the semitendinosus tendon or actually sees slight flexion of the knee take place.

Achilles' Tendon Reflex (S1)

The **Achilles tendon reflex** represents the **S1 nerve root**. This reflex may be elicited in the patient who is seated with the legs dangling comfortably off the end or side of the examination table. The examiner gently dorsiflexes the foot to place the Achilles tendon under tension, and then strikes the Achilles about 3 cm above the calcaneus using the flat end of the reflex hammer (Fig. 9–24*A*).

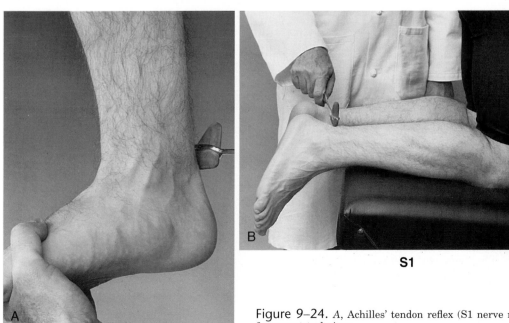

S1

Figure 9–24. *A*, Achilles' tendon reflex (S1 nerve root). *B*, Reinforcement technique.

In most patients, this action produces a visible twitch of the ankle into plantar flexion. As with other deep tendon reflexes, a unilateral decrease in the magnitude of or disappearance of the Achilles reflex suggests a lower motor neuron lesion. The most common cause of this picture is a herniated L5-S1 disk impinging the ipsilateral S1 nerve root. Bilateral hyperreflexia suggests the possibility of an upper motor neuron lesion.

If the examiner experiences difficulty in eliciting the Achilles tendon reflex, the use of **reinforcement** techniques is often helpful. A convenient method for reinforcing the Achilles tendon reflex is to ask the patient to kneel on the examination table with the feet projecting a few inches past the end or side (see Fig. 9–24*B*). The examiner then strikes each Achilles in turn as already described. This technique brings out the Achilles tendon reflex in the vast majority of individuals.

Pathologic Reflexes

If undue briskness of the Achilles or the patellar tendon reflexes leads the examiner to suspect the presence of an upper motor neuron lesion, the provocative tests for **ankle clonus** and the **Babinski sign** should be carried out. The details of these procedures are described in Chapter 8, Cervical and Thoracic Spine. It is important to remember that the spinal cord usually ends at the inferior margin of the L1 vertebra. Distal to this level, the nerve roots that constitute the cauda equina function very much like peripheral nerves. Thus, for an upper motor neuron picture to occur, a lesion must typically be situated at the L1 level or higher.

NERVE TENSION TESTS

An important component of the lumbar spine examination is to determine whether evidence of nerve root compression exists. Nerve root compression is usually considered probable when stretching the peripheral nerve associated with the nerve root in question reproduces pain in the distribution of that nerve. The most important peripheral nerves deriving from the lumbar and the sacral nerve roots are the femoral and the sciatic nerves. The **femoral nerve** runs down the anteromedial aspect of the thigh and is formed by the L2, L3, and L4 nerve roots. The **sciatic nerve** runs down the posterior thigh and is formed by the L4, L5, S1, S2, and S3 nerve roots.

Straight-Leg Raising Test

The **straight-leg raising test** is the most well-known nerve tension test for the lumbar spine. The test is performed with the patient lying in a comfortable supine position with the head and pelvis flat. While full knee extension is maintained, one of the patient's feet is slowly lifted off the table. The limb is progressively elevated until maximal hip flexion is reached or the patient asks the examiner to stop owing to pain (Fig. 9–25). The angle formed by the lower limb and the examination table at the point of maximal elevation is noted, and the procedure is repeated with the opposite limb.

In a normal patient, straight-leg raising of 70° to 90° should be possible and may be accompanied by a feeling of tightness in the posterior thigh. In the presence of **sciatica**, the angle of hip flexion is reduced and the patient reports shooting pain radiating down the posterior thigh and often into the lower leg along the distribution of the sciatic nerve. Straight-leg raising stretches the **L5 and S1 nerve roots** 2 mm to 6 mm, but it puts little tension on the more proximal nerve roots. An abnormal straight-leg raising test, therefore, suggests a lesion of either the L5 or the S1 nerve root. Beyond 70° of hip flexion, deformation of the sciatic nerve occurs beyond the spine. Sciatic pain that is reproduced only with hip flexion beyond 70°, therefore, suggests the possibility of sciatic nerve compression outside the spinal canal. If the patient with limited straight-leg raising reports tightness in the posterior thigh rather than sciatica, hamstring tightness is the probable cause. Hamstring tightness may be associated with a wide variety of conditions, including spondylolysis. **Lasegue's test**, discussed later, does not exacerbate the dis-

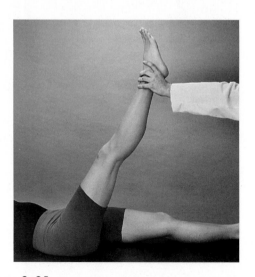

Figure 9–25. Straight-leg raising test.

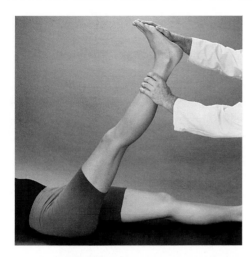

Figure 9–26. Lasegue's test.

comfort of hamstring tightness the way it exacerbates sciatica.

Crossed Straight-Leg Raising Test

Performing the straight-leg raising test on the side opposite that of the sciatica is called the **crossed straight-leg raising test**. For example, if a patient complains of right-sided sciatica, the examiner performs a straight-leg raising test on the patient's left side. If this maneuver reproduces or exacerbates the patient's right-sided sciatica, the result is extremely sensitive and specific for a herniated **L5-S1** or **L4-L5 lumbar disk**. In one study, 97% of patients who had a positive crossed straight-leg raising test and underwent surgery had surgically confirmed disk herniations.

Lasegue's Test

Lasegue's test is a progression of the straight-leg raising test. To perform **Lasegue's test**, the examiner carries out the straight-leg raising test, pausing when the patient complains of reproduction of his or her typical sciatic pain. While maintaining the degree of hip flexion at which sciatic pain is induced, the examiner passively dorsiflexes the foot of the leg being raised (Fig. 9–26). This maneuver further deforms the sciatic nerve. If the patient's radicular pain is exacerbated, the diagnosis of sciatica is strengthened. Lasegue's test may also reproduce radicular pain in some cases of lumbar disk herniation in which the straight-leg raising test is otherwise negative. The results of both the straight-leg raising test and the Lasegue test are abnormal in most cases of lumbar disk herniation, however.

Bowstring Sign

MacNab described another confirmatory test for sciatic nerve tension known as the **bowstring sign**. To elicit the bowstring sign, the examiner again begins by performing the straight-leg raising test to the point of reproduction of the patient's radicular pain. The knee is then flexed 90°, which usually relieves the patient's symptoms. Digital pressure is then applied to the popliteal fossa over the posterior aspect of the sciatic nerve (Fig. 9–27). If this again reproduces the patient's radicular pain, the impression of sciatica is further confirmed.

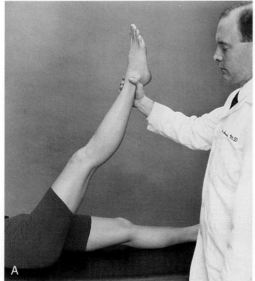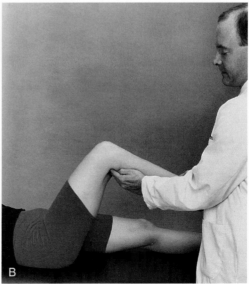

Figure 9–27. *A* and *B*, Bowstring sign.

Slump Test

The **slump test** is really a variant of the straight-leg raising and Lasegue tests performed in the seated position. The slump test is a progressive series of maneuvers designed to place the sciatic nerve roots under increasing tension. The patient begins the slump test sitting on the side of the examination table with the back straight, looking straight ahead (Fig. 9–28A). The patient is then encouraged to slump, allowing the thoracic and lumbar spines to collapse into flexion while still looking straight ahead (Fig. 9–28B). The next step is to fully flex the cervical spine (Fig. 9–28C). The patient is then instructed to extend one knee, thus performing a straight-leg raise (Fig. 9–28D). The patient then dorsiflexes the foot on the same side, thus duplicat-

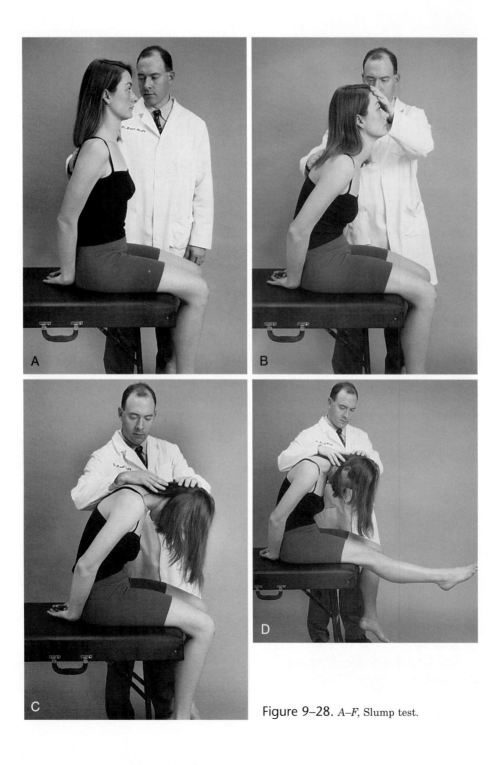

Figure 9–28. *A–F,* Slump test.

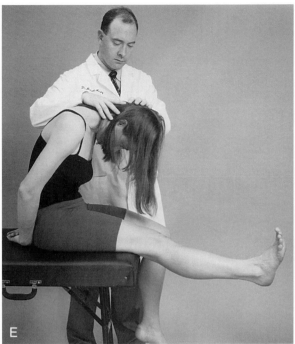

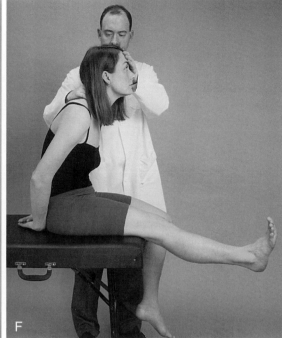

Figure 9–28 *Continued*

ing the Lasegue test (Fig. 9–28*E*). The process is then repeated with the opposite lower extremity.

At each stage in the procedure, the patient informs the examiner what is being felt and whether radicular pain is produced. Many normal individuals feel tightness in the lower back and the thigh with this series of maneuvers. Reproduction of familiar radicular pain, as in the straight-leg raising, Lasegue, and crossed straight-leg raising tests, is highly suggestive of sciatic nerve root tension. Subsequent extension of the neck relaxes the spinal cord and may thus relieve nerve tension (see Fig. 9–28*F*).

Femoral Nerve Stretch Test

As noted, the straight-leg raising test and its variants do not place significant tension on the nerve roots above L5. Although compression of the upper lumbar nerve roots is not common, it does occur. Herniations of the L3-L4 disk commonly compress the L4 nerve root. The **femoral nerve stretch test** is designed to assess compression of the **L2, L3, or L4 nerve roots**. To perform the femoral nerve stretch test, the patient is positioned prone on the examination table with the knee flexed to at least 90°. The

patient's hip is then extended passively by lifting the thigh off the examination table (Fig. 9–29). In the normal patient, this induces only a mild feeling of tightness in the anterior thigh. When one of the nerve roots that contribute to the femoral nerve is compressed, this maneuver reproduces the patient's radicular pain in the anterior thigh.

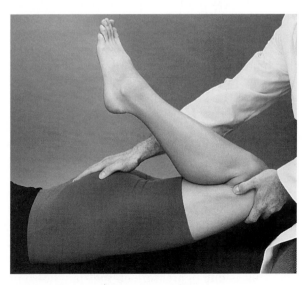

Figure 9–29. Femoral nerve stretch test.

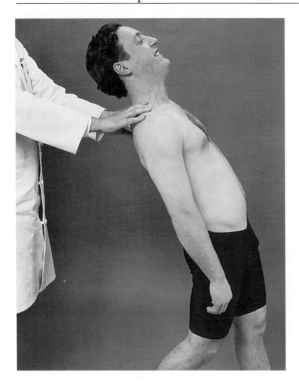

Figure 9–30. Single leg hyperextension test.

MISCELLANEOUS SPECIAL TESTS

Single Leg Hyperextension Test

It has already been noted that hyperextension of the lumbar spine is often painful in the presence of *spondylolysis*. The **single leg hyperextension test** has been described as a more specific test to detect the presence of spondylolysis and to suggest which side is involved in the process. To perform the single leg hyperextension test, the patient is asked to stand in the straddle position with one lower limb extended behind the other. The patient is then instructed to lean back as far as possible, and the examiner assists the patient in achieving the maximal hyperextension of the spine possible without falling over (Fig. 9–30). The procedure is then repeated with the position of the lower limbs reversed. In the presence of unilateral spondylolysis, hyperextension tends to exacerbate the patient's pain and the pain tends to be more severe when the lower limb on the affected side is extended posteriorly.

Valsalva's Maneuver

The **Valsalva maneuver** is designed to increase intrathecal pressure and therefore exacerbate pain that is due to pressure on the spinal cord or its nerve roots. To perform the Valsalva maneu-ver, the patient is instructed to bear down as if attempting to have a bowel movement (Fig. 9–31). If pain is present owing to pressure on the spinal cord or the nerve roots, this maneuver usually exacerbates the pain. Pain from other causes should not be affected by the Valsalva maneuver.

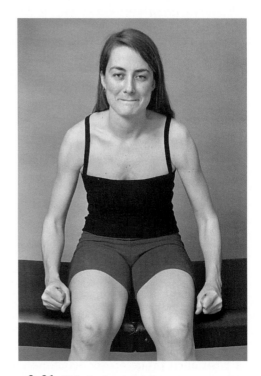

Figure 9–31. Valsalva's maneuver.

NONORGANIC SIGNS OF WADDELL

Waddell's nonorganic signs, already discussed in Chapter 8, Cervical and Thoracic Spine, were actually originally described in conjunction with the lumbar spine. They are helpful signals to alert the examiner to the possibility of nonorganic pathology or organic symptoms that are being enhanced by nonorganic factors.

EXAMINATION OF OTHER AREAS AND SYSTEMS

Pain due to lumbar spine pathology frequently radiates to the pelvis, the posterior hip, or the thigh. In the case of lumbar disk disease, back pain may sometimes be completely absent, with the patient sensing pain only in the sciatic notch and the posterior thigh areas. Patients with this clinical picture often believe that they have a painful hip joint or a hamstring strain. Complete investigation of potential lumbar spine pathology, therefore, often includes evaluation of the **sacroiliac joint,** the **sacrum** and the **pelvis,** the **hip** joint, and the **thigh.** The details of these related examinations are described in Chapter 5, Pelvis, Hip, and Thigh.

Because the symptoms of *claudication* due to peripheral vascular disease are similar to those of *pseudoclaudication* associated with spinal stenosis, an examination of the **peripheral circulation** of the lower extremities is often a necessary adjunct to the lumbar spine examination. Finally, the examiner must always remember that pathology of the **abdomen** or the **retroperitoneum** may present with back pain and must be alert for symptoms or signs that might indicate a disease process in one of these areas.

The physical findings in common conditions of the lumbar spine are summarized in Table 9–2.

TABLE 9–2.
PHYSICAL FINDINGS IN COMMON CONDITIONS OF THE LUMBAR SPINE

Herniated Lumbar Disk (Herniated Nucleus Pulposus)

Reproduction or exacerbation of sciatic symptoms with nerve tension tests (straight-leg raising, Lasegue's test, slump test, bowstring sign)
Reproduction of sciatica with flexion of the lumbar spine
Reproduction of sciatica with crossed straight-leg raising test (highly specific)
Sciatic notch tenderness
Lumbar muscle spasm or list away from the involved nerve root (variable)
Neurologic deficit in the distribution of the involved nerve root (variable)
Exacerbation of pain by Valsalva's maneuver

Spinal Stenosis

Loss of normal lumbar lordosis
Passive spine extension reproduces leg symptoms
Sciatic notch tenderness
Motor or sensory deficit (variable)
Abnormal straight-leg raising test (infrequent)

Spondylolysis

Lumbar tenderness at the level of involvement (variable)
Decreased lumbar lordosis (variable)
Hamstring tightness with straight-leg raising test
Pain exacerbated by hyperextension of the lumbar spine (passive extension, active extension, single leg extension test) (frequent)
Signs of associated spondylolisthesis, if present

Spondylolisthesis

Signs of spondylolysis (see above)
Visible or palpable lumbar step-off (more severe cases)
Sciatic notch tenderness (variable)
Motor or sensory deficit (variable)

Lumbar Fracture

Tenderness at the level of injury
Localized swelling and hematoma or ecchymosis
Lower motor neuron deficit owing to injury to the cauda equina or the nerve roots (variable)
Upper motor neuron deficit if lesion above the level of the cauda equina

Lumbar Spondylosis

Decreased range of motion
Pain exacerbated by motion (variable)
Localized or diffuse tenderness (variable)

Low Back Strain

Paraspinous muscle tenderness
Paraspinous muscle spasm (variable)
Symptoms exacerbated by forward flexion
List (variable)
Normal neurologic examination

Bibliography

Apley AG: A System of Orthopaedics and Fractures, 4th ed. London, Butterworths, 1973.
Beetham WP, Polley HF, Stocumb CH, Weaver WF: Physical Examination of the Joints. Philadelphia, WB Saunders, 1965.
Borenstein DG, Weisel SW: Low Back Pain: Medical Diagnosis and Comprehensive Management. Philadelphia, WB Saunders, 1989.
Breig A, Troup JDG: Biomechanical considerations in the straight-leg-raising test. Spine. 1979;4:242–250.

Christodoulides AN: Ipsilateral sciatica on femoral nerve stretch test is pathognomonic of an L4/5 disc protrusion. J Bone Joint Surg Br. 1989;71:88–89.
Dyck P: The femoral nerve traction test with lumbar disc protrusion. Surg Neurol. 1976;6:163–66.
Dyck P: Lumbar nerve root: the enigmatic eponyms. Spine. 1984;9:3–6.
Estridge MN, Rouhe SA, Johnson NG: The femoral stretching test. J Neurosurg. 1982;57:813–817.
Foerster O: The dermatomes in man. Brain. 1933;56:1–39.
Forst JJ: Contribution a L'Etude Clinique de la Sciatique. [thesis], Thes No. 33. Paris, 1881.
Hoppenfeld S, ed: Physical Examination of the Spine and Extremities. New York, Appleton-Century-Crofts, 1976.

Beevor's sign A sign of the asymmetric loss of thoracic nerve root motor function, consisting of the deviation of the umbilicus away from the dermatome innervated by the injured root when the patient attempts to perform a modified situp.

benediction hand A deformity that may be produced by a high ulnar nerve palsy in which the little finger and the ring finger are clawed.

biceps instability test A provocative test designed to induce subluxation or dislocation of the long head biceps tendon from the intertubercular groove.

Bouchard's nodes Arthritic enlargement of the proximal interphalangeal joints of the fingers.

bounce home test (see passive extension test of the knee)

boutonnière deformity A complex deformity of the finger in which a flexion deformity of the proximal interphalangeal joint is combined with a hyperextension deformity of the distal interphalangeal joint.

bowstring sign A confirmatory progression of the straight-leg raising test in which the patient's symptoms are alleviated by flexing the knee to relax tension on the nerve roots and then reproduced by directly compressing the sciatic nerve in the popliteal fossa.

broad-based gait A gait abnormality in which the width of the patient's stance is increased owing to balancing difficulties during single leg stance.

bunion A forefoot deformity characterized by an enlarged prominence on the medial aspect of the head of the first metatarsophalangeal joint.

bunionette, tailor's bunion A forefoot deformity characterized by an enlarged prominence on the lateral aspect of the head of the fifth metatarsal.

Bunnell-Littler test A manipulative test to distinguish among different possible causes of restricted flexion of the interphalangeal joints of the fingers, including intrinsic muscle tightness.

calcaneus contracture, calcaneus deformity An ankle joint contracture in which the ankle is fixed in dorsiflexion.

callus, callosity Thickened cornified skin on the foot that reflects areas of greater weightbearing or pressure.

capillary refill A method of assessing the circulation to a finger or a toe according to the speed with which normal color returns to the digit after blanching.

carpal bossing Benign bony prominences that can form on the dorsum of the proximal ends of the metacarpals.

carpal tunnel compression test A provocative test for carpal tunnel syndrome in which the examiner compresses the median nerve at the entrance to the carpal tunnel in an attempt to reproduce symptoms of tingling or numbness in the median nerve distribution.

carrying angle The normally valgus alignment of the elbow, created by the axis of the humerus and the axis of the forearm.

caudal Toward the distal end of the spine.

Childress' test A provocative test to induce the pain associated with a meniscus tear by having the patient duck walk.

Chopart's joint An alternative term that refers collectively to the joints between the talus and calcaneus and the distal tarsal bones.

circumduction test A provocative test for posterior shoulder instability that attempts to induce a posterior subluxation by passively circumducting the patient's shoulder.

claw hand A hand deformity in which all fingers are hyperextended at the metacarpophalangeal joints and flexed at the interphalangeal joints, usually owing to combined median and ulnar nerve palsies.

claw toe A toe deformity in which both the proximal and the distal interphalangeal joints are held in an abnormal amount of flexion; usually multiple toes are involved.

clonus Rhythmic involuntary flexion and extension of the ankle induced by a sudden forced dorsiflexion; increased clonus is a sign of an upper motor neuron neurologic lesion.

contralateral On the opposite side of the body.

coxalgic gait (see abductor limp)

Craig's test, Ryder's method for measuring femoral anteversion A clinical test for estimating femoral anteversion by comparing the position of the greater trochanter with the flexion axis of the knee.

cranial Toward the proximal end of the spine.

crepitus A palpable and occasionally audible sensation of crackling or grating produced by the rubbing together of two irregular surfaces, such as fractured bone fragments or degenerated articular cartilage.

cross-chest adduction or cross-body adduction   A test in which the patient is asked to adduct the shoulder by reaching across the chest to touch the opposite shoulder; this maneuver often irritates a painful acromioclavicular joint.

crossed straight-leg raising test   A variation of the straight-leg raising test that is performed on the leg opposite the side of suspected lower lumbar radiculopathy; it is thought to be highly specific for a herniated L5-S1 or L4-L5 disk.

cubitus valgus   Valgus deformity of the elbow.

cubitus varus, gunstock deformity   Varus deformity of the elbow.

distraction test   A followup to the axial compression test of the cervical spine in which the neck is distracted in an attempt to alleviate the symptoms of nerve root compression.

dorsal   Related to the dorsum or posterior aspect of the hand or of any other part of the body.

dorsiflexion   An alternative term for extension of the wrist or the ankle.

drawer test of the shoulder   A passive test for the assessment of shoulder laxity in which the patient's humeral head is grasped and translated both anteriorly and posteriorly.

drop foot gait, steppage gait   A gait abnormality associated with weakness of ankle dorsiflexion, in which the patient lifts the knee of the involved leg higher than normal during swing phase and may allow the foot to slap against the ground at heel strike.

droparm sign, droparm test   The patient's inability to prevent the abducted arm from falling uncontrollably toward the side when the patient attempts to lower the arm in a controlled manner.

dropback phenomenon   The tendency of the tibia to sublux posteriorly in relation to the distal femur when the knee is in a position of 90° flexion in a supine patient; a sign of posterior cruciate ligament injury.

dropped knuckle   A loss of the normal dorsal prominence of a metacarpal head owing to a fracture of the metacarpal neck or shaft.

dynamic posterior shift test   A manipulative and provocative test in which passive tightening of the hamstrings is used to reduce posterior or posterolateral subluxation of the knee with a sudden shift.

elbow flexion test   A provocative test for ulnar nerve compression at the elbow in which prolonged passive elbow flexion is used to elicit the patient's neurologic symptoms.

Ely's test   A manipulative test to detect contracture of the rectus femoris muscle.

equinus contracture, equinus deformity   An ankle joint contracture in which the ankle is fixed in plantar flexion.

extension   Motion in a limb, a digit, or the spine that tends to straighten the involved body segment or, in the case of the shoulder and the hip, to move the limb posterior to the trunk in the sagittal plane.

extension lag   The situation in which a joint, most commonly the knee, can be fully extended passively but not actively.

external rotation   Axial rotation at a joint that tends to rotate the distal limb away from the midline when the patient is viewed from the anterior position.

external rotation test   A manipulative test for detecting abnormal posterolateral laxity of the knee by demonstrating a unilateral increase in passive external rotation.

FABER test   (see Patrick's test)

Fairbanks' apprehension test   (see patellar apprehension test)

femoral anteversion, femoral retroversion   The angle between the femoral neck and a plane defined by the shaft of the femur and the flexion axis of the knee; in anteversion, the femoral neck angles anteriorly; in retroversion, it angles posteriorly.

femoral nerve stretch test   A provocative test designed to demonstrate compression of the L2, L3, or L4 nerve roots by passively extending the prone patient's hip and flexing the knee on the involved side.

Finkelstein's test   A provocative test in which flexion of the thumb and ulnar deviation of the wrist are used to elicit the pain of deQuervain's tenosynovitis.

first metatarsal rise test   A manipulative test to detect posterior tibial tendon dysfunction by producing passive inversion of the heel and observing whether the first metatarsal remains in contact with the ground.

flat back deformity   Pathologic, usually iatrogenic, straightening of the normal thoracic kyphosis or the normal lumbar lordosis.

flexion   Motion in a limb, a digit, or the spine that tends to bend the involved body segment or, in the case of the shoulder and the hip, to move the limb anterior to the trunk in the sagittal plane.

flexion contracture   The condition in which normal extension of a joint is prevented by soft tissue contractures or other abnormalities.

flexed knee gait   A gait abnormality in which the knee does not extend normally during ambulation.

flexion-rotation drawer test   A variation of the pivot shift test designed to be less provocative by inducing a subluxation and a reduction of the knee that are gentler than in the classic pivot shift test.

fluid wave (visible, palpable)   A method for detecting an effusion in the knee in which the fluid is squeezed into the suprapatellar pouch and then forced back down along the sides of the patella.

foot drop   Weakness or paralysis of the muscles that produce ankle dorsiflexion.

forefoot abductus, forefoot abduction   A foot deformity in which the forefoot appears deviated laterally in relation to the hindfoot.

forefoot adductus, forefoot adduction   A foot deformity in which the forefoot appears deviated medially in relation to the hindfoot.

formication sign   (see Tinel's sign)

Froment's sign   Flexion of the interphalangeal joint of the thumb during Froment's test, owing to unconscious substitution of the flexor pollicis longus for the weakened adductor pollicis; usually a sign of ulnar nerve injury.

Froment's test   A resistive test to evaluate the strength of key pinch, an action powered in the thumb primarily by the adductor pollicis.

fulcrum test   A provocative test for stress fractures of the femoral shaft in which the examiner bends the patient's thigh over the edge of the examination table in an attempt to elicit pain.

Gaenslen's test   A provocative test for sacroiliac joint pain in which the joint is stressed by hyperextending the ipsilateral hip off the side of the examination table.

genu recurvatum   Hyperextension of the knee beyond the neutral position.

genu valgum   A valgus deformity of the knee(s).

genu varum   A varus deformity of the knee(s).

gibbus   A sharply angled kyphosis.

glove or stocking sensory loss   A circumferential sensory deficit in the entire limb distal to a certain point, typical of diabetic sensory neuropathy, reflex sympathetic dystrophy, and nonorganic disorders.

gluteus maximus lurch   A gait abnormality in which the patient locks the hip in extension as the contralateral limb is advanced for the next step; a sign of gluteus maximus weakness.

Godfrey's test   A method of demonstrating the dropback phenomenon by flexing the hips and knees to 90° in the supine, relaxed patient.

grind test   A provocative test for arthritis of the basilar joint of the thumb in which the first metacarpal is rotated against the trapezium in an attempt to produce painful grinding.

gunstock deformity   (see cubitus varus)

Haglund's deformity, pump bump   An abnormal enlargement of the posterior aspect of the calcaneal tuberosity and the associated overlying soft tissue.

hallux rigidus   Reduced or absent motion in the first metatarsophalangeal joint.

hallux valgus   Valgus deformity at the first metatarsophalangeal joint, so that the great toe deviates away from the midline.

hallux varus   Varus deformity at the first metatarsophalangeal joint, so that the great toe deviates toward the midline.

Halsted's test   A provocative test for thoracic outlet syndrome, in which downward traction on the patient's arm is combined with positioning of the head in an attempt to obliterate the radial pulse.

hammer toe   A toe deformity consisting of hyperextension of the metatarsophalangeal and the distal interphalangeal joints combined with hyperflexion of the proximal interphalangeal joint; usually involves a single digit.

Hawkins' impingement reinforcement test   A test for rotator cuff impingement in which the shoulder is flexed 90° and maximally internally rotated.

Heberden's nodes   Arthritic enlargement of the distal interphalangeal joints of the fingers.

heloma durum (hard corn)   A hard collection of dense compacted keratotic tissue that occurs over pressure areas on the toes.

heloma molle (soft corn) A soft hyperkeratosis characteristically located in the web spaces between the toes.

Homans' test, Homans' sign A provocative test for deep vein thrombosis of the calf in which the ankle is passively dorsiflexed in an attempt to reproduce or aggravate the patient's pain.

hyperabduction test A screening test for thoracic outlet syndrome in which the patient's radial pulse is palpated as the arms are abducted.

hyperextension Extension of a joint beyond the neutral position.

hyperlordosis, swayback deformity A spinal deformity consisting of excessive lordosis of the lumbar spine.

iliopsoas sign Pain in the iliopsoas sheath produced by forcefully externally rotating the hip in the figure-four position.

in-facing patellae (see squinting patellae)

internal rotation Axial rotation that tends to rotate the distal limb toward the midline when the patient is viewed from the anterior position.

in-toeing, pigeon-toed deformity The condition in which a patient's feet angle toward each other when he or she is standing or walking.

inversion stress test, varus stress test of the ankle A manipulative test to detect abnormal varus laxity in the ankle joint; primarily a test of calcaneofibular ligament function.

ipsilateral On the same side of the body.

jerk test of the knee A variation of the pivot shift test that begins with the knee in flexion instead of in extension.

jerk test of the shoulder A provocative test for posterior shoulder instability in which the shoulder is flexed 90° and the arm is then pushed posteriorly.

Jobe's test, supraspinatus isolation test A resistive test for the shoulder, designed to isolate supraspinatus function as much as possible, performed with the shoulder in a position of 90° abduction and maximal internal rotation in a plane 30° anterior to the coronal plane.

kyphosis A spinal curve in the sagittal plane that is convex posteriorly; the normal contour of the thoracic spine.

Lachman's test A manipulative test for detecting abnormal anterior laxity in the knee performed in a position of mild flexion; primarily a test of anterior cruciate ligament integrity.

Lasegue's test A progression of the straight-leg raising test in which the patient's ankle is passively dorsiflexed to increase tension on the lower lumbar nerve roots.

lateral bending Spinal movement consisting of bending to the side in the coronal plane.

lateral pelvic compression test A manipulative screening test for pathology of the major joints of the pelvic ring performed by pressing downward on one iliac crest while the patient is lying on the opposite side.

lateral rotation Spinal motion consisting of rotation to one side or the other in the transverse plane.

lateral scapular slide A soft tissue contracture, typically seen in athletes who throw, that draws the scapula of the dominant shoulder away from the midline.

leg length discrepancy (functional or apparent) The situation in which the actual length of the patient's two lower limbs is identical, but other factors such as joint or muscle contractures cause one of the limbs to function or appear as if it were shorter or longer than the other.

leg length discrepancy (true) The situation in which an actual difference exists between the length of a patient's two lower limbs, as measured from the hip joint to the plantar surfaces of the feet.

Lhermitte's maneuver A provocative test performed by asking the seated patient to maximally flex the cervical and thoracic spine.

Lhermitte's sign The production of distal paresthesias in multiple extremities or the trunk in response to Lhermitte's maneuver, thought to be indicative of spinal stenosis and resulting spinal cord compression.

Lisfranc's joint An alternative term that refers collectively to the tarsometatarsal joints of the foot.

list A functional spinal deformity consisting of a pure planar shift to one side in the coronal plane.

load-and-shift test A method of assessing the passive anterior and posterior laxity of the shoulder, similar to the drawer test of the shoulder; the examiner may apply an axial load to the humerus to increase the sense of subluxation as the humeral head is shifted.

long finger extension test   A provocative test for radial tunnel syndrome in which the patient is asked to extend the long finger against resistance in an attempt to reproduce the patient's symptoms.

long finger proximal interphalangeal joint flexion test   A provocative test for median nerve compression by the flexor digitorum superficialis in which the patient is asked to flex the proximal interphalangeal joint of the long finger against resistance in an attempt to reproduce the patient's symptoms.

lordosis   A spinal curve in the sagittal plane that is concave posteriorly; the normal contour of the cervical and the lumbar spines.

Losse's test   A variation of the pivot shift test that uses direct pressure behind the head of the fibula to produce a subluxation of the knee.

lunotriquetral ballottement test   A manipulative test that attempts to detect abnormal laxity between the lunate and the triquetrum.

mallet finger   Inability to actively extend the distal interphalangeal joint of the finger, usually owing to rupture or avulsion of the extensor digitorum communis insertion.

mallet toe   A toe deformity consisting of an isolated abnormal flexion deformity of the distal interphalangeal joint of the involved toe.

McMurray's test   A provocative test to elicit pain and clicking associated with a torn meniscus by passively manipulating a hyperflexed knee.

metatarsus primus varus   A forefoot deformity in which the first metatarsal deviates medially; usually associated with hallux valgus.

midcarpal instability test   A manipulative and provocative test in which the examiner attempts to induce a subluxation at the midcarpal joint of the wrist.

Morton's test   A manipulative and provocative test for the detection of interdigital neuromas performed by compressing the metatarsal heads and observing for a palpable click or reproduction of the patient's pain.

Mulder's click   A sign of interdigital neuroma in which a palpable click is produced by compressing the neuroma between the adjacent metatarsal heads.

Neer's impingement sign   The production of pain by maximal passive forward flexion of the shoulder, considered a sign of rotator cuff impingement.

Neer's impingement test   A followup to Neer's impingement sign, in which anesthetic is injected in the subacromial space to see if the pain of the impingement sign is eliminated.

nonradicular sensory loss   A sensory deficit in a distribution overlapping more than one dermatome.

Ober's test   A manipulative test to detect contracture of the iliotibial tract.

O'Brien's test   A provocative test that may elicit pain associated with an injured acromioclavicular joint or a torn glenoid labrum.

opposition   A complex motion of the thumb in which the thumb abducts and rotates (pronates) at the basilar joint, so that the volar surface of the tip of the thumb touches that of the tip of the little finger.

out-facing patellae   A variation in rotational alignment of the lower limbs in which the patellae angle away from each other when the patient stands with the feet pointing straight forward.

out-toeing, slew-footed deformity   The condition in which a patient's feet angle away from each other when he or she is standing or walking.

painful arc syndrome, sign   Subjective or objective evidence of pain experienced by a patient during active abduction of the shoulder, usually in an arc including the 90° abducted position and typically caused by rotator cuff disease.

palmar abduction   A movement in which the thumb moves away from the rest of the hand in a plane perpendicular to the plane of the palm.

palmar adduction   A movement in which the thumb moves toward the rest of the hand in a plane perpendicular to the plane of the palm.

palmar flexion   An alternative term for flexion of the wrist.

passive extension test of the knee, bounce home test   A provocative test to induce the pain associated with a displaced bucket handle tear of a meniscus by passively extending the knee past the point of comfort.

passive range of motion (PROM)   The arc through which a joint can be moved by another individual or the muscles from another part of the patient's body.

patella alta   A high riding patella, caused by a relatively long patellar tendon.

patella baja, patella infra   A low riding patella, caused by a relatively short patellar tendon.

patellar apprehension test, Fairbanks' apprehension test A provocative test designed to simulate an episode of patellar subluxation or dislocation by passively pushing the patella laterally as the knee is passively flexed.

patellar glide test A manipulative test to demonstrate passive patellar mobility by passively pushing the patella medially and laterally in the relaxed patient.

patellar grind test (active, passive) Methods of demonstrating patellar crepitus using active quadriceps contraction or passive direct pressure on the patella as the knee is taken through a range of motion.

patellar tracking The path followed by the patella during active knee extension.

Patrick's test, FABER test A provocative test for sacroiliac joint pain in which the sacroiliac joint is stressed by forcefully externally rotating the hip in the figure-four position.

pectus carinatum A thoracic deformity in which the sternum is abnormally convex.

pectus excavatum A thoracic deformity in which the sternum is abnormally concave.

pelvic extension Rotation of the pelvis around a transverse axis that causes the superior pelvis to rotate anteriorly and the inferior pelvis to rotate posteriorly.

pelvic flexion Rotation of the pelvis around a transverse axis in which the superior pelvis rotates posteriorly while the inferior pelvis rotates anteriorly.

pelvic obliquity The situation in which the two sides of the patient's pelvis are not level with each other when the patient is standing.

pelvic rotation Rotation of the pelvis in the coronal or transverse planes during gait.

peroneal tendon instability test An active provocative test to induce and detect peroneal tendon instability by asking the patient to actively rotate the foot and ankle using a circular motion.

pes cavus A foot deformity characterized by an abnormally high longitudinal arch.

pes planus A foot deformity characterized by an abnormally low or absent longitudinal arch.

Phalen's test A provocative test for carpal tunnel syndrome in which the wrist is held in a flexed position for a minute in an attempt to elicit the patient's symptoms.

Phelps' test A clinical test for contractures of the gracilis muscle that compares the magnitude of passive hip abduction possible in different positions of knee flexion.

piano key test A manipulative test to detect abnormal laxity of the distal radioulnar joint of the wrist.

pigeon-toed deformity (see in-toeing)

piriformis test A manipulative test for contracture of the piriformis muscle or sciatic nerve irritation owing to compression by the piriformis.

pivot shift test A manipulative and provocative test for demonstrating the rotatory subluxation that is often associated with anterior cruciate ligament injury.

pivot shift test of the elbow (see posterolateral rotatory instability test)

posterolateral rotatory instability test, pivot shift test of the elbow A provocative test designed to induce an episode of posterolateral rotatory subluxation of the elbow, usually manifested by the creation of apprehension in the conscious patient.

plantar flexion An alternative term for flexion of the ankle, the toes, and the other joints of the foot toward the plantar surface.

plantar reflex The response of the toes, either dorsiflexion or plantar flexion, to stroking the sole of the foot firmly.

Popeye's deformity The bunching together of the biceps brachii muscle seen after rupture of the long head of the biceps tendon.

posterior drawer test of the knee A manipulative test for detecting abnormal posterior laxity in the knee by pushing posteriorly on the tibia with the knee flexed 90°; primarily a test of posterior cruciate ligament integrity.

posterolateral drawer sign A method of demonstrating increased posterolateral laxity of the knee by performing the posterior drawer test with the patient's foot externally rotated.

pronation Rotation of the forearm so that the palm faces downward; by extension, analogous rotation in other parts of the body.

pubic symphysis stress test A provocative test for detecting instability or pain associated with the pubic symphysis performed by attempting to create a shearing motion at the symphysis with direct manipulation

pump bump (see Haglund's deformity)

Q angle, quadriceps angle The angle formed between a line from the anterior superior iliac spine to the center of the patella and a line from the center of the patella to the center of the tibial tubercle when the patient is standing with the feet in a neutral position.

quadriceps active drawer test A method of demonstrating posterior subluxation of the knee by eliciting a contraction of the quadriceps muscle, thus producing a visible reduction of the subluxation.

radial Related to the lateral side of the hand or the forearm, on which the radius and thumb are located.

radial abduction A movement in which the thumb moves away from the rest of the hand within the plane of the palm.

radial deviation A motion of the wrist produced by bending the hand toward the radial side of the forearm.

radicular sensory loss A sensory deficit in a distribution corresponding to a specific dermatome.

range of motion (ROM) The arc through which a joint passes during movement.

release test A further followup to the apprehension and relocation tests of the shoulder in which the direct posterior pressure on the patient's arm is released to see whether the patient's pain or apprehension returns.

relocation test A followup test to the apprehension test for anterior shoulder instability in which a direct posterior force is applied to the patient's arm in an attempt to eliminate the associated pain or apprehension.

resting position The position that a limb or joint assumes when the muscle forces acting on it are fully relaxed.

reverse Phalen's test A provocative test for carpal tunnel syndrome in which the wrist is held in an extended position for a minute in an attempt to elicit the patient's symptoms.

reverse pivot shift test A dynamic test to demonstrate abnormal posterolateral laxity of the knee by inducing a posterolateral subluxation followed by a sudden reduction.

rheumatoid nodules Rubbery subcutaneous nodules that may occur in rheumatoid arthritis.

rocker bottom foot An extreme foot deformity in which the bottom of the foot has a convex appearance instead of the normal concave longitudinal arch.

Roos' test A provocative test for thoracic outlet syndrome in which the patient is asked to exercise the ipsilateral hand while the shoulder is abducted in an attempt to reproduce the patient's symptoms.

Ryder's method for measuring femoral anteversion (see Craig's test)

scaphoid shift test, Watson's test A manipulative and provocative test for scapholunate instability in which the examiner attempts to produce a subluxation of the proximal pole of the scaphoid with respect to the distal radius.

Schober's test, modified Schober's test Methods of assessing flexion of the spine by measuring the apparent change in length between the extended and the flexed positions.

scoliosis A complex helical deformity of the spine in which a curve in the coronal plane is combined with abnormal rotation of the vertebrae in the transverse plane.

seated leg raising test A variant of the straight-leg raising test performed with the patient in the seated position.

short leg gait A number of gait abnormalities that may be seen in conjunction with a leg length discrepancy.

shuck test A manipulative and provocative test for instability or degeneration of the basilar joint of the thumb in which the first metacarpal is passively translated in relation to the trapezium.

shuffling gait A gait abnormality in which the feet are dragged on the ground during the swing phase.

silver fork deformity, Velpeau's deformity A posttraumatic deformity in which the distal radius and the hand appear dorsally displaced with respect to the rest of the forearm.

single leg hyperextension test A provocative test designed to exacerbate the pain of spondylolysis by having the patient hyperextend the lumbar spine while the ipsilateral lower limb is extended behind the patient.

slap foot gait A gait abnormality in which the feet strike the ground in a violent, unpredictable manner.

slew-footed deformity (see out-toeing)

slump test A series of maneuvers designed to demonstrate tension on the lower lumbar nerve roots that incorporates elements of the straight-leg raising test and Lasegue's test and is performed in the seated position.

snapping hip The sensation of soft tissue snapping or shifting during movement of the hip, most commonly caused by the iliotibial tract or the iliopsoas tendon.

snapping scapula A phenomenon in which retraction and protraction of the scapula produce a palpable and often audible grating between the scapula and the underlying chest wall.

sniffing position A postural deformity of the cervical spine in which the face of the patient appears to be thrust anteriorly.

soft spot of the elbow The most common site for aspiration or injection of the elbow, located in the center of a triangle formed by the radial head, the lateral epicondyle, and the tip of the olecranon.

soft spot of the shoulder A point on the posterior shoulder over the superior portion of the glenohumeral joint.

Speed's test A provocative test for biceps tendon pain in which the shoulder is flexed against resistance with the forearm supinated.

splayfoot A forefoot deformity in which the metatarsals deviate excessively from each other.

Sprengel's deformity A congenital deformity in which the scapula is usually abnormally small and displaced proximal to its normal location on the posterior chest wall.

Spurling's test A provocative test designed to exacerbate encroachment of a cervical nerve root at the neural foramen by extension and rotation of the neck toward the involved side.

squinting patellae, in-facing patellae A variation in rotational alignment of the lower limbs in which the patellae angle toward each other when the patient stands with the feet pointing straight forward.

step-off deformity A lumbar spine deformity in which a visible or palpable step or shelf is present between two vertebrae owing to a high grade spondylolisthesis.

steppage gait (see drop foot gait)

step-up–step-down test A method of eliciting patellofemoral crepitus by having the patient climb up and down from a stepstool.

stiff knee gait A gait abnormality in which the patient attempts to prevent normal flexion and extension of the knee during ambulation.

Stinchfield's test A provocative test designed to elicit hip joint pain requiring the patient to perform an active straight-leg raise with the ipsilateral knee locked in extension.

straight-leg raising test A provocative test designed to exacerbate the symptoms of lower lumbar radiculopathy by passively flexing the patient's hip with the knee extended.

sulcus sign The appearance of a transverse sulcus between the humeral head and the lateral acromion when the arm is pulled distally, a sign of inferior laxity of the shoulder.

supination Rotation of the forearm so that the palm faces upward; by extension, analogous rotation in other parts of the body.

supraspinatus isolation test (see Jobe's test)

swan neck deformity A complex deformity of the finger in which a hyperextension deformity of the proximal interphalangeal joint is combined with a flexion deformity of the distal interphalangeal joint.

swayback deformity (see hyperlordosis)

tailor's bunion (see bunionette)

tenodesis effect Involuntary passive extension or flexion of the fingers associated with flexion or extension of the wrist, respectively, owing to the intrinsic tone of the musculotendinous units.

Thomas' test A clinical method for measuring flexion and extension of the hip that uses the contralateral limb to lock the pelvis in flexion and thus prevent compensatory motion of the lumbar spine.

Thompson's test A manipulative test to detect Achilles' tendon rupture by squeezing the patient's calf and observing for the normal associated plantar flexion response.

tibia vara A varus deformity (bowing) of the tibia.

tibial torsion Twisting of the tibia about its longitudinal axis, as judged by the difference between the flexion axis of the knee and the flexion axis of the ankle joint.

Tinel's sign, formication sign A sign of nerve compression, injury, or regeneration after injury in which tapping over the nerve at the site of involvement produces characteristic paresthesias or dysesthesias in the distribution of the nerve.

Tinel's test   Tapping over a nerve with the tip of the long finger in an attempt to elicit Tinel's sign.

too-many-toes sign   A sign of unilateral pes planus, classically caused by posterior tibial tendon dysfunction, in which more toes than usual can be seen in the involved foot when the patient is viewed from behind.

total active elevation   An alternative method of assessing shoulder motion, measured by asking the patient to raise the arm as far as possible in the plane in which it is most comfortable.

transillumination   A method of identifying a ganglion cyst by its ability to transmit light in a characteristic manner.

Trendelenburg's gait   A gait abnormality in which the patient's pelvis sags when the patient lifts the uninvolved limb to take a step, usually caused by gluteus medius weakness.

Trendelenburg's sign   Sagging of the pelvis during single-leg standing; a sign of gluteus medius weakness.

Trendelenburg's test   A provocative test for gluteus medius weakness or hip joint pain in which the patient is asked to stand on one leg at a time.

triangular fibrocartilage complex compression test   A provocative test to elicit painful clicking and popping in the presence of a triangular fibrocartilage complex (TFCC) tear.

tripod sign   The observation that passive extension of the knee in a seated patient causes the patient's trunk to fall backwards; usually a sign of hamstring tightness or sciatica.

tubercle-sulcus angle   The angle between a line drawn from the center of the patella to the center of the tibial tubercle and a second line perpendicular to the floor when the patient is in a seated position.

ulnar   Related to the medial side of the hand or the forearm, on which the ulna and the little finger are located.

ulnar deviation   A motion of the wrist produced by bending the hand toward the ulnar side of the forearm.

ulnar nerve compression test of the elbow   A provocative test for ulnar neuropathy at the elbow in which prolonged passive elbow flexion is combined with digital pressure over the cubital tunnel.

ulnar nerve compression test of the wrist   A provocative test for ulnar nerve compression at the wrist in which the nerve is compressed at a point just radial to the pisiform bone in an attempt to reproduce the patient's symptoms.

upper limb tension tests (ULTT)   A series of provocative tests that seeks to reproduce or exacerbate neurologically based symptoms in the upper extremity by placing progressive tension on the cervical nerve roots and the associated peripheral nerves.

valgus stress test of the elbow   A manipulative test for abnormal valgus laxity of the elbow.

valgus stress test of the knee   A manipulative test for detecting increased valgus laxity of the knee; primarily a test of the medial collateral ligament complex.

valgus thrust   A gait abnormality in which the knee is thrust into a position of increased valgus alignment when the limb is in single leg stance.

Valsalva's maneuver   A provocative maneuver designed to increase intrathecal pressure and thereby exacerbate pain due to spinal cord or nerve root compression by asking the patient to bear down as if attempting to have a bowel movement.

varus recurvatum test   A method of demonstrating abnormal posterolateral laxity of the knee in the supine patient by grasping the patient's great toe and raising the leg from the examination table.

varus recurvatum thrust   A gait abnormality in which the knee is thrust into a varus and hyperextended (recurvatum) position during single leg stance.

varus stress test of the ankle   (see inversion stress test)

varus stress test of the elbow   A manipulative test to assess abnormal varus laxity of the elbow

varus stress test of the knee   A manipulative test for detecting increased varus laxity in the knee; primarily a test of the lateral collateral ligament complex.

varus thrust   A gait abnormality in which the knee is thrust into a position of increased varus alignment when the limb is in single leg stance.

Velpeau's deformity   (see silver fork deformity)

volar, palmar   Related to the anterior surface of the hand, on which the palm is located.

voluntary dislocation of the shoulder A phenomenon in which the patient is able to demonstrate the active ability to sublux or dislocate the shoulder.

Waddell's nonorganic signs A set of five physical signs, originally described by Waddell in patients with unsuccessful back surgery, that suggest the possibility of nonorganic pathology being responsible for the patient's symptoms; the signs are nonanatomic tenderness, the simulation sign, the distraction sign, a regional sensory or motor disturbance, and overreaction.

Watson's test (see scaphoid shift test)

Wilson's test A manipulative, provocative test to elicit the pain of osteochondritis dissecans of the knee by impinging the anterior cruciate ligament against the osteochondritis dissecans lesion using passive internal rotation of the tibia.

windlass effect The coupled, involuntary heel inversion and accentuation of the longitudinal arch that normally occur when a person rises up on the toes.

windswept deformity The situation in which a patient has a varus deformity in one knee and a valgus deformity in the other.

winging of the scapula The tendency of the medial border of the scapula to stand out from the underlying chest wall, most commonly due to weakness of the serratus anterior muscle.

Wright's maneuver A provocative test for thoracic outlet syndrome in which the examiner attempts to eliminate the patient's radial pulse by abducting the shoulder to 90° and externally rotating the arm.

Yeoman's test A provocative test in which resisted extension of the hip is used to elicit the pain of gluteus maximus tendinitis.

Yergason's test A provocative test for biceps tendon pain in which the patient is asked to simultaneously flex the elbow and supinate the forearm against resistance.

Note: Page numbers in *italics* refer to illustrations; page numbers followed by t refer to tables.